Instructor's Resource Manual for

HEALTH ASSESSMENT IN NURSING

SECOND EDITION

Incorporating Test Bank and Transparency Masters

Instructor's Resource Manual for

HEALTH ASSESSMENT IN NURSING

SECOND EDITION

Incorporating Test Bank and Transparency Masters

Patricia Dillon, RN, MSN
Nursing Instructor
Gwynedd Mercy College
Gwynedd Valley, Pa.

Patricia Gonce Morton, RN, PhD
Assistant Professor
School of Nursing
The University of Maryland
Baltimore

Springhouse Corporation
Springhouse, Pennsylvania

Staff

Executive Director, Editorial
Stanley Loeb

Director of Trade and Textbooks
Minnie B. Rose, RN, BSN, MEd

Art Director
John Hubbard

Associate Acquisitions Editor
Betsy Steinmetz

Editor
Nancy Priff

Copy Editor
Pamela Wingrod

Designers
Stephanie Peters (associate art director),
Julie Carleton Barlow (book designer)

Manufacturing
Deborah Meiris (manager), T.A. Landis, Anna Brindisi

Production Coordinator
Caroline Lemoine

Printed in the United States of America.
ISBN 0-87434-426-3

RTAIM-2E-020593

Table of Contents

Advisory Board

A Note To The Instructor

Health Assessment in Nursing, Second Edition provides an organized, comprehensive approach to the teaching and learning of nursing health assessment. This *Instructor's Resource Manual and Test Bank* is designed to help the instructor present the textbook information and evaluate student understanding of this information. It can be used by instructors in virtually all types of nursing education programs, including Diploma, Associate Degree, Bachelor of Science in Nursing (BSN), and Nurse Practitioner programs, and in classroom and clinical laboratory settings.

Reflecting the contents of *Health Assessment in Nursing, Second Edition,* this manual is organized into 5 units and 22 chapters. Unit One explores the nurse's role in assessment, including discussions of the nursing process and of nursing and medical collaboration. Unit Two centers on general assessment skills, including obtaining a health history and developing physical assessment skills. Unit Three addresses the assessment of activities of daily living, sleep and wakefulness patterns, and nutritional status. Unit Four covers the assessment of specific body systems, structures, and organs. Unit Five presents guidelines for special assessments, including complete and partial assessments as well as perinatal and neonatal assessments.

For the instructor's convenience, the chapters in this manual are presented in a standard format. Each begins with an overview that highlights key concepts. Next are suggested lecture topics and critical thinking activities that help develop effective teaching and learning strategies for specific chapter topics. To enhance teaching effectiveness, the suggested lecture topics include cross-references to the appropriate transparency masters and the pages of the Photo Gallery in the text. Three types of student study questions follow.

The manual includes the study questions from the textbook, which are answered here; a test bank of multiple-choice questions, which are not in the textbook; and a quiz bank of matching and true or false questions, which also are not in the textbook. Answers for the test bank and quiz bank questions are accompanied by textbook page numbers should the student need to look again at a fuller explanation. Answers for the test bank questions also include rationales. For the instructor's convenience, test and quiz questions also are provided on a reproducible page, without accompanying answers or rationales.

Appropriate chapters in this manual contain two guides that the instructor can teach from or photocopy and distribute to students for laboratory use:

• *Skills laboratory guide: Health history* lists important questions that the student should ask a client during a health history interview.

• *Skills laboratory guide: Physical assessment* identifies assessment techniques for each body area, along with special considerations and normal findings.

In the appendix, the *Skills Laboratory Assessment Guide* features a formatted reproducible page that encourages student practice in documenting health history and physical assessment findings. This page will be useful to the student during each textbook chapter on assessing a body area or body system.

The manual concludes with a group of transparency masters, each bearing a descriptive title and chapter reference. The instructor should review the masters when preparing to teach each chapter so that appropriate visual aids can be incorporated into the lecture.

1

Assessment and the Nursing Process

Overview

The primary focus of nursing today is client health—the highest level of physical, emotional, spiritual, and social functioning. Because nurses care for clients of many ages in a wider variety of health care settings than in the past, nurses have diverse roles and increased responsibilities. They are accountable legally and ethically to the public for their actions in these various roles. To meet the diverse roles of nursing and ensure continuity of practice, the nursing profession has developed a system that considers all factors that affect the client. This holistic approach is called the nursing process. Derived from the scientific method of problem solving, the nursing process has five steps. Chapter 1 describes the problem-solving methods and theories as they relate to the nursing process, and then discusses each step of the nursing process. It covers the following information:

- Reflexive problem solving refers to decisions that the nurse makes automatically without analyzing or individualizing the situation.
- The trial-and-error method of problem solving involves random thinking. It lets the nurse develop creative responses to problems without the restrictions of the other problem-solving methods.
- With the intuitive method, the nurse uses insight into the client's characteristics and emotions or conditions to solve a problem.
- Based on critical thinking, the scientific problem-solving method requires the nurse to identify the general problem,

collect data, formulate hypotheses, plan ways to test the hypothetical solutions, implement the tests, and interpret the results.
- To develop nursing process flexibility, the nurse should use all four problem-solving methods.
- The nursing process steps are assessment, nursing diagnosis, planning, implementation, and evaluation.
- Assessment refers to the collection of subjective data (obtained from the client and family using interviewing techniques) and objective data (obtained through physical assessment techniques and diagnostic studies). It provides a basis for identifying problems and serves as a baseline against which to compare further assessments. The nurse should record the data systematically.
- Nursing diagnosis is the statement of actual or potential health problems that can be resolved, diminished, or otherwise changed by nursing interventions. Labels assigned to specific nursing diagnoses have been standardized by the North American Nursing Diagnosis Association (NANDA) into a taxonomy of nursing diagnostic categories to ensure that all nurses use the same terminology. Each nursing diagnosis has three parts: problem, etiology, and signs and symptoms.
- Planning allows the nurse to develop a course of action that will help the client achieve improved or optimal functioning. Effective planning includes determining priorities, setting goals, and selecting interventions that will help the client attain short- and long-term goals. The nursing care plan becomes part of the client's record and is used to direct the client's nursing care.

- Implementation requires the nurse to work with the client and significant others to perform the designated interventions. Interventions fall into three categories: interdependent, dependent, or independent.
- Evaluation involves examination of the client's progress toward established goals. It should occur constantly during implementation so the nurse can determine if the selected interventions are helping the client meet the desired goals.

Suggested lecture topics

- Explain the four problem-solving techniques, using the reflexive, trial-and-error, intuitive, and scientific approaches in nursing situations.
- Discuss the steps of the nursing process and, using a nursing care plan, explain how to use the process. (For a visual aid, see the transparency master *The nursing process and scientific method.*)
- Differentiate between subjective and objective assessment data.
- Explain how to create a three-part nursing diagnosis statement, using a sample data base containing subjective and objective assessment data.
- Demonstrate how to write measurable goals for a sample nursing care plan.

Suggested critical thinking activities

- Have the students describe how to use each of the four problem-solving methods in four clinical situations.
- Give the students a written data base containing subjective and objective assessment findings. Ask them to differentiate between subjective and objective findings and to explain their choices.
- Have the students apply the nursing process to a case study. Remind them to formulate a three-part nursing diagnosis and to set measurable goals.

Student study questions and answers

The following study questions are taken from text page 19 of Chapter 1, Assessment and the Nursing Process. Their answers are based on information in that chapter.

1. Roy Likowski has come to the emergency department complaining of severe chest pain. He states, "It feels as if an elephant is sitting on my chest. I'm having trouble breathing. It's probably just indigestion." You note that Mr. Likowski is pale, diaphoretic (perspiring), and restless. Mrs. Likowski tells you that her husband has been feeling this way for the last 3 hours.
- Which of the above data are considered subjective; which are objective?
- What further data related to Mr. Likowski's condition should you obtain from the primary source and from the secondary source?

- Using the NANDA nursing diagnosis list, which three nursing diagnoses (potential or actual) could be included in Mr. Likowski's care plan?

Answer
Subjective data
- "It feels as if an elephant is sitting on my chest. I'm having trouble breathing. It's probably just indigestion." Any other statements made by Mr. Likowski that indicate his perception of his condition also would provide subjective data.
Objective data
- Pallor, diaphoresis, restlessness, and any other available physical assessment data.
Further primary source data (data obtained from Mr. Likowski)
- The nurse should ask Mr. Likowski such questions as "Do you have any other discomfort? Have you ever had this type of discomfort before? Did you take any medication to relieve this pain? If so, what and when? Do you have any allergies?" The nurse also should obtain any other information that could clarify the presenting problem and should save nonessential questions for later.
Further secondary source data (data obtained from Mrs. Likowski)
- She may be able to answer questions about the onset and duration of the pain, Mr. Likowski's state of health, and the family's financial and social situation—questions that Mr. Likowski may not be able to answer at this time.
Examples of possible nursing diagnoses
- Altered cardiopulmonary tissue perfusion related to myocardial ischemia
- Anxiety related to hospitalization
- Anxiety related to possible myocardial infarction
- Decreased cardiac output related to myocardial ischemia
- Knowledge deficit related to medical condition
- Pain related to myocardial ischemia.

2. Amy Kline, age 3, was admitted to the pediatric orthopedic unit. Although she has a fractured right femur and severe discomfort, she is alert and oriented. The nursing diagnosis assigned to Amy is "Pain related to fracture."
- What data should you obtain immediately from Amy's parents on admission? Give rationales for your choices.
- During which step of the nursing process will you set goals with Amy's parents?
- What additional information do you need to establish goals with Amy's parents?
- What short-term and long-term goals could you construct related to the established nursing diagnosis? (List one of each.)

Answer
- Data obtained from Amy's parents on admission: level of pain, any other discomfort, medication taken, any history of chronic illness, and family members or caregivers avail-

able. Data should be pertinent to Amy's immediate needs. When her pain is under control and she is stable, other information can be obtained.
• Goal setting occurs during planning, after the nurse has collected data and assigned nursing diagnoses.
• Additional information needed for goal setting: Amy's normal activity levels, her perceptions of her present illness, any physical or emotional factors that may affect her recovery, the anticipated length of her hospitalization, and her anticipated level of recovery. Goal setting usually deals with realistic time frames, the level of wellness that can be achieved, and the client's perception of these factors.
• Short-term goal: Amy will report that her pain level has diminished within 4 hours. Long-term goal: Amy will be free of pain by the time of her discharge.

3. As a home health care nurse, you visit Robert Dunn who has recently been diagnosed with insulin-dependent diabetes mellitus. He is obese and denies knowledge of his correct dietary or medication regimen. The following nursing care plan was established for Mr. Dunn. Unfortunately, multiple errors occur in this plan as written. How would you rewrite this care plan to correct the errors? (Give rationales for your corrections.)

Problem	Goals	Interventions
Diabetes	Client will not have any complications. Client will learn about his disease.	1. Give insulin. 2. Watch for complications. 3. Teach him about diabetes. 4. Teach his wife.

• What assessments should you make to evaluate Mr. Dunn's progress toward the established goals?
• What are correct nursing actions if the identified problems are resolved? If they are unresolved?

Answer
Weaknesses of the proposed care plan
Problem
No nursing diagnosis is provided. "Diabetes" is a medical diagnosis referring to the client's physical problem, not his response to that problem, which is in the realm of nursing. Based on the information given, correct nursing diagnoses for this client are: Knowledge deficit related to medical condition; Knowledge deficit related to dietary requirements; Knowledge deficit related to medication administration; and Altered nutrition: more than body requirements, related to imbalance of intake and expenditures.
Goals
• Goals must be specific and measurable, and they must include outcome criteria and a time frame that is realistic for the client and for the behavior desired.
• The goals must relate to the nursing diagnosis. None of these characteristics are present in the goals as written.

Interventions
• These are nursing activities that will facilitate goal achievement. The selected interventions must be client-centered, specific, creative, and consistent with the established medical regimen.
Sample corrected care plans, developing two nursing diagnoses
Nursing diagnosis
Knowledge deficit related to correct information about insulin administration
Goals
• The client will verbalize correct information about insulin administration and diet within 1 day after a diabetic instruction class on these topics.
Interventions
1. Schedule the client and wife for diabetic instruction class.
2. Provide the client with "take-home" instructional materials about insulin administration and dietary requirements for diabetics.
3. Schedule 15 minutes during day and evening shifts to review basic information with the client and wife.
4. Encourage the client and wife to ask questions about his condition.
5. Introduce the client to other clients with similar conditions.
6. Inform the client of diabetic services available in the community, such as those of the American Diabetes Association.
Nursing diagnosis
Altered nutrition: more than body requirements, related to imbalance of intake and expenditures
Goals
• The client will maintain a daily caloric intake of 1,200 calories as indicated by the dietitian within 2 days after nutritional counseling.
• The client will lose 2 lb/week for a total 40-lb weight loss in 5 months.
Interventions
1. Monitor caloric intake with the client and dietitian through use of a calorie count with each meal.
2. Record the client's weight every other day at the same time on the same scale.
3. Establish a nonfood reward system with the client, and reward the client for each 2-lb weight loss.
4. Inform the client of weight-loss support groups in the community, such as Weight Watchers and Overeaters Anonymous.
• The evaluation step should be performed at the time specified for goal achievement in the nursing care plan or by health care facility policy.
• The nurse should reassess Mr. Dunn continually to identify new dysfunctional areas and to determine progress made on previously identified areas.
• According to health care facility policy, the nurse should note the resolution of identified problems on the nursing

care plan and in the client's chart, including the date of resolution and any pertinent information about the status of the problem. If the client's problem is unresolved, the nurse should reassess the client, apply the nursing process again, and revise the nursing care plan.

4. As a visiting nurse, you are caring for Mr. Jones, who is on bedrest at home after sustaining a closed head injury and bilateral fractured wrists. He tells you his concerns about missing work and his related financial needs. He is the only employed family member.
• What assessments would you make when visiting the Jones family?
• Which nursing diagnoses pertain to Mr. Jones and his family?
• Which factors help you establish priorities among the identified problem areas?

Answer
Assessments
The nurse should perform a physical assessment of affected systems, particularly the nervous system. The nurse also should assess Mr. Jones's financial and social situations, then determine his specific concerns, available support systems, and his perception of a solution to his current problem. This information will help the visiting nurse to contact appropriate community resources who can assist the client.
Sample nursing diagnoses
• Impaired home maintenance management related to head and wrist injuries
• Impaired physical mobility related to casts on wrists
• Powerlessness related to inability to work or care for self
• Dressing and grooming self-care deficit related to bilateral wrist fractures
• Impaired tissue integrity related to prolonged bedrest
• Self-esteem disturbance related to inability to work.
Priorities
• Life-threatening physical needs take precedence, followed by other needs as identified by the client and caregiver. In Mr. Jones's case, after his physical needs have been met, the next priority is to deal with his financial concerns, then his psychosocial needs related to self-esteem and power. Alleviation of Mr. Jones's financial concerns may relieve or prevent potential difficulties related to self-esteem and power.

Questions, answers, and rationales

1. Michael Jones, age 50, is admitted to the emergency department because he has had chest pain for the past 2 hours. The nurse immediately assesses Mr. Jones's vital signs and takes an electrocardiogram (ECG), following the facility's protocol for clients with chest pain. These actions are examples of which problem-solving method?
(a) Intuitive
(b) Reflexive
(c) Trial-and-error
(d) Scientific
Correct answer: (b), see text page 4. The reflexive method is based on ritualistic thinking that results in an automatic response, such as following a standard protocol.

2. What does the nurse do during the assessment step of the nursing process?
(a) Collects data
(b) Identifies nursing diagnoses
(c) Plans care
(d) Establishes outcome criteria
Correct answer: (a), see text page 6. Assessment, the first step of the nursing process, is the collection of relevant data from various sources.

3. Which data about Mr. Jones are subjective?
(a) Vital signs
(b) ECG patterns
(c) Serum enzyme levels
(d) Mr. Jones's description of chest pain
Correct answer: (d), see text page 7. Subjective data, referred to as symptoms, come directly from the client. They usually are recorded as direct quotations reflecting the client's opinions or feelings about the situation.

4. The nurse examines Mr. Jones's past medical records. Which type of data does the nurse obtain from such records?
(a) Primary source
(b) Historical
(c) Secondary source
(d) Subjective source
Correct answer: (c), see text page 7. Secondary sources of data include family members, friends, coworkers, and community service groups; health history and physical assessment reports; and other members of the health care team.

5. The nurse uses the nursing process to formulate Mr. Jones's plan of care. Which problem-solving method serves as the basis for the nursing process?
(a) Reflexive
(b) Trial-and-error
(c) Intuitive
(d) Scientific
Correct answer: (d), see text page 5. Based on critical thinking and a systematic approach, the scientific method of problem solving is the basis of the nursing process.

6. Andrea Smith, age 40, returns from the recovery room after a cholecystectomy. Her vital signs are stable, but the nurse feels that "something is just not right." Which problem-solving method is the nurse using?
(a) Reflexive
(b) Trial-and-error
(c) Intuitive
(d) Scientific
Correct answer: (c), see text page 4. The intuitive method of problem solving is based on insight related to appreciative thinking—an increased perception about a client, the client's values or beliefs, or a situation.

7. Ms. Smith's postoperative assessment includes auscultation of breath and bowel sounds. Which type of data does the nurse obtain with these techniques?
(a) Subjective
(b) Objective
(c) Secondary source
(d) Medical
Correct answer: (b), see text page 7. Physical assessment techniques and diagnostic studies provide objective data, which reflect findings without interpretation.

8. Which of Ms. Smith's assessment findings is considered a symptom?
(a) Vital signs
(b) Reports of incisional pain
(c) Breath and bowel sounds
(d) Serum electrolyte levels
Correct answer: (b), see text page 3. A symptom is an indication of a disease or change in condition as perceived subjectively by the client.

9. The nurse's assessment of Ms. Smith includes primary source data. Which of the following sources is considered primary?
(a) Family members
(b) The primary physician
(c) The client
(d) Previous medical records
Correct answer: (c), see text page 7. Primary source data are obtained directly from the client.

10. Which of the following is an appropriate nursing diagnosis for Ms. Smith?
(a) Ineffective breathing pattern related to guarded respirations caused by pain
(b) Hypoventilation related to surgical incision
(c) Tachypnea
(d) Shortness of breath related to pain
Correct answer: (a), see text page 9. A complete nursing diagnosis has three parts: the first part identifies the actual or potential problem, based on the NANDA taxonomy; the second states the etiology; and the third records the signs and symptoms and other data that are essential to the diagnosis.

11. Ms. Smith may have several actual or potential problems, which the nurse must prioritize as part of the planning stage of care. Which problem would have the highest priority?
(a) Altered role performance
(b) Knowledge deficit
(c) High risk for infection
(d) Pain
Correct answer: (d), see text pages 13 and 14. When prioritizing the client's problems, the nurse should address physiologic needs before others. In this case, pain is an actual physiologic problem, which takes priority over potential physiologic problems and developmental or situational problems.

12. Which other action must the nurse take during the planning stage of Ms. Smith's care?
(a) Develop goals
(b) Record data
(c) Implement interventions
(d) Formulate data
Correct answer: (a), see text page 12. During the planning phase of the nursing process, the nurse determines priorities, develops short-term and long-term goals, and selects appropriate interventions to achieve these goals.

13. Jacob Brown, age 70, is admitted to the hospital with aspiration pneumonia. After assessing Mr. Brown, the nurse assigns a nursing diagnosis of Ineffective airway clearance related to thickened secretions and fatigue. Based on this nursing diagnosis, which goal would be most appropriate?
(a) The client's breathing will be normal.
(b) The client will have clear breath sounds by discharge.
(c) The client will state that his breathing feels better before discharge.
(d) The client will cough.

Correct answer: (b), see text pages 14 and 16. The goal—the desired outcome of nursing care—should be realistic and measurable. The goal should identify the desired client behavior, criteria for measurement, appropriate time frame, and conditions under which the behavior should occur.

14. The nurse monitors Mr. Brown's hydration. This action is an example of which type of intervention?
(a) Independent
(b) Dependent
(c) Interdependent
(d) Collaborative
Correct answer: (a), see text page 17. Monitoring hydration status is an independent intervention, which does not require a physician's order to be implemented because its execution is suited to the nurse's education and knowledge.

15. During which step of the nursing process might the nurse revise Mr. Brown's care plan?
(a) Assessment
(b) Planning
(c) Implementation
(d) Evaluation
Correct answer: (d), see text page 18. During evaluation, the final step of the nursing process, the nurse determines the extent to which the client has met established goals. An unmet or partially met goal requires the nurse to reexamine the available data and revise the care plan.

16. Sally Liddel, age 42, is admitted to the orthopedic unit with low back pain. After assessing Ms. Liddel, the nurse formulates a nursing diagnosis. What are the components of a nursing diagnosis?
(a) Problem statement, etiology, and signs and symptoms
(b) Medical diagnosis, problem, and signs and symptoms
(c) Etiology, signs and symptoms, and interventions
(d) Signs and symptoms, conditions, and treatment
Correct answer: (a), see text page 14. The PES method for developing a nursing diagnosis requires a problem statement followed by the etiology and signs and symptoms.

17. In the nursing diagnosis, what do the signs and symptoms represent?
(a) Actual or potential health concern
(b) Possible cause of the problem
(c) Cluster of cues that help define the diagnosis
(d) Outcome criteria to be used in the care plan
Correct answer: (c), see text page 14. Signs and symptoms identify the cluster of cues that define a diagnostic label or problem statement applicable to a particular client.

18. Louise Jenkins, a 55-year-old, obese black woman, is admitted to the medical unit with hypertension. While assessing Ms. Jenkins, the nurse performs a venipuncture to obtain laboratory specimens, as ordered. This action is an example of which type of intervention?
(a) Independent
(b) Dependent
(c) Interdependent
(d) Collaborative
Correct answer: (b), see text page 17. Dependent interventions are activities the nurse performs at the direct request of a physician to help fulfill the medical regimen.

19. The nurse records subjective and objective assessment data for Ms. Jenkins. Which data about Ms. Jenkins are subjective?
(a) Body weight of 257 lb
(b) Total hemoglobin of 12.5 g/dl
(c) "I'm worried about my weight."
(d) Blood pressure of 150/98 mm Hg
Correct answer: (c), see text page 3. Subjective data are obtained from the client's description of a problem and are recorded in the client's words.

20. Which nursing diagnostic label is most appropriate for Ms. Jenkins?
(a) Obesity
(b) Poor dietary habits
(c) Excessive calorie intake
(d) Altered nutrition: more than body requirements
Correct answer: (d), see text pages 10 and 11. NANDA-approved nursing diagnostic labels include Altered nutrition: more than body requirements and Altered nutrition: less than body requirements.

Test bank for Chapter 1, Assessment and the Nursing Process

1. Michael Jones, age 50, is admitted to the emergency department because he has had chest pain for the past 2 hours. The nurse immediately assesses Mr. Jones's vital signs and takes an electrocardiogram (ECG), following the facility's protocol for clients with chest pain. These actions are examples of which problem-solving method?
(a) Intuitive
(b) Reflexive
(c) Trial-and-error
(d) Scientific

2. What does the nurse do during the assessment step of the nursing process?
(a) Collects data
(b) Identifies nursing diagnoses
(c) Plans care
(d) Establishes outcome criteria

3. Which data about Mr. Jones are subjective?
(a) Vital signs
(b) ECG patterns
(c) Serum enzyme levels
(d) Mr. Jones's description of chest pain

4. The nurse examines Mr. Jones's past medical records. Which type of data does the nurse obtain from such records?
(a) Primary source
(b) Historical
(c) Secondary source
(d) Subjective source

5. The nurse uses the nursing process to formulate Mr. Jones's plan of care. Which problem-solving method serves as the basis for the nursing process?
(a) Reflexive
(b) Trial-and-error
(c) Intuitive
(d) Scientific

6. Andrea Smith, age 40, returns from the recovery room after a cholecystectomy. Her vital signs are stable, but the nurse feels that "something is just not right." Which problem-solving method is the nurse using?
(a) Reflexive
(b) Trial-and-error
(c) Intuitive
(d) Scientific

7. Ms. Smith's postoperative assessment includes auscultation of breath and bowel sounds. Which type of data does the nurse obtain with these techniques?
(a) Subjective
(b) Objective
(c) Secondary source
(d) Medical

8. Which of Ms. Smith's assessment findings is considered a symptom?
(a) Vital signs
(b) Reports of incisional pain
(c) Breath and bowel sounds
(d) Serum electrolyte levels

9. The nurse's assessment of Ms. Smith includes primary source data. Which of the following sources is considered primary?
(a) Family members
(b) The primary physician
(c) The client
(d) Previous medical records

10. Which of the following is an appropriate nursing diagnosis for Ms. Smith?
(a) Ineffective breathing pattern related to guarded respirations caused by pain
(b) Hypoventilation related to surgical incision
(c) Tachypnea
(d) Shortness of breath related to pain

11. Ms. Smith may have several actual or potential problems, which the nurse must prioritize as part of the planning stage of care. Which problem would have the highest priority?
(a) Altered role performance
(b) Knowledge deficit
(c) High risk for infection
(d) Pain

12. Which other action must the nurse take during the planning stage of Ms. Smith's care?
(a) Develop goals
(b) Record data
(c) Implement interventions
(d) Formulate data

13. Jacob Brown, age 70, is admitted to the hospital with aspiration pneumonia. After assessing Mr. Brown, the nurse assigns a nursing diagnosis of Ineffective airway clearance related to thickened secretions and fatigue. Based on this nursing diagnosis, which goal would be most appropriate?
(a) The client's breathing will be normal.
(b) The client will have clear breath sounds by discharge.
(c) The client will state that his breathing feels better before discharge.
(d) The client will cough.

14. The nurse monitors Mr. Brown's hydration. This action is an example of which type of intervention?
(a) Independent
(b) Dependent
(c) Interdependent
(d) Collaborative

15. During which step of the nursing process might the nurse revise Mr. Brown's care plan?
(a) Assessment
(b) Planning
(c) Implementation
(d) Evaluation

16. Sally Liddel, age 42, is admitted to the orthopedic unit with low back pain. After assessing Ms. Liddel, the nurse formulates a nursing diagnosis. What are the components of a nursing diagnosis?
(a) Problem statement, etiology, and signs and symptoms
(b) Medical diagnosis, problem, and signs and symptoms
(c) Etiology, signs and symptoms, and interventions
(d) Signs and symptoms, conditions, and treatment

17. In the nursing diagnosis, what do the signs and symptoms represent?
(a) Actual or potential health concern
(b) Possible cause of the problem
(c) Cluster of cues that help define the diagnosis
(d) Outcome criteria to be used in the care plan

18. Louise Jenkins, a 55-year-old, obese black woman, is admitted to the medical unit with hypertension. While assessing Ms. Jenkins, the nurse performs a venipuncture to obtain laboratory specimens, as ordered. This action is an example of which type of intervention?
(a) Independent
(b) Dependent
(c) Interdependent
(d) Collaborative

19. The nurse records subjective and objective assessment data for Ms. Jenkins. Which data about Ms. Jenkins are subjective?
(a) Body weight of 257 lb
(b) Total hemoglobin of 12.5 g/dl
(c) "I'm worried about my weight."
(d) Blood pressure of 150/98 mm Hg

20. Which nursing diagnostic label is most appropriate for Ms. Jenkins?
(a) Obesity
(b) Poor dietary habits
(c) Excessive calorie intake
(d) Altered nutrition: more than body requirements

2

Nursing and Medicine: A Collaborative Approach

Overview

Chapter 2 presents the historical development of nursing as a profession. It compares the medical and nursing professions and discusses their similarities and differences in health care delivery, which are based on each profession's health care goals. These similarities and differences provide the basis for defining nursing actions as independent, dependent, or interdependent. The chapter discusses the effects of collaboration (communication and joint decision making between nurses and physicians) on health care and outlines strategies for successful nurse-physician collaboration. It covers the following information:

• The development of professional nursing began in the mid-1800s when Florence Nightingale first clearly delineated the nurse's role. She emphasized skilled observation and stated that the goal of "sick nursing" and "health nursing" was to put people "in the best possible conditions for Nature to restore or preserve health."

• In this century, nursing leaders developed the rudiments of the nursing process, as well as numerous philosophies and definitions of nursing. They also began to focus attention on the nurse's independent functions.

• Years of debate on the use of nursing diagnoses culminated in 1973 with the First National Conference on Classification of Nursing Diagnoses. As a result of this conference, nurses today routinely use nursing diagnoses to describe client responses and to help plan appropriate nursing interventions.

• The professional relationship between nurses and physicians has changed significantly throughout this century. Now, as equal partners in health care provision, nurses and physicians share the same professional goal—to provide the best possible client care.

• Today's nursing model emphasizes independent and collaborative practice. The National Joint Practice Commission, an inter-professional organization established by the American Nurses' Association (ANA) and the American Medical Association (AMA), has identified five elements that promote nurse-physician collaboration in hospitals: the use of primary nursing, integrated client records, individual decision-making by nurses, a joint practice committee, and joint care reviews.

• Nurses can use several strategies to increase collaboration: communication, professional accountability, competence, and trust in the nurse-physician partnership.

Suggested lecture topics

• Discuss and compare the historical development of nursing and medical practice from the time of Hippocrates and Nightingale to the present.

• Describe the development of nursing diagnoses and the accepted functional patterns for grouping nursing diagnoses.

• Define and give examples of strategies for successful nurse-physician collaboration, highlighting areas of independent and interdependent practice.

Suggested critical thinking activities

- Have the students formulate different goals for a sample client based on the tenets of three different nursing theorists.
- Using a case study, have the students identify dependent, independent, and interdependent nursing roles.
- Ask the students to identify factors in a particular clinical setting that could foster or inhibit nurse-physician collaboration.

Student study questions and answers

The following study questions are taken from text page 31 of Chapter 2, Nursing and Medicine: A Collaborative Approach. Their answers are based on information in that chapter.

1. Experts credit the origin of professional nursing to Florence Nightingale in the 1860s. How has the focus of nursing evolved from its original form to its present form? (Include definitions developed by Nightingale, Brown, Henderson, and the American Nurses' Association.)

Answer
- In her 1893 paper "Sick Nursing and Health Nursing," Florence Nightingale differentiated between "sick nursing," which requires professional training, and "health nursing," which every woman provides for her family. This was the first attempt to distinguish between trained and untrained nurses. According to Nightingale, the goal of both types of nursing is to put people "in the best possible conditions for Nature to restore or to preserve health—to prevent or cure disease or injury."
- In the late 1940s, Esther Brown, a layperson who headed a national committee to study society's need for nursing, defined nursing as "an art and a science which involves the whole patient—body, mind, and spirit; promotes his spiritual, mental, and physical health by teaching and by example; stresses health education and health preservation, as well as ministration to the sick; involves the care of the patient's environment—social and spiritual as well as physical; and gives health service to the family and community as well as to the individual."
- The next major revision of the definition of nursing came in 1966, when nursing theorist Virginia Henderson presented a definition that was accepted by the International Congress of Nursing: The unique function of the nurse is to assist the individual, sick or well, in the performance of those activities contributing to health or its recovery (or to peaceful death) that he would perform unaided if he had the necessary strength, will, or knowledge. And to do this in such a way as to help him gain independence as rapidly as possible.
- In 1980, the ANA responded to the continuing development of nursing models and theories by defining nursing and its scope of practice as "the diagnosis and treatment of human responses to actual or potential health problems."

2. Nightingale described observation as an essential nursing skill. How does observation, as described by Nightingale, relate to today's nursing process?

Answer
As defined by the ANA, the nursing process consists of five steps—assessment, diagnosis, planning, implementation or intervention, and evaluation. Observation, as initially described by Nightingale, is one of the key elements of assessment. Today, observation has been more explicitly defined as inspection and interview, and skilled observation remains an essential nursing tool.

3. Give an example of a collaborative problem. How does it differ from a nursing diagnosis?

Answer
Here are several examples:
- In a client with pneumonia, the collaborative problem could be "Potential complication: hypoxemia." The nursing diagnosis might be "Impaired gas exchange related to immobility."
- In a client with diabetes mellitus, the collaborative problem could be "Potential complication: hypoglycemia" or "Potential complication: hyperglycemia." The nursing diagnosis might be "Altered nutrition: more than body requirements, related to intake in excess of activity expenditures."
- In a client who has chest tubes in place, the collaborative problem could be "Potential complication: pneumothorax." The nursing diagnosis might be "Impaired physical mobility related to presence of chest tubes."
- Collaborative problems, which frequently result from physiologic complications, result in interdependent interventions. Nursing diagnoses lead to independent nursing interventions.

4. What are the elements of collaboration between physicians and nurses?

Answer
According to the National Joint Practice Commission, the elements of nurse-physician collaboration include:
- *Primary nursing.* Nursing with little or no delegation of nursing tasks to others. One nurse is responsible for a client's comprehensive care.
- *Integrated client records.* Interdisciplinary client progress notes that combine nurse and physician observations, judgments, and actions and provide a formal means of nurse-physician communication about client care.

- *Individual decision-making by nurses.* Ability to exercise independent judgment and initiate care based on that judgment. Decisions must lie within the scope of nursing practice.
- *Joint practice committee.* A committee of nurses and physicians that monitors nurse-physician relationships and recommends actions that support collaboration.
- *Joint care reviews.* Monthly review of client charts by a review committee of nurses and physicians to evaluate collaborative care.

5. In 1981, the National Joint Practice Commission reported that collaboration between nursing and medicine was necessary to meet the goal of improved client care. What actions can nurses and physicians take to foster effective collaboration?

Answer
Effective nurse-physician collaboration requires four basic actions:
- expert communication skills
- professional accountability
- competence
- trust in the nurse-physician partnership.

Questions, answers, and rationales

1. Sam Bolton, age 50, is admitted to the coronary care unit with an acute myocardial infarction. Which type of approach is the nurse most likely to take toward Mr. Bolton's health?
(a) Disease-oriented
(b) Holistic
(c) Crisis-oriented
(d) Curative
Correct answer: (b), see text page 22 and 26. Today's nurses commonly take a holistic approach toward health, addressing the client, environment, family, and community.

2. The nurse and the physician assess Mr. Bolton. How do nursing models differ from medical models?
(a) Nursing models emphasize the human response to illness.
(b) Nursing models emphasize the cure of disorders.
(c) Nursing models focus on disease diagnosis and treatment.
(d) Nursing models focus on high-quality client care.
Correct answer: (a), see text page 23. Both models focus on high-quality client care. However, nursing models tend to emphasize the human response to illness; medical models tend to emphasize the cure of diseases.

3. Which nursing theorist would promote adaptation in caring for Mr. Bolton?
(a) Hildegarde Peplau
(b) Dorothy Johnson
(c) Martha Rogers
(d) Sister Callista Roy
Correct answer: (d), see text page 24. Roy's nursing theory promotes adaptation in each adaptive mode (physiologic needs, self-concept, role function, and interdependence) to contribute to the client's quality of life, health, and death with dignity.

4. Which nursing theorist would take a self-care-oriented approach toward Mr. Bolton's health care?
(a) Florence Nightingale
(b) Virginia Henderson
(c) Dorothea Orem
(d) Rosemary Parse
Correct answer: (c), see text page 24. Orem states that the goal of nursing is to teach and manage continuous self-care to help clients sustain life and health.

5. Theorist Jean Watson believed that nursing had which goal?
(a) To substitute for client deficits
(b) To promote harmonious interaction between man and environment
(c) To guide the client in choosing among the possibilities in the changing health process
(d) To help the client gain self-knowledge, control, and self-healing and restore a sense of harmony
Correct answer: (d), see text page 24. Watson also states that the goal of nursing is to protect, enhance, and preserve humanity through transpersonal human-to-human communications by helping the client find meaning in illness, suffering, pain, and existence.

6. Martin Woods, age 81, is admitted to the orthopedic unit with a fractured left femur. The physician orders traction until Mr. Woods is cleared for surgery. If an interdependent approach to care is used for Mr. Woods, nursing interventions should have which characteristic?
(a) They should contradict medical treatment.
(b) They should be based solely on the physician's orders.
(c) They should be totally independent from the physician's orders.
(d) They should complement the medical treatment.
Correct answer: (d), see text page 30. An interdependent approach to care provides nursing interventions and medical treatments that complement each other.

7. Which example best represents a collaborative problem for Mr. Woods?
(a) Immobility
(b) Fractured left femur
(c) Potential complication: fracture deformity
(d) Potential for impaired skin integrity related to immobility
Correct answer: (c), see text pages 30 and 31. Collaboration is required for this problem; the physician and nurse must perform interdependent interventions to prevent the complication.

8. Which nursing intervention for Mr. Woods would be considered collaborative?
(a) Providing frequent skin care
(b) Applying and maintaining traction
(c) Applying sheepskin to the bed
(d) Maintaining proper alignment of fractured leg
Correct answer: (b), see text page 31. Collaborative nursing interventions involve carrying out physician's orders, such as the order for traction. The other interventions are independent ones.

9. Which strategy is the most essential for promoting a collaborative nurse-physician relationship?
(a) Trust
(b) Accountability
(c) Communication
(d) Competence
Correct answer: (c), see text pages 27 and 28. Communication is most essential because it promotes nurse-physician understanding and improves health care. In collaborative practice, the nurse and physician must clearly understand each other's roles, responsibilities, and care plans.

10. Which type of nursing would best foster a collaborative nurse-physician relationship in providing Mr. Woods's care?
(a) Primary nursing
(b) Team nursing
(c) Functional nursing
(d) Extended nursing
Correct answer: (a), see text page 28. Primary nursing fosters a collaborative relationship by providing direct communication between the primary nurse and physician, client care coordination by one person, nursing autonomy, shared accountability with the physician, fewer errors in care, and increased client satisfaction.

11. Gunther Jorgensen, age 74, is admitted for tests to rule out cerebrovascular accident. When caring for Mr. Jorgensen, the nurse may adhere to one of many models of nursing. According to Rosemary Parse's model, what is the goal of nursing?
(a) To provide the best possible conditions for nature to restore or preserve health
(b) To substitute for what clients lack in physical strength, knowledge, or will
(c) To restore, preserve, or attain the client's behavioral system balance and dynamic stability
(d) To guide the client in choosing among the possibilities in the changing health process
Correct answer: (d), see text page 24. Parse states that the goal of nursing is to guide the client in choosing among the possibilities in the changing health process.

12. In Dorothy Johnson's model, what is the goal of nursing?
(a) To promote harmonious interaction between man and the environment
(b) To substitute for what clients lack in physical strength, knowledge, or will
(c) To restore, preserve, or attain the client's behavioral system balance and dynamic stability
(d) To guide the client in choosing among the possibilities in the changing health process
Correct answer: (c), see text page 24. Johnson believes that the goal of nursing is to restore, preserve, or attain the client's behavioral system balance and dynamic stability at the highest possible level.

13. Based on Martha Rogers's model, what is the goal of nursing?
(a) To promote harmonious interaction between man and the environment
(b) To substitute for what clients lack in physical strength, knowledge, or will
(c) To restore, preserve, or attain the client's behavioral system balance and dynamic stability
(d) To guide the client in choosing among the possibilities in the changing health process
Correct answer: (a), see text page 24. Rogers asserts that the goal of nursing is to promote harmonious interaction between man and the environment, to strengthen the integrity and coherence of the human field, and to direct the patterning of human and environmental fields to realize maximum human potential.

14. For a theorist like Virginia Henderson, what is nursing's goal?
(a) To promote harmonious interaction between man and the environment
(b) To substitute for what clients lack in physical strength, knowledge, or will
(c) To restore, preserve, or attain the client's behavioral system balance and dynamic stability
(d) To guide the client in choosing among the possibilities in the changing health process
Correct answer: (b), see text page 24. Henderson states that the goal of nursing is to substitute for what clients lack in physical strength, knowledge, or will to help them become whole or independent.

15. Florence Nightingale's model included which goal of nursing?
(a) To help move the client's personality and other human processes toward creative, productive, personal, and community living
(b) To teach and manage continuous self-care to help clients sustain life and health
(c) To restore, preserve, or attain the client's behavioral system balance and dynamic stability
(d) To put clients in the best possible conditions for nature to restore or preserve health
Correct answer: (d), see text page 24. The founder of modern nursing, Nightingale wrote that the goal of nursing is to put clients in the best possible conditions for nature to restore or preserve health.

16. Myrtle Downing, age 69, is admitted to the critical care unit with uncontrolled hypertension. After assessing Ms. Downing, the nurse formulates appropriate nursing diagnoses, which must fall into one of the approved functional patterns for grouping nursing diagnoses. Which of the following is a functional pattern?
(a) Health promotion pattern
(b) Sociocultural pattern
(c) Human response pattern
(d) Cognitive-perceptual pattern
Correct answer: (d), see text page 25. Functional patterns include health-perception–health-management, nutritional-metabolic, elimination, activity-exercise, sleep-rest, cognitive-perceptual, self-perception–self-concept, role-relationship, sexuality-reproductive, coping–stress-tolerance, and value belief patterns.

17. To provide the highest-quality care for Ms. Downing, the nurse works with the physician in a collaborative relationship. Which of the following is an element of collaboration?
(a) Independent decision-making by the nurse
(b) Separate nurse and physician notes on client progress
(c) Regular audits by an independent health care consultant
(d) Committee of administrators to referee problems
Correct answer: (a), see text page 28. Elements of collaboration include primary nursing, integrated client records, independent decision-making by nurses, joint practice committee of nurses and physicians, and joint care reviews by nurses and physicians.

18. Which strategy might the nurse use to increase collaboration with the physician?
(a) Realism
(b) Holistic care
(c) Accountability
(d) Health promotion
Correct answer: (c), see text page 28. To increase collaboration, nurses can use several strategies, including communication, accountability, competence, and trust.

19. Roberta Evans, age 55, visits her nurse practitioner for an annual check-up. When caring for Ms. Evans, the nurse may draw on one of many nursing theories. What are the key concepts of most nursing theories?
(a) Man or person, health, illness, and health care
(b) Man or person, environment, health, and nurse
(c) Health, illness, health restoration, and caring
(d) Health, environment, disease, and treatment
Correct answer: (b), see text page 21. Nursing theories include several key concepts: man or person (individual with biophysical, emotional, psychological, intellectual, social, cultural, and spiritual aspects), environment (external conditions that affect life and development), health (optimal physical, social, and emotional functioning of an individual), and nurse.

20. The nurse also practices according to ANA guidelines. What is the ANA's definition of nursing?
(a) Diagnosis and treatment of human responses to actual or potential health problems
(b) Diagnosis and treatment designed to cure or alleviate disease
(c) Process of assisting the client to improved health
(d) Process of meeting the client's physical, psychosocial, cultural, and spiritual needs
Correct answer: (a), see text page 23. The ANA defines nursing and its scope of practice as "the diagnosis and treatment of human responses to actual or potential health problems."

Test bank for Chapter 2, Nursing and Medicine: A Collaborative Approach

1. Sam Bolton, age 50, is admitted to the coronary care unit with an acute myocardial infarction. Which type of approach is the nurse most likely to take toward Mr. Bolton's health?
(a) Disease-oriented
(b) Holistic
(c) Crisis-oriented
(d) Curative

2. The nurse and the physician assess Mr. Bolton. How do nursing models differ from medical models?
(a) Nursing models emphasize the human response to illness.
(b) Nursing models emphasize the cure of disorders.
(c) Nursing models focus on disease diagnosis and treatment.
(d) Nursing models focus on high-quality client care.

3. Which nursing theorist would promote adaptation in caring for Mr. Bolton?
(a) Hildegarde Peplau
(b) Dorothy Johnson
(c) Martha Rogers
(d) Sister Callista Roy

4. Which nursing theorist would take a self-care-oriented approach toward Mr. Bolton's health care?
(a) Florence Nightingale
(b) Virginia Henderson
(c) Dorothea Orem
(d) Rosemary Parse

5. Theorist Jean Watson believed that nursing had which goal?
(a) To substitute for client deficits
(b) To promote harmonious interaction between man and environment
(c) To guide the client in choosing among the possibilities in the changing health process
(d) To help the client gain self-knowledge, control, and self-healing and restore a sense of harmony

6. Martin Woods, age 81, is admitted to the orthopedic unit with a fractured left femur. The physician orders traction until Mr. Woods is cleared for surgery. If an interdependent approach to care is used for Mr. Woods, nursing interventions should have which characteristic?
(a) They should contradict medical treatment.
(b) They should be based solely on the physician's orders.
(c) They should be totally independent from the physician's orders.
(d) They should complement the medical treatment.

7. Which example best represents a collaborative problem for Mr. Woods?
(a) Immobility
(b) Fractured left femur
(c) Potential complication: fracture deformity
(d) Potential for impaired skin integrity related to immobility

8. Which nursing intervention for Mr. Woods would be considered collaborative?
(a) Providing frequent skin care
(b) Applying and maintaining traction
(c) Applying sheepskin to the bed
(d) Maintaining proper alignment of fractured leg

9. Which strategy is the most essential for promoting a collaborative nurse-physician relationship?
(a) Trust
(b) Accountability
(c) Communication
(d) Competence

10. Which type of nursing would best foster a collaborative nurse-physician relationship in providing Mr. Woods's care?
(a) Primary nursing
(b) Team nursing
(c) Functional nursing
(d) Extended nursing

11. Gunther Jorgensen, age 74, is admitted for tests to rule out cerebrovascular accident. When caring for Mr. Jorgensen, the nurse may adhere to one of many models of nursing. According to Rosemary Parse's model, what is the goal of nursing?
(a) To provide the best possible conditions for nature to restore or preserve health
(b) To substitute for what clients lack in physical strength, knowledge, or will
(c) To restore, preserve, or attain the client's behavioral system balance and dynamic stability
(d) To guide the client in choosing among the possibilities in the changing health process

12. In Dorothy Johnson's model, what is the goal of nursing?
(a) To promote harmonious interaction between man and the environment
(b) To substitute for what clients lack in physical strength, knowledge, or will
(c) To restore, preserve, or attain the client's behavioral system balance and dynamic stability
(d) To guide the client in choosing among the possibilities in the changing health process

13. Based on Martha Rogers's model, what is the goal of nursing?
(a) To promote harmonious interaction between man and the environment
(b) To substitute for what clients lack in physical strength, knowledge, or will
(c) To restore, preserve, or attain the client's behavioral system balance and dynamic stability
(d) To guide the client in choosing among the possibilities in the changing health process

14. For a theorist like Virginia Henderson, what is nursing's goal?
(a) To promote harmonious interaction between man and the environment
(b) To substitute for what clients lack in physical strength, knowledge, or will
(c) To restore, preserve, or attain the client's behavioral system balance and dynamic stability
(d) To guide the client in choosing among the possibilities in the changing health process

15. Florence Nightingale's model included which goal of nursing?
(a) To help move the client's personality and other human processes toward creative, productive, personal, and community living.
(b) To teach and manage continuous self-care to help clients sustain life and health
(c) To restore, preserve, or attain the client's behavioral system balance and dynamic stability
(d) To put clients in the best possible conditions for nature to restore or preserve health

16. Myrtle Downing, age 69, is admitted to the critical care unit with uncontrolled hypertension. After assessing Ms. Downing, the nurse formulates appropriate nursing diagnoses, which must fall into one of the approved functional patterns for grouping nursing diagnoses. Which of the following is a functional pattern?
(a) Health promotion pattern
(b) Sociocultural pattern
(c) Human response pattern
(d) Cognitive-perceptual pattern

17. To provide the highest-quality care for Ms. Downing, the nurse works with the physician in a collaborative relationship. Which of the following is an element of collaboration?
(a) Independent decision-making by the nurse
(b) Separate nurse and physician notes on client progress
(c) Regular audits by an independent health care consultant
(d) Committee of administrators to referee problems

18. Which strategy might the nurse use to increase collaboration with the physician?
(a) Realism
(b) Holistic care
(c) Accountability
(d) Health promotion

19. Roberta Evans, age 55, visits her nurse practitioner for an annual check-up. When caring for Ms. Evans, the nurse may draw on one of many nursing theories. What are the key concepts of most nursing theories?
(a) Man or person, health, illness, and health care
(b) Man or person, environment, health, and nurse
(c) Health, illness, health restoration, and caring
(d) Health, environment, disease, and treatment

20. The nurse also practices according to ANA guidelines. What is the ANA's definition of nursing?
(a) Diagnosis and treatment of human responses to actual or potential health problems
(b) Diagnosis and treatment designed to cure or alleviate disease
(c) Process of assisting the client to improved health
(d) Process of meeting the client's physical, psychosocial, cultural, and spiritual needs

3

The Health History

Overview

Chapter 3 discusses the major source of subjective data in assessing a client's health status—the comprehensive health history, which guides the nurse through the physical assessment and provides insight for identifying actual and potential problems. After describing the essential components of the health history, the chapter discusses communication skills and gives examples of effective and ineffective interviewing techniques. It describes the interview process and explains how to modify the health history for pediatric, pregnant, elderly, and disabled clients. The chapter then discusses how to document health history findings. It covers the following information:

• The nursing health history takes a holistic view of the client and provides insights into actual or potential health problems. This allows the nurse to develop an individualized care plan and provides an opportunity for client teaching.

• The nursing health history consists of five major components: biographic data, health and illness patterns, health promotion and protection patterns, role and relationship patterns, and a summary of health history data.

• Biographic data identify the client and provide important sociocultural information. They include the client's name, address, telephone number, contact person, sex, age, birth date, Social Security number, place of birth, race, nationality, cultural background, marital status, names of persons living with the client, education, religion, and occupation.

• Health and illness patterns provide an overview of the client's general health status. This part of the health history covers the client's reasons for seeking health care, current health status, past health status, family health status, status of physiologic systems, and developmental considerations.

• Health promotion and protection patterns cover what the client does or does not do to stay healthy, including health beliefs; personal habits; and sleep and wake, exercise and activity, recreation, nutrition, stress and coping, socioeconomic, environmental health, and occupational health patterns.

• Role and relationship patterns reflect the client's psychosocial health. Assessment of this area involves investigation of the client's self-concept, cultural influences, spiritual and religious influences, family role and relationship patterns, sexual and reproductive patterns, social support patterns, and emotional health status.

• The summary of health history data reviews all interview findings, including normal findings that are pertinent to assessment of an ill client. For a well client, it summarizes the client's health promotion and protection patterns, along with health education needs.

• To obtain a complete and accurate health history, the nurse needs a basic knowledge of pathophysiology and psychosocial principles, of interpersonal and communication skills, and of the therapeutic use of self.

• During the health history interview, the nurse should try to make the client feel comfortable, respected, and trusting. Effective interviewing techniques include offering general leads, restating, reflecting, verbalizing the implied meaning, focusing the discussion, placing a problem or event in proper sequence, encouraging client participation, providing clarification or consensual validation, presenting reality, making observations, giving information, using silence, and summarizing.

• Ineffective interviewing techniques include asking why or how questions, using probing and persistent questioning, using inappropriate language, giving advice, giving false

Skills laboratory guide: Health history

This form may be used in laboratory simulations and in clinical settings to obtain a complete health history. It should guide the students' health history interview and help organize and document their findings.

BIOGRAPHIC DATA

Name:	Race:
Address:	Nationality:
Home phone:	Culture:
Work phone:	Marital status:
Sex:	Dependents:
Age:	Contact person:
Birth date:	Education:
Social Security number:	Religion:
Place of birth:	Occupation:

HEALTH AND ILLNESS PATTERNS

Reason for seeking health care:

Current health status:

Past health status:

Family health status:

Status of physiologic systems:
- General state of health:
- Skin, hair, and nails:
- Head and neck:
- Nose and sinuses:
- Mouth and throat:
- Eyes:
- Ears:

- Respiratory system:
- Cardiovascular system:
- Breasts:
- Gastrointestinal system:
- Urinary system:
- Reproductive system:
- Nervous system:
- Musculoskeletal system:
- Immune system and blood:
- Endocrine system:

Developmental considerations:

HEALTH PROMOTION AND PROTECTION PATTERNS

Health beliefs:

Personal habits:

Sleep and wake patterns:

Exercise and activity patterns:

Recreational patterns:

Nutritional patterns:

Stress and coping patterns:

Socioeconomic patterns:

Environmental health patterns:

Occupational health patterns:

ROLE AND RELATIONSHIP PATTERNS

Self-concept:

Cultural influences:

Spiritual and religious influences:

Family role and relationship patterns:

Sexuality and reproductive patterns:

Social support patterns:

Emotional health status:

SUMMARY OF HEALTH HISTORY DATA

Significant findings:

---

reassurance, changing the subject, interrupting, using clichés or stereotyped responses, giving excessive approval or agreement, jumping to conclusions, using defensive responses, making too many literal responses, and asking leading questions.

- The nurse must modify the health history somewhat for a pediatric, pregnant, elderly, or disabled client. For example, a pediatric client's history would include questions about childhood diseases and immunizations; an elderly client's history would substitute questions about current health problems and medications.

- The nurse must document health history information clearly, concisely, and objectively. This documentation should contain no opinions or biases.
- The health history format and recommendations in this chapter are suggestions, not dictums. Obtaining a health history is a process with few absolutes; experience helps the nurse develop an effective interviewing style. Therapeutic use of self, the single most important interviewing skill, will help the nurse develop a trusting relationship with the client and express concern for the client as an individual.

Suggested lecture topics

- Discuss the major components of a nursing health history, providing sample questions for each component.
- Describe factors that influence nurse-client communication, including feelings and behaviors that may aid or impede the health history interview.
- Discuss health history modifications for pediatric, pregnant, elderly, and disabled clients.

Suggested critical thinking activities

- Ask two students to role-play a health history interview based on a case study. Have the other students analyze the communication techniques used, the information gathered, and the accuracy of the documentation.
- Pair the students and have them obtain health history information from each other and document their findings, using the Skills Laboratory Guide: Health History.
- Have the students obtain and document health history information for an ill client in a clinical setting.

Student study questions and answers

The following study questions are taken from text page 69 of Chapter 3, The Health History. Their answers are based on information in that chapter.

1. What are the five major components of the nursing health history? What information is included in each component?

Answer
The major components of the nursing health history are:
- Biographic data, including the client's name; address; telephone number; contact person; sex; age and birth date; Social Security number; place of birth; race, nationality, and cultural background; marital status and names of persons living with the client; education; religion; and occupation

- Health and illness patterns, including the client's reason for seeking health care; current, past, and family health status; status of physiologic systems; and developmental considerations
- Health promotion and protection patterns, including health beliefs; personal habits; and sleep and wake, exercise and activity, recreation, nutrition, stress and coping, socioeconomic, environmental health, and occupational health patterns
- Role and relationship patterns, including self-concept; cultural, spiritual, and religious influences; family role and relationship patterns; sexuality and reproductive patterns; social support patterns; and emotional health status
- Summary of health history data, including a review of all pertinent findings.

2. What is the significance of the nursing health history to the overall health assessment process?

Answer
The nursing health history, the major source of subjective data about a client's health status, serves as a guide to the subsequent physical assessment by identifying and providing insight into actual or potential health problems. It also gives the nurse an opportunity to establish a rapport with the client, to orient the client to the total health assessment process, and to identify areas in which the client needs education or support.

3. What are the major factors critical to a nurse's success in obtaining a meaningful and reliable health history?

Answer
Factors for a successful health history interview fall into three basic areas: characteristics associated with the nurse, characteristics associated with the client, and characteristics associated with the interview setting. Nursing characteristics include communication and interpersonal skills; self-awareness; knowledge of pathophysiology and the psychosocial factors that may affect a client's health status; and therapeutic use of self. Client characteristics include expectations of the history-taking process; behavioral factors; cultural and ethnic factors; and the client's developmental status. Characteristics of the interview setting include physical comfort, privacy, and psychological comfort.

4. How would you compare effective and ineffective interviewing techniques? Provide sample dialogues that illustrate two effective techniques and two ineffective techniques.

Answer
- Effective interviewing techniques are those that help the nurse obtain the maximum amount of information on the

client's health status. Such techniques include offering the client general leads, such as "Tell me more about your work-related stress" or "Describe how the pain in your leg feels"; placing a problem (or an event) in proper sequence by asking, for example, "Did you feel dizzy before or after you fell, or both?"; and making observations, such as "I notice that you've been yawning a lot. Are you feeling tired now?" Additional techniques include restating, reflecting, verbalizing the implied meaning, focusing the discussion, encouraging client participation, encouraging client evaluation, clarification or consensual validation, presenting reality, giving information, using silence, and summarizing.

• Ineffective interviewing techniques are those that make the client feel uncomfortable or block the client's attempts to provide information. Examples include asking why or how questions, such as "Why don't you stop smoking?" or "How did you come to that conclusion?"; using inappropriate language in such statements as "If you can't micturate, you may need a catheter"; and using clichés or stereotyped responses, such as "Every cloud has a silver lining" or "Cheer up. Things always look better in the morning." Other ineffective interviewing techniques include using probing, persistent questioning; giving advice; giving false reassurance; changing the subject or interrupting; giving excessive approval or agreement; jumping to conclusions; using defensive responses; making too many literal responses; and asking leading questions.

5. How does the content of a health history differ for an elderly client and a pediatric client? How do interviewing techniques differ for these clients?

Answer

• In contrast to the interview of a younger adult, an elderly client's interview seeks more specific information about potential problems experienced by elderly clients, including changes in sensory ability, such as vision and hearing; changes in the musculoskeletal system, such as decreased mobility; changes in the ability to carry out activities of daily living; and adjustment to losses in family and social support systems. In general, the history should focus on current problems rather than past ones. When assessing an elderly client's past health status and status of physiologic systems, the nurse may use more direct and closed-ended questions to clarify large amounts of data and to prevent the client from losing focus or rambling. Role and relationship patterns require in-depth assessment. Questions about family and social support systems should be sensitive to the many losses that an elderly client normally experiences as part of the aging process.

• The general interview format for an elderly client remains the same as for a younger adult, but the nurse needs to use interviewing strategies that accommodate the client's needs and general state of health. The nurse should remember to avoid stereotyping the elderly client as someone who is ill, confused, or nonproductive.

• The pediatric health history differs in content and interviewing strategies. The content of a young child's history should include detailed information about prenatal and perinatal status, such as the mother's health during pregnancy, length of labor, type of delivery, and the infant's health during the perinatal period. Information about developmental milestones, school performance, behavior, and discipline also should be assessed. Also, the nurse should obtain detailed information about communicable childhood illnesses and immunizations.

• Interview strategies vary with the pediatric client's developmental status. A parent or guardian usually accompanies a young child, and the nurse should obtain most of the history data from this secondary source. When interviewing a parent about a child's health, the nurse should try to determine whether the parent has realistic expectations about the child's behavior and development. When interviewing a school-age child or an adolescent, the nurse should direct part or all of the interview to the client, asking questions geared to the client's level of understanding. The nurse also needs to assure an adolescent client that all information will be strictly confidential, and should ask if the client wants a parent present during the interview.

Questions, answers, and rationales

1. Joseph Walsh, age 50, is brought to the emergency department because he has had chest pain for the past hour. The nurse should employ "therapeutic use of self" when interviewing Mr. Walsh. Which technique enhances the nurse's therapeutic use of self?
(a) Giving false reassurance
(b) Giving advice
(c) Giving recognition
(d) Giving excessive approval
Correct answer: (c), see text page 37. "Therapeutic use of self" refers to using interpersonal skills in a healing way to help the client. Three important techniques for enhancing the nurse's therapeutic use of self are exhibiting empathy, demonstrating acceptance, and giving recognition.

2. The nurse begins to assess Mr. Walsh. Which assessment component is the major source of subjective data about Mr. Walsh's health status?
(a) Laboratory study results
(b) Health history
(c) Physical assessment
(d) Electrocardiogram
Correct answer: (b), see text page 34. The health history provides subjective data; the physical assessment and diagnostic studies provide objective data.

3. The physician and the nurse take a health history from Mr. Walsh. Which factor does the nursing health history assess that the medical one does not?
(a) Family health history
(b) Status of body systems
(c) Impact of illness on the client and family
(d) Current health status
Correct answer: (c), see text pages 35 and 36. Unlike the physician, the nurse takes a health history to assess the impact of illness on the client and the family and to identify educational and discharge planning needs.

4. Which section of the health history identifies Mr. Walsh's support systems?
(a) Biographic data
(b) Health and illness patterns
(c) Health promotion and protection patterns
(d) Role and relationship patterns
Correct answer: (d), see text page 37. Role and relationship patterns assess the client's self-concept; cultural, spiritual, and religious influences; family role and relationship, sexuality and reproductive, and social support patterns; and emotional health status.

5. Which section of the health history is most useful in identifying contributing risk factors of cardiovascular disease, such as diet, activity, and stress?
(a) Biographic data
(b) Health and illness patterns
(c) Health promotion and protection patterns
(d) Role and relationship patterns
Correct answer: (c), see text page 36. Assessment of health promotion and protection patterns focuses on health beliefs; personal habits; and sleep and wake, exercise and activity, recreational, nutritional, stress and coping, socioeconomic, environmental health, and occupational health patterns.

6. Which questions provide the most useful information about Mr. Walsh's chest pain?
(a) Open-ended
(b) Closed-ended
(c) Leading
(d) Probing, persistent
Correct answer: (a), see text page 44. Open-ended questions permit more subtle and flexible responses and usually result in the most useful information.

7. Which question would be most useful when assessing Mr. Walsh's chest pain?
(a) "Are you having chest pain?"
(b) "Is the chest pain constant?"
(c) "Is the chest pain sharp?"
(d) "What does the pain feel like?"
Correct answer: (d), see text page 44. Open-ended questions usually provide more useful information and give clients the feeling that they are actively participating in and have some control over the interview. Closed-ended questions limit clients to yes or no responses.

8. While assessing Mr. Walsh, the nurse asks, "The pain radiates to your arm, correct?" This is an example of which type of question?
(a) Open-ended
(b) Leading
(c) Probing
(d) Reflective
Correct answer: (b), see text page 42. A leading question suggests the "right" answer by its phrasing. The nurse should avoid this type of question because it may force the client to supply the expected response rather than an honest one.

9. During which phase of the interview with Mr. Walsh should the nurse explain the purpose of the health history?
(a) Introductory
(b) Working
(c) Termination
(d) Evaluation
Correct answer: (a), see text page 42. During the introductory phase, the nurse should put the client at ease and explain the purpose and desired outcome of the health history.

10. While taking Mr. Walsh's health history, the nurse develops a genogram. What is the purpose of the genogram?
(a) To identify potential or undetected physiologic disorders
(b) To identify genetic and familial health problems
(c) To identify the chief complaint
(d) To identify chronic disorders
Correct answer: (b), see text page 47. Because it organizes family history data, the genogram is used to identify any actual or potential genetic and familial health problems.

11. Which section of the health history helps assess potential or undetected physiologic disorders?
(a) Biographic data
(b) Current health status
(c) Status of physiologic systems
(d) Developmental considerations
Correct answer: (c), see text page 47. The status of physiologic systems provides data about the client's past and current physiologic status, which helps identify potential or undetected physiologic disorders.

12. Joey Dwyer, age 9, is admitted to the pediatric surgical unit after sustaining a fractured tibia from a fall. Joey complains of leg pain. What is the most effective way to assess the severity of this pain?
(a) Ask him what it feels like.
(b) Ask him what makes it feel better.
(c) Ask him to rate the pain on a scale of 1 to 10, with 10 being the worst.
(d) Ask him what makes it feel worse.
Correct answer: (c), see text page 46. All of these questions would help assess Joey's pain in general, but rating the pain on a scale of 1 to 10 is the most effective way to assess its severity.

13. Which component of the health history usually is longer for a pediatric client than an adult?
(a) Status of physiologic systems
(b) Past health status
(c) Family health status
(d) Developmental considerations
Correct answer: (d), see text page 48. Because rapid physical and psychological changes in children affect growth and development, the developmental section of a child's health history usually is more detailed than an adult's.

14. After assessing Joey, the nurse obtains additional information from Joey's mother to prevent misunderstanding. What is this interviewing technique called?
(a) Clarification
(b) Restating
(c) Summarizing
(d) Reflecting
Correct answer: (a), see text pages 35 and 40. Clarification is a technique that involves obtaining additional information to make something clear or understandable.

15. Katie Smith is 2 months pregnant. Her initial prenatal visit includes a detailed health history. Which component of her history should the nurse analyze closely?
(a) Biographic data
(b) Cultural background
(c) Family history
(d) Developmental history
Correct answer: (c), see text page 64. The nurse should analyze the client's family history for evidence of genetic diseases.

16. During which phase of Ms. Smith's health history should the nurse summarize important interview points?
(a) Introductory phase
(b) Planning phase
(c) Working phase
(d) Termination phase
Correct answer: (d), see text page 43. During the termination phase of the interview, the nurse summarizes important points, informs the client about interview results, explains how the physical assessment will be conducted, and discusses follow-up plans.

17. Patricia Bowen, age 75, is admitted to the medical-surgical unit because of uncontrolled diabetes. When assessing this elderly client, the nurse should place extra emphasis on which component of the health history?
(a) Developmental considerations
(b) Childhood illnesses
(c) Biographic data
(d) Role and relationship patterns
Correct answer: (d), see text page 65. The nurse should assess role and relationship patterns thoroughly for an elderly client because losses associated with aging and changed social roles may affect the client's health status.

18. While assessing Ms. Bowen's socioeconomic patterns, the nurse discovers she is on a fixed income. Which section of the health history addresses socioeconomic patterns?
(a) Biographic data
(b) Health and illness patterns
(c) Health promotion and protection patterns
(d) Role and relationship patterns
Correct answer: (c), see text page 36. Health promotion and protection patterns include socioeconomic patterns, along with health beliefs; personal habits; and sleep and wake, exercise and activity, recreational, nutritional, stress and coping, environmental health, and occupational health patterns.

19. Ms. Bowen tells the nurse that she is afraid because her brother died from diabetic complications, and then asks if she is going to die. What would be the nurse's best response?
(a) "Everything will be okay."
(b) "Don't worry!"
(c) "Where there's life, there's hope."
(d) "This must be frightening for you. Would you like to talk about it?"
Correct answer: (d), see text page 41. The nurse should avoid giving false reassurance or using clichés. An answer that focuses on the client's feelings is more therapeutic.

20. Ms. Bowen says, "The last time I was in the hospital, the nurses took forever to answer my call light." What would be the nurse's best response?
(a) "I'm sure no one meant to ignore you."
(b) "The nurses must have been very busy."
(c) "That must have been a difficult experience."
(d) "Don't worry. It won't happen this time."
Correct answer: (c), see text page 41. Focusing on the client's feelings is more therapeutic than using defensive responses or giving false reassurance.

Test bank for Chapter 3, The Health History

1. Joseph Walsh, age 50, is brought to the emergency department because he has had chest pain for the past hour. The nurse should employ "therapeutic use of self" when interviewing Mr. Walsh. Which technique enhances the nurse's therapeutic use of self?
(a) Giving false reassurance
(b) Giving advice
(c) Giving recognition
(d) Giving excessive approval

2. The nurse begins to assess Mr. Walsh. Which assessment component is the major source of subjective data about Mr. Walsh's health status?
(a) Laboratory study results
(b) Health history
(c) Physical assessment
(d) Electrocardiogram

3. The physician and the nurse take a health history from Mr. Walsh. Which factor does the nursing health history assess that the medical one does not?
(a) Family health history
(b) Status of body systems
(c) Impact of illness on the client and family
(d) Current health status

4. Which section of the health history identifies Mr. Walsh's support systems?
(a) Biographic data
(b) Health and illness patterns
(c) Health promotion and protection patterns
(d) Role and relationship patterns

5. Which section of the health history is most useful in identifying contributing risk factors of cardiovascular disease, such as diet, activity, and stress?
(a) Biographic data
(b) Health and illness patterns
(c) Health promotion and protection patterns
(d) Role and relationship patterns

6. Which questions provide the most useful information about Mr. Walsh's chest pain?
(a) Open-ended
(b) Closed-ended
(c) Leading
(d) Probing, persistent

7. Which question would be most useful when assessing Mr. Walsh's chest pain?
(a) "Are you having chest pain?"
(b) "Is the chest pain constant?"
(c) "Is the chest pain sharp?"
(d) "What does the pain feel like?"

8. While assessing Mr. Walsh, the nurse asks, "The pain radiates to your arm, correct?" This is an example of which type of question?
(a) Open-ended
(b) Leading
(c) Probing
(d) Reflective

9. During which phase of the interview with Mr. Walsh should the nurse explain the purpose of the health history?
(a) Introductory
(b) Working
(c) Termination
(d) Evaluation

10. While taking Mr. Walsh's health history, the nurse develops a genogram. What is the purpose of the genogram?
(a) To identify potential or undetected physiologic disorders
(b) To identify genetic and familial health problems
(c) To identify the chief complaint
(d) To identify chronic disorders

11. Which section of the health history helps assess potential or undetected physiologic disorders?
(a) Biographic data
(b) Current health status
(c) Status of physiologic systems
(d) Developmental considerations

12. Joey Dwyer, age 9, is admitted to the pediatric surgical unit after sustaining a fractured tibia from a fall. Joey complains of leg pain. What is the most effective way to assess the severity of this pain?
(a) Ask him what it feels like.
(b) Ask him what makes it feel better.
(c) Ask him to rate the pain on a scale of 1 to 10, with 10 being the worst.
(d) Ask him what makes it feel worse.

13. Which component of the health history usually is longer for a pediatric client than an adult?
(a) Status of physiologic systems
(b) Past health status
(c) Family health status
(d) Developmental considerations

14. After assessing Joey, the nurse obtains additional information from Joey's mother to prevent misunderstanding. What is this interviewing technique called?
(a) Clarification
(b) Restating
(c) Summarizing
(d) Reflecting

15. Katie Smith is 2 months pregnant. Her initial prenatal visit includes a detailed health history. Which component of her history should the nurse analyze closely?
(a) Biographic data
(b) Cultural background
(c) Family history
(d) Developmental history

16. During which phase of Ms. Smith's health history should the nurse summarize important interview points?
(a) Introductory phase
(b) Planning phase
(c) Working phase
(d) Termination phase

17. Patricia Bowen, age 75, is admitted to the medical-surgical unit because of uncontrolled diabetes. When assessing this elderly client, the nurse should place extra emphasis on which component of the health history?
(a) Developmental considerations
(b) Childhood illnesses
(c) Biographic data
(d) Role and relationship patterns

18. While assessing Ms. Bowen's socioeconomic patterns, the nurse discovers she is on a fixed income. Which section of the health history addresses socioeconomic patterns?
(a) Biographic data
(b) Health and illness patterns
(c) Health promotion and protection patterns
(d) Role and relationship patterns

19. Ms. Bowen tells the nurse that she is afraid because her brother died from diabetic complications, and then asks if she is going to die. What would be the nurse's best response?
(a) "Everything will be okay."
(b) "Don't worry!"
(c) "Where there's life, there's hope."
(d) "This must be frightening for you. Would you like to talk about it?"

20. Ms. Bowen says, "The last time I was in the hospital, the nurses took forever to answer my call light." What would be the nurse's best response?
(a) "I'm sure no one meant to ignore you."
(b) "The nurses must have been very busy."
(c) "That must have been a difficult experience."
(d) "Don't worry. It won't happen this time."

4

Physical Assessment Skills

Overview

Chapter 4 presents the physical assessment skills that provide the objective data base. It discusses the four physical assessment techniques along with the equipment necessary to perform them. Then it describes approaches to physical assessment, including special considerations for pediatric, pregnant, elderly, and disabled clients. The chapter also explores three of the four main parts of physical assessment: the general survey, vital signs, and height and weight measurements. It includes the following information:

- Basic assessment equipment includes the thermometer, stethoscope, sphygmomanometer, visual acuity charts, penlight or flashlight, measuring tape, pocket ruler, marking pencil, and a scale. Other basic equipment, such as tongue depressor, safety pins, cotton balls, examination gloves, and water-soluble lubricant, also may be used.
- Advanced assessment equipment includes an ophthalmoscope, nasoscope, otoscope, and tuning fork.
- The four basic assessment techniques are inspection, palpation, percussion, and auscultation.
- Inspection, in which the nurse observes the client critically and objectively, is an ongoing process that may be performed directly or indirectly.
- Palpation uses the sense of touch and commonly is performed with inspection. Light palpation lets the nurse assess surface characteristics, such as skin temperature, texture, consistency, warmth, mobility, and tenderness. Deep palpation, which can be performed single-handedly or bimanually, lets the nurse assess organ size and shape, rebound tenderness, and abnormalities, such as tumors or masses. Ballottement involves gentle, repetitive bouncing of tissues against the hand.

- Percussion requires the nurse to use hearing and touch to determine the density of the underlying organs, elicit tenderness, or assess reflexes. The basic percussion methods include indirect, direct, and blunt percussion. Normal percussion sounds include resonance, tympany, dullness, flatness, and hyperresonance.
- Auscultation involves listening to body sounds, usually through a stethoscope. The nurse should determine the intensity, pitch, and duration and check the frequency of recurring sounds.
- Depending on the client's condition and the clinical setting, the nurse may perform a complete or modified assessment. To enhance the effectiveness of either type of assessment, the nurse should maintain a professional attitude, communicate effectively, and use a systematic approach.
- The nurse should tailor the assessment to the client's developmental status, making adjustments as needed for a pediatric, pregnant, elderly, or disabled client.
- The general survey is a brief summary of the nurse's first impressions of the client. It should list the client's sex, race, and apparent age and should include descriptions of any signs of distress as well as the client's facial characteristics; body type, posture, and movements; speech; dress, grooming, and personal hygiene; and psychological state. It also should describe any developmental, cultural, and ethnic considerations. The nurse should document general survey findings in one short paragraph.
- Vital sign measurements help monitor vital body functions. Vital signs include temperature, pulse, respirations, and blood pressure. The nurse should document vital signs accurately and completely.

• Height and weight measurements provide more specific information about the client's general health and nutritional status.

Suggested lecture topics

• Demonstrate how to use a stethoscope, sphygmomanometer, visual acuity chart, ophthalmoscope, nasoscope, otoscope, and tuning fork.
• Demonstrate the techniques of inspection, palpation, percussion, and auscultation. (For visual aids, see the transparency masters *Light palpation, Deep palpation, Light and deep ballottement, Indirect percussion, Direct percussion,* and *Blunt percussion.)*
• Discuss how to tailor assessment to the client's developmental status.
• Demonstrate how to take and record vital signs and height and weight measurements.
• Demonstrate how to record a general survey accurately.

Suggested critical thinking activities

• Pair the students and have them take vital signs, obtain height and weight measurements, and perform a general survey on each other. Have them document and discuss their findings.
• Have the paired students practice on each other using the physical assessment equipment.
• Have the paired students practice inspection, palpation, percussion, and auscultation on each other. Then have them critique each other's technique.
• Ask the students to identify three alterations to make when assessing a pediatric, pregnant, elderly, or disabled client.

Student study questions and answers

The following study questions are taken from text page 102 of Chapter 4, Physical Assessment Skills. Their answers are based on information in that chapter.

1. What is the overall purpose of the physical assessment? What is the purpose of the general survey and what does it contribute to the physical assessment?

Answer
The physical assessment allows the nurse to obtain objective data about the client. It includes the general survey, vital sign measurements, height and weight measurements, and physical examination. The general survey is a one-paragraph statement of the nurse's initial impressions of the client's physical and psychological health. It identifies problems that may need exploration and helps convey key information so subsequent caregivers will know if the client's behavior or appearance has changed significantly.

The survey may include comments about facial and body characteristics, dress and manner, speech, mental state, and signs of distress. It may include normal and abnormal findings.

2. What equipment should you expect to gather for a basic assessment? How would you use this equipment?

Answer
The complete collection of basic physical assessment equipment (and its uses) includes:
• a thermometer to measure the client's body temperature
• a stethoscope to listen to heart, lung, and bowel sounds and to obtain blood pressure and pulse measurements
• a sphygmomanometer to measure blood pressure
• a visual acuity chart to assess far and near vision
• a penlight or flashlight to evaluate pupillary responses and to assess hard-to-see areas, such as the oral or nasal structures
• a measuring tape to determine the length, width, and circumference of body parts and to assess gradual anatomic changes, such as leg swelling
• a pocket ruler to measure diaphragmatic excursion and liver size
• scales to measure the client's height and weight
• a wooden tongue depressor to assess the gag reflex and reveal the pharynx
• safety pins to test how well a client differentiates between sharp and dull pain
• cotton balls to check for fine-touch sensitivity
• common, easily identified substances, such as ground coffee and vanilla extract, to evaluate smell and taste sensations
• a water-soluble lubricant and disposable latex gloves for rectal and vaginal assessment, for touching any open lesions or wounds, and for handling body fluids.

3. A caring, supportive approach will enhance the assessment's effectiveness. What techniques can you use to put the client at ease and reduce stress during the assessment?

Answer
To enhance the client's comfort and the assessment's effectiveness, follow the guidelines below:
• Introduce yourself.
• Dress professionally.
• Address the client by title and last name.
• Explain what will occur during the assessment.
• Make sure the room is well lighted.
• Gather all equipment before the assessment.
• Ask the client to void before assessment begins.
• Work at a pace suitable to the client's age or health status.
• Respect the client's comfort and privacy.

- Warn the client before performing a procedure that may cause discomfort.
- Use warmth, empathy, and effective communication skills during the assessment.
- Wash your hands before and after the assessment.
- By using these techniques, the nurse can establish a trusting relationship with the client. This reduces the stressfulness of the experience for the client, enhances cooperation, and promotes the efficiency of the assessment.

4. Several factors characterize a well-documented physical assessment. What are these factors and their importance?

Answer
- A well-documented physical assessment is objective, clear, concise, and complete. It focuses on what was found, rather than what was done. It highlights salient findings and must be legible. The nurse should describe abnormal findings in terms of color, shape, texture, and other characteristics, and should document size in millimeters or centimeters. Drawings may be used to pinpoint location. The nurse should use specific descriptions instead of relative terms, such as "average," "good," or "negative."
- The written record of physical assessment is a legal document. It provides important health information about the client and shows the nursing actions that were performed. Following the guidelines above ensures complete and accurate documentation.

5. Physical assessment of a pediatric client differs greatly from that of the adult. How would you describe these differences?

Answer
The nurse should assess a pediatric client with the parents present, and vary the approach and technique depending on the client's age and developmental level. Different equipment must be used, and the nurse must keep in mind different vital sign parameters, such as the higher pulse and respiratory rates found in infants. To ensure proper evaluation, the nurse needs to know the general developmental abilities of each age-group and should document physical growth and cognitive development. For small children, games help make the experience pleasant. Distressing portions of the assessment, such as eye and ear examinations, should be performed last. During the assessment, the nurse should note parent-child interactions, reassure the parents about the child's development, and answer questions.

Questions, answers, and rationales

1. Margie Martin, age 22, is scheduled for her yearly physical examination. Which physical assessment technique does the nurse use when touching Ms. Martin to feel vibrations and locate body structures?
(a) Inspection
(b) Palpation
(c) Percussion
(d) Auscultation
Correct answer: (b), see text page 83. During palpation, the nurse touches the client's body to feel pulsations and vibrations, to locate body structures, and to assess such characteristics as size, texture, warmth, mobility, and tenderness.

2. Which characteristic should the nurse check with the dorsal surface of the hand when assessing Ms. Martin's skin?
(a) Crepitus
(b) Texture
(c) Tenderness
(d) Warmth
Correct answer: (d), see text page 82. The back, or dorsal surface, of the hand can best feel for warmth.

3. Which part of the hand should the nurse use to assess for palpable vibrations, such as fremitus?
(a) Dorsal surface
(b) Fingertips
(c) Ulnar surface
(d) Finger pads
Correct answer: (c), see text page 82. The ulnar surface, or ball, of the hand is best for detecting thrills (fine vibrations over the precordium), fremitus (tremulous vibrations over the chest wall), and vocal vibrations through the chest wall.

4. Ms. Martin's complete physical assessment should include which main component?
(a) Electrocardiogram
(b) Laboratory test results
(c) 24-hour dietary recall
(d) General survey
Correct answer: (d), see text page 71. The physical assessment has four main parts: the general survey, vital sign measurements, assessment of height and weight, and physical examination.

5. Tom Turner, age 14, is brought to the emergency department by his parents. His chief complaint is abdominal pain. Which nursing action is appropriate during abdominal assessment?
(a) Palpate the painful area first.
(b) Begin the assessment with deep palpation.
(c) Palpate for rebound tenderness.
(d) Avoid tender areas until the end of the assessment.
Correct answer: (d), see text page 87. If possible, the nurse should avoid touching tender or painful areas until the end of the assessment. Before assessing these areas, the nurse should warn the client.

6. The nurse assesses Tom's abdomen with light palpation. Which technique is used in light palpation?
(a) Indenting the skin ½″ to ¾ ″ with the fingertips
(b) Indenting the skin 1″ to 2″ with the fingertips
(c) Indenting the skin 1″ using a bimanual approach
(d) Indenting the skin 1″, then releasing the pressure
Correct answer: (a), see text page 84. To perform light palpation, the nurse presses gently on the skin with the tips and pads of the fingers, indenting it ½″ to ¾″.

7. The nurse could use deep palpation to assess Tom's abdomen. What is the major purpose of deep palpation?
(a) To assess skin turgor
(b) To assess organs
(c) To assess temperature
(d) To assess hydration
Correct answer: (b), see text page 84. Deep palpation involves indenting the skin about 1½″ to assess underlying structures and organs, such as the kidneys, spleen, or uterus.

8. Because Tom's chief complaint is abdominal pain, the nurse should assess for rebound tenderness. Which technique is used to elicit rebound tenderness?
(a) Press firmly with one hand, remove it quickly, and note tenderness upon release.
(b) Note tenderness over an area during light palpation.
(c) Press firmly with one hand, release pressure while maintaining fingertip contact with the skin, and note tenderness upon release.
(d) Note tenderness over an area during deep ballottement.
Correct answer: (a), see text page 84. Rebound tenderness is elicited by firmly pressing with one hand, removing the hand quickly, and noting tenderness upon release; it may indicate peritonitis when elicited in the abdomen.

9. Which special consideration should the nurse give the adolescent client?
(a) Having parents present during the examination
(b) Helping the client undress
(c) Instructing the client on sexual growth and development
(d) Recognizing the client's increased sense of modesty
Correct answer: (d), see text page 89. Adolescents are more independent than younger children and have an increased sense of modesty. Providing privacy and expressing willingness to answer questions related to sexuality are helpful approaches.

10. The nurse uses indirect percussion to assess Tom's abdomen. What is the purpose of percussion?
(a) To assess areas of tenderness
(b) To assess organ and tissue density
(c) To assess areas of inflammation
(d) To assess skin turgor
Correct answer: (b), see text page 83. Upon percussion, organs and tissues produce sounds of varying loudness, pitch, and duration, depending on their density.

11. Randolph Smith, age 70, is admitted to the hospital with uncontrolled hypertension and angina. Because of Mr. Smith's age, the nurse should keep which special consideration in mind during his assessment?
(a) Talk in a loud voice.
(b) Shorten the assessment.
(c) Allow extra time for each assessment step.
(d) Call the client by his first name.
Correct answer: (c), see text page 89. Special considerations for an elderly client include addressing the client respectfully, providing simple instructions, and allowing extra time for each assessment step.

12. Mr. Smith's initial assessment includes vital sign measurements. Which characteristic should the nurse note when assessing Mr. Smith's pulse?
(a) Amplitude
(b) Timing in the cardiac cycle
(c) Intensity
(d) Pitch
Correct answer: (a), see text page 96. When assessing the client's pulse, the nurse should note the rate, rhythm, and amplitude. The amplitude may be documented with a numerical scale or descriptive term.

13. When auscultating Mr. Smith's heart sounds, the nurse uses a stethoscope with a bell and a diaphragm. Which statement about this type of stethoscope is correct?
(a) The bell is best for detecting high-pitched sounds.
(b) The diaphragm is best for detecting high-pitched sounds.
(c) The bell is best for detecting thrills.
(d) The diaphragm is best for detecting low-pitched sounds.
Correct answer: (b), see text page 73. The diaphragm is best for detecting high-pitched sounds; the bell, for detecting low-pitched sounds.

14. What is the correct technique for using the bell of the stethoscope?
(a) Do not touch the bell during auscultation.
(b) Hold the bell lightly with one finger.
(c) Apply light pressure and tilt the bell up slightly.
(d) Hold the bell firmly against the client's chest.
Correct answer: (b), see text page 73. The bell should be heavy enough to stay in place when held lightly with one finger.

15. How should the nurse determine the proper cuff size to use in taking Mr. Smith's blood pressure?
(a) Wrap the cuff around the limb; the uninflated bladder should cover about three-quarters of the limb circumference.
(b) Measure the arm about 1″ above the antecubital space.
(c) Wrap the cuff around the limb; the uninflated bladder should cover about one-third of the limb circumference.
(d) Use a bladder 6″ long (the proper size for an older adult).
Correct answer: (a), see text page 76. To determine the proper cuff size, the nurse wraps the cuff around the client's arm or leg with the bladder uninflated; the bladder should cover about three-quarters of the limb circumference.

16. What should the nurse do to avoid misreading the blood pressure in the auscultatory gap?
(a) Inflate the cuff to 200 mm Hg.
(b) Measure the blood pressure in both arms.
(c) Inflate the cuff 30 mm Hg over the point at which the palpated pulse disappeared.
(d) Take the blood pressure with the client in different positions.
Correct answer: (c), see text page 100. To avoid underestimating the systolic or overestimating the diastolic reading in the auscultatory gap, the nurse should inflate the cuff at least 30 mm Hg over the point at which the palpated pulse first disappeared.

17. After measuring Mr. Smith's blood pressure, the nurse should document which phases of pulse sounds?
(a) I, II, and III
(b) I, III, and V
(c) I, IV, and V
(d) I, III, and IV
Correct answer: (c), see text page 99. The American Heart Association recommends documenting phases I, IV, and V of pulse sounds.

18. The nurse also must assess Mr. Smith's temperature. Which route should the nurse avoid because of Mr. Smith's cardiac disorder?
(a) Oral
(b) Axillary
(c) Rectal
(d) Oto-tympanic
Correct answer: (c), see text page 94. The rectal route is contraindicated in a client with a cardiac disorder, such as angina, because it may stimulate the vagus nerve, possibly leading to vasodilation and a decreased heart rate.

19. Patty Walsh, age 6, has a persistent productive cough caused by mycoplasma pneumonia. During vital sign measurement, the nurse assesses Patty's respiratory movements. Which muscles do children normally use to breathe?
(a) Accessory
(b) Thoracic
(c) Abdominal
(d) Intercostal
Correct answer: (c), see text page 98. Normally, men and children use abdominal muscles to breathe; women, thoracic muscles.

20. When percussing Patty's chest, the nurse elicits dullness over the affected area. Which sound normally would be elicited over healthy lung tissue?
(a) Resonance
(b) Hyperresonance
(c) Tympany
(d) Dullness
Correct answer: (a), see text page 86. Resonance, a percussion sound normally heard over healthy lung tissue, is moderate to loud in intensity, low-pitched, of long duration, and hollow-sounding.

Test bank for Chapter 4, Physical Assessment Skills

1. Margie Martin, age 22, is scheduled for her yearly physical examination. Which physical assessment technique does the nurse use when touching Ms. Martin to feel vibrations and locate body structures?
(a) Inspection
(b) Palpation
(c) Percussion
(d) Auscultation

2. Which characteristic should the nurse check with the dorsal surface of the hand when assessing Ms. Martin's skin?
(a) Crepitus
(b) Texture
(c) Tenderness
(d) Warmth

3. Which part of the hand should the nurse use to assess for palpable vibrations, such as fremitus?
(a) Dorsal surface
(b) Fingertips
(c) Ulnar surface
(d) Finger pads

4. Ms. Martin's complete physical assessment should include which main component?
(a) Electrocardiogram
(b) Laboratory test results
(c) 24-hour dietary recall
(d) General survey

5. Tom Turner, age 14, is brought to the emergency department by his parents. His chief complaint is abdominal pain. Which nursing action is appropriate during abdominal assessment?
(a) Palpate the painful area first.
(b) Begin the assessment with deep palpation.
(c) Palpate for rebound tenderness.
(d) Avoid tender areas until the end of the assessment.

6. The nurse assesses Tom's abdomen with light palpation. Which technique is used in light palpation?
(a) Indenting the skin ½" to ¾ " with the fingertips
(b) Indenting the skin 1" to 2" with the fingertips
(c) Indenting the skin 1" using a bimanual approach
(d) Indenting the skin 1", then releasing the pressure

7. The nurse could use deep palpation to assess Tom's abdomen. What is the major purpose of deep palpation?
(a) To assess skin turgor
(b) To assess organs
(c) To assess temperature
(d) To assess hydration

8. Because Tom's chief complaint is abdominal pain, the nurse should assess for rebound tenderness. Which technique is used to elicit rebound tenderness?
(a) Press firmly with one hand, remove it quickly, and note tenderness upon release.
(b) Note tenderness over an area during light palpation.
(c) Press firmly with one hand, release pressure while maintaining fingertip contact with the skin, and note tenderness upon release.
(d) Note tenderness over an area during deep ballottement.

9. Which special consideration should the nurse give the adolescent client?
(a) Having parents present during the examination
(b) Helping the client undress
(c) Instructing the client on sexual growth and development
(d) Recognizing the client's increased sense of modesty

10. The nurse uses indirect percussion to assess Tom's abdomen. What is the purpose of percussion?
(a) To assess areas of tenderness
(b) To assess organ and tissue density
(c) To assess areas of inflammation
(d) To assess skin turgor

11. Randolph Smith, age 70, is admitted to the hospital with uncontrolled hypertension and angina. Because of Mr. Smith's age, the nurse should keep which special consideration in mind during his assessment?
(a) Talk in a loud voice.
(b) Shorten the assessment.
(c) Allow extra time for each assessment step.
(d) Call the client by his first name.

12. Mr. Smith's initial assessment includes vital sign measurements. Which characteristic should the nurse note when assessing Mr. Smith's pulse?
(a) Amplitude
(b) Timing in the cardiac cycle
(c) Intensity
(d) Pitch

13. When auscultating Mr. Smith's heart sounds, the nurse uses a stethoscope with a bell and a diaphragm. Which statement about this type of stethoscope is correct?
(a) The bell is best for detecting high-pitched sounds.
(b) The diaphragm is best for detecting high-pitched sounds.
(c) The bell is best for detecting thrills.
(d) The diaphragm is best for detecting low-pitched sounds.

14. What is the correct technique for using the bell of the stethoscope?
(a) Do not touch the bell during auscultation.
(b) Hold the bell lightly with one finger.
(c) Apply light pressure and tilt the bell up slightly.
(d) Hold the bell firmly against the client's chest.

15. How should the nurse determine the proper cuff size to use in taking Mr. Smith's blood pressure?
(a) Wrap the cuff around the limb; the uninflated bladder should cover about three-quarters of the limb circumference.
(b) Measure the arm about 1″ above the antecubital space.
(c) Wrap the cuff around the limb; the uninflated bladder should cover about one-third of the limb circumference.
(d) Use a bladder 6″ long (the proper size for an older adult).

16. What should the nurse do to avoid misreading the blood pressure in the auscultatory gap?
(a) Inflate the cuff to 200 mm Hg.
(b) Measure the blood pressure in both arms.
(c) Inflate the cuff 30 mm Hg over the point at which the palpated pulse disappeared.
(d) Take the blood pressure with the client in different positions.

17. After measuring Mr. Smith's blood pressure, the nurse should document which phases of pulse sounds?
(a) I, II, and III
(b) I, III, and V
(c) I, IV, and V
(d) I, III, and IV

18. The nurse also must assess Mr. Smith's temperature. Which route should the nurse avoid because of Mr. Smith's cardiac disorder?
(a) Oral
(b) Axillary
(c) Rectal
(d) Oto-tympanic

19. Patty Walsh, age 6, has a persistent productive cough caused by mycoplasma pneumonia. During vital sign measurement, the nurse assesses Patty's respiratory movements. Which muscles do children normally use to breathe?
(a) Accessory
(b) Thoracic
(c) Abdominal
(d) Intercostal

20. When percussing Patty's chest, the nurse elicits dullness over the affected area. Which sound normally would be elicited over healthy lung tissue?
(a) Resonance
(b) Hyperresonance
(c) Tympany
(d) Dullness

5

Activities of Daily Living and Sleep Patterns

Overview

A balance between daily activities and sleep is vital in promoting and maintaining physiologic and psychosocial health. Chapter 5 explains how the nurse can assess the client's ability to perform activities of daily living (ADLs) and to achieve and maintain restful sleep patterns. It also discusses factors that affect ADLs and sleep patterns. The chapter covers the following information:

• ADLs are the activities necessary to develop physiologic and psychosocial well-being. These include five components: personal care, family responsibility, work or school, recreation, and socialization. A client's ability to perform necessary ADLs depends on several factors: age, developmental status, culture, physiologic health, cognitive function, psychosocial function, stress level, and biological rhythms.

• Assessment evaluates a client's functional level and identifies actual and potential health problems related to ADLs. Ideally, the nurse assesses the client at home, using interview techniques and observation to gather information on activities associated with personal care, family responsibility, work or school, recreation, and socialization.

• To determine a client's personal care status, the nurse first assesses mobility and then evaluates the client's ability to prepare and eat meals and to perform elimination, personal hygiene, and dressing and grooming activities. When assessing the client's family responsibilities, the nurse must keep in mind that those responsibilities depend on the client's developmental status and family role. The nurse also determines the nature and demands of the client's work or schoolwork and investigates the client's play or recreational activities and socialization activities.

• To assess sleep patterns, the nurse must identify factors that affect sleep, distinguish between normal and abnormal sleep patterns, and know when to refer a client for further evaluation. Factors affecting sleep patterns include the client's age, exercise level, personal habits, diet, environment, and mood. Throughout the night, two types of sleep occur: rapid eye movement (REM) sleep and non-rapid eye movement (NREM) sleep. The length and pattern of these types of sleep vary among clients.

• During the general health assessment, the nurse gathers information about the client's usual patterns of sleep and activity. The assessment includes basic questions about the client's age, normal sleeping environment, and time of sleep and awakening. If the client reports a sleep problem, the nurse obtains more detailed information. A client with a sleep disorder may yawn frequently and have pale skin, dark circles under the eyes, and puffy eyelids.

Suggested lecture topics

• Discuss factors affecting ADLs and explain how to assess a client's ADLs.

• Discuss which ADLs are appropriate for different age-groups.

• Describe sleep cycles and the factors affecting sleep.

• Identify the physiologic and psychological changes that result from sleep deprivation.

Suggested critical thinking activities

• Pair the students and have them assess and then discuss each other's ADLs.
• Have the students describe their sleep patterns and compare them to the patterns of different age-groups.
• Have the students identify factors that may aid or interrupt sleep for a hospitalized client in a case study.
• Have the students identify personal stressors and appropriate coping mechanisms.

Student study questions and answers

The following study questions are taken from text page 121 of Chapter 5, Activities of Daily Living and Sleep Patterns. Their answers are based on information in that chapter.

1. Ralph Thompson, age 55, comes to the clinic for a follow-up evaluation of hypertension. During the visit, he mentions difficulty sleeping at night. What data should you obtain to assess Mr. Thompson's sleeping problem?

Answer
Ask Mr. Thompson if he has difficulty falling asleep or staying asleep. Assess his problems, habits, mood, stress level, snoring, and use of medications that might interfere with sleep. Ask if he is excessively sleepy during the day. Determine if he sleeps normally, but at an inappropriate time of day. Ask if he sleepwalks, experiences night terrors, or makes unexplained movements or noises at night. Assess factors that influence sleep: age, exercise, smoking, caffeine, alcohol, diet, environment, and emotions.

2. Ms. Jenkins brings her daughter Cindy, age 8, to the clinic for a routine checkup. During the interview, Ms. Jenkins expresses concern that, for the past several weeks, Cindy has "moped around the house" instead of engaging in normal play. When Cindy does play with her friends, the activity usually ends prematurely because of fighting. What factors should you explore to discover the reasons for Cindy's changed pattern of play? Why are these factors important? How would you document your findings?

Answer
• Age and developmental status. An 8-year-old usually enjoys various interests and play activities. At this age, a child likes to compete and play games, but usually requires supervision in play. Assess the type of play in which the child participates and how peers are involved in that play so that you can determine if the activities are appropriate for the child's age.

Skills laboratory guide: Health history

Activities of daily living and sleep patterns are two components of the health promotion and protection patterns section of the health history. To collect information about these components, ask questions about personal care activities, family responsibility activities, work and school activities, recreational activities, socialization activities, and sleep-wake patterns. Sample questions from each category are listed below.

PERSONAL CARE ACTIVITIES

• Do you have difficulty standing, walking, or climbing stairs?
• Can you open packages and containers?
• Can you use the toilet alone, or do you require assistance?
• Do you have any problems with personal hygiene or bathing?
• Do you have any difficulties with dressing or grooming yourself?

FAMILY RESPONSIBILITY ACTIVITIES

• What are your living arrangements?
• Do you have any problems with food management, such as shopping or food preparation?
• Are you having any difficulties managing your money, such as getting to a bank?

WORK AND SCHOOL ACTIVITIES

• What does your typical day involve?
• What is your work schedule like?
• Do you have any difficulties balancing school activities with other life responsibilities?

RECREATIONAL ACTIVITIES

• What do you do when you're not working or in school?
• How much recreational time do you have in a day and in a week?
• How often do you get physical exercise?

SOCIALIZATION ACTIVITIES

• What kinds of things do you do when you are alone?
• Do you have many close friends?
• Do you belong to any social groups, such as clubs or church groups?

SLEEP-WAKE PATTERNS

• What time do you usually go to bed?
• Do you fall asleep easily?
• Do you feel rested when you awaken in the morning?

• Culture. Culture influences the types of play in which a child participates. In different cultures, play may be mostly an outdoor activity or may involve little adult supervision. Ask the child's mother what type of play she encourages and what her role is in the child's play.
• Physiologic health. A child with a physical disorder may not have the energy to participate in usual play activities. Fatigue or illness may contribute to changes in play pat-

terns. Gather data about any actual or potential physiologic health problems that may interfere with the child's usual play.

• Cognitive function. Problems with cognitive function may influence the child's ability to think, to pay attention, or to remember. The problem may manifest itself during play or school. Ask Ms. Jenkins about Cindy's ability to concentrate and remember and about her school performance.

• Psychosocial function. The ability to establish relationships with others, to communicate, and to fulfill role expectations influences a person's psychosocial health. Problems in any of these areas may manifest themselves during play. Ask about Cindy's relationships with family members, with teachers, and with peers. Also explore her position in the family and her communication patterns with family members, teachers, and peers.

• Stress level. A child may feel stress, but may not be able to verbalize it; instead, the child may exhibit behavioral changes. Explore with the child and the mother any possible stressors in the child's life, such as a new sibling, the loss of a friend or pet, or expectations regarding school. Try to assess potential stressors from the child's viewpoint.

• Biological rhythms. A child needs a balance between sleep and activity. An 8-year-old should get 9 to 11 hours of sleep a night. During waking hours, the child should have time not only for school, but also for play and exercise. Ask about the child's sleep patterns, including questions about hours of sleep per night, usual bedtime, bedtime routine, usual awakening time, and any problems associated with sleep (such as nightmares or bed wetting). Then evaluate the balance between sleep and daily activities.

• Documentation of findings could appear as follows: "Cindy Jenkins, age 8, is brought to the clinic by her mother, who is concerned because Cindy has been 'moping around the house' for the past few weeks. Although the child plays with friends, the play usually ends in fights." Document additional information based on your assessment of Cindy's developmental status, culture, physiologic health, cognitive function, psychosocial function, stress level, and biological rhythms.

3. How do sleep patterns change with age?

Answer
Sleep patterns change over the life span. An infant sleeps 16 to 20 hours a day and shifts into different sleep stages every 20 to 35 minutes. In an infant age 6 months, total sleep time decreases to about 13 hours a day and begins with NREM sleep rather than REM sleep. Total sleep time decreases from age 4 (10 to 12 hours) to age 10 (9 to 10 hours). During adolescence, total sleep time decreases to about 7.5 hours and remains at that level until about age 50. However, the amount of sleep in each stage shifts. After age 35, the amount of Stage 3 and 4 sleep decreases. Adults under age 60 may have difficulty falling asleep, but, once asleep, have no

difficulty staying asleep. The need for sleep does not decrease with age. After age 60, a client has more Stage 1 and 2 sleep and less deep sleep. After age 70, sleep patterns usually include daytime naps.

4. What factors are important when assessing a client with a sleep pattern disturbance?

Answer
Ask if the client has difficulty falling asleep and staying asleep. Find out if the client is excessively sleepy during the day. Determine if the client sleeps normally, but at inappropriate times. Ask if the client sleepwalks, experiences night terrors or enuresis, or makes unexplained movements or noises at night. Also ask about factors that influence sleep: age, exercise, smoking, caffeine, alcohol, diet, environment, and emotions.

5. Regina Johnson, age 68, was diagnosed with Parkinson's disease a year ago. She tells you she is having difficulty dressing herself. What questions would you ask to assess her ability to perform ADLs?

Answer:
The nurse could ask the following questions to assess Ms. Johnson's ability to perform ADLs:

• Are your difficulties with dressing more pronounced on the left or right side or in the upper or lower part of your body? Can you fasten buttons, snaps, and zippers?

• Is dressing easier with certain types of clothing? If so, which kinds?

• What are your usual bathing habits? Do you have any problems with personal hygiene or bathing? Can you get in and out of a tub or shower? Can you care for your teeth, hair, and nails?

• Can you open packages or containers? Can you use utensils for eating? Can you cut your food? Do you have any problems feeding yourself?

Questions, answers, and rationales

1. Kate Jones, age 50, comes to the clinic for a follow-up evaluation of her hypertension. The nurse assesses Ms. Jones's health promotion and protection patterns, including ADLs and sleep patterns. Which factor would influence Ms. Jones's ADLs?
(a) Occupation
(b) Environment
(c) Culture
(d) Diet
Correct answer: (c), see text page 105. These factors affect a person's interest in and ability to perform ADLs: age and developmental status, culture, physiologic health, cognitive function, stress level, and biological rhythms.

2. To assess Ms. Jones's personal care ability, the nurse should use which question?
(a) "What are your living arrangements?"
(b) "What do you do when you're not working?"
(c) "What kinds of things do you do when you're alone?"
(d) "Do you have any problems with dressing?"
Correct answer: (d), see text pages 107 and 108. Personal care activities address meal preparation and consumption, elimination, personal hygiene, and dressing and grooming.

3. The nurse asks Ms. Jones how she feels about retirement. This question helps assess which ADLs?
(a) Socialization activities
(b) Family responsibility activities
(c) Work and school activities
(d) Recreational activities
Correct answer: (c), see text page 109. Work and school activities focus on work demands, views of retirement, and school concerns.

4. To improve her cardiovascular status, Ms. Jones has begun an exercise program. What should the nurse tell Ms. Jones about exercise and sleep?
(a) Vigorous exercise before retiring may inhibit sleep.
(b) Sporadic exercise before retiring induces sleep.
(c) Regular exercise inhibits sleep.
(d) Sporadic exercise induces sleep.
Correct answer: (a), see text page 113. Regular or sporadic exercise tends to have little effect on sleep. However, vigorous exercise before retiring may inhibit sleep by causing pain or aching muscles.

5. Ms. Jones also is beginning a weight reduction program. Which effect does diet have on sleep?
(a) A person gaining weight tends to sleep for shorter periods but more deeply than normal.
(b) A person losing weight tends to sleep for shorter periods and may have more fragmented sleep.
(c) A person losing weight tends to sleep longer and deeper than normal.
(d) Diet has little or no effect on sleep-wake patterns.
Correct answer: (b), see text page 113. A person gaining weight may sleep longer and deeper than normal; a person losing weight may sleep for shorter periods and may have more fragmented sleep.

6. Julie Newman, age 22, is a nurse who works a night shift every 3 weeks. Shift work can disrupt the circadian rhythm. How long is the usual cycle for the circadian rhythm?
(a) 8 hours
(b) 10 hours
(c) 12 hours
(d) 24 hours
Correct answer: (d), see text page 107. The circadian rhythm, a type of biological rhythm, operates on a cycle of approximately 24 hours.

7. Maria Palino, age 25, has just given birth to a girl. What should the nurse tell Ms. Palino about her infant's sleeping pattern?
(a) Infants normally have 10 to 14 hours of consolidated sleep daily.
(b) Infants normally have 16 to 20 hours of consolidated sleep daily.
(c) Infants normally have 10 to 14 hours of fragmented sleep daily.
(d) Infants normally have 16 to 20 hours of fragmented sleep daily.
Correct answer: (d), see text page 112. Infants, particularly neonates, usually sleep 16 to 20 hours daily; their sleep is not confined to one period (consolidated), but is fragmented with frequent nocturnal awakenings.

8. Ellen Carver brings her son, Robert, age 3, to the pediatrician for his yearly check-up. When the nurse assesses Robert's sleep and wakefulness patterns, Ms. Carver expresses concern that he still takes an afternoon nap. How should the nurse respond to this statement?
(a) "This is a normal sleep pattern for a 3-year-old."
(b) "He shouldn't need an afternoon nap anymore."
(c) "He probably should take a morning nap as well."
(d) "He must need to sleep longer at night."
Correct answer: (a), see text page 112. By age 3, a child's sleep usually is consolidated into one period at night and an afternoon nap; afternoon naps may continue until about age 5.

9. Ms. Carver also expresses concern that Robert still wets the bed. The nurse should tell her that enuresis is considered abnormal after the child reaches which age?
(a) 2
(b) 3
(c) 4
(d) 5
Correct answer: (d), see text page 115. Although most children gain bladder control by age 3 to 4, experts do not consider enuresis abnormal in children under age 5.

10. Joe Jarvis, age 40, comes to the physician's office with complaints about sleeping difficulties. What is the average amount of sleep for healthy adults of Mr. Jarvis's age?
(a) 6.5 hours
(b) 7 hours
(c) 7.5 hours
(d) 8 hours
Correct answer: (c), see text page 111. On the average, healthy adults between ages 20 and 50 sleep approximately 7.5 hours each night and do not require daytime naps.

11. At Mr. Jarvis's age, he is most likely to experience which sleeping difficulty?
(a) Difficulty falling asleep
(b) Difficulty staying asleep
(c) Night terrors
(d) Somnambulism
Correct answer: (a), see text page 112. Adults under age 60 may complain of problems falling asleep, but usually do not have difficulty staying asleep.

12. Non-rapid eye movement (NREM) sleep usually occurs in how many stages?
(a) One
(b) Two
(c) Four
(d) Five
Correct answer: (c), see text page 112. NREM sleep occurs in four stages that progress from light to deep sleep.

13. Which stage accounts for the highest percentage of nightly sleep?
(a) Stage 2
(b) Stage 3
(c) Stage 4
(d) Stage 5
Correct answer: (a), see text page 112. Stage 2 sleep constitutes approximately 50% of nightly sleep.

14. Which response would be most likely to occur if Mr. Jarvis were awakened during stage 4 sleep?
(a) He would state he felt awake.
(b) He would awaken immediately and be alert.
(c) He would be able to recall his dreams.
(d) He would be difficult to arouse.
Correct answer: (d), see text page 112. During stages 3 and 4 sleep (delta sleep), people are difficult to arouse and, once awake, may need a few moments to become alert and oriented.

15. During which type of sleep does dreaming occur?
(a) REM sleep
(b) NREM sleep
(c) Delta sleep
(d) Transition sleep
Correct answer: (a), see text page 112. During REM sleep, a person experiences dreams, thinks illogical and bizarre thoughts, and cannot move voluntarily.

16. Mr. Jarvis's health history reveals that he smokes. How may cigarette smoking affect sleep?
(a) It should have no effect on sleep.
(b) It may reduce the amount of time needed to fall asleep.
(c) It may produce a deeper sleep for longer periods.
(d) It may cause lighter sleep with more frequent arousals.
Correct answer: (d), see text page 113. Smoking increases the amount of time needed to fall asleep and causes lighter sleep with more frequent arousals.

17. Mr. Jarvis also has a high caffeine intake. How may this affect his sleep?
(a) It should have no effect on sleep.
(b) It may increase sleep latency and reduce total sleep time.
(c) It may increase sleep latency and total sleep time.
(d) It may decrease sleep latency and total sleep time.
Correct answer: (b), see text page 113. A single cup of coffee before bedtime is unlikely to disrupt sleep, but two or more cups increase sleep latency and reduce total sleep time.

18. Mr. Jarvis tells the nurse that lately he has tried drinking alcohol before bedtime to help him sleep. The nurse should tell him that alcohol ingestion has which effect on sleep?
(a) It increases deep sleep.
(b) It increases REM activity.
(c) It fragments REM sleep.
(d) It increases sleep latency.
Correct answer: (c), see text page 113. Alcohol ingestion decreases REM sleep and makes it more fragmented and alters arousal patterns.

19. Mr. Jarvis tells the nurse that he snores. Which sleep disorder is associated with snoring?
(a) Sleep apnea
(b) Insomnia
(c) Bruxism
(d) Somnambulism
Correct answer: (a), see text page 117. Snoring often accompanies sleep apnea. The loudness of snoring is a rough indication of the problem's severity.

20. Margaret Brennan, age 73, is a recent widow who has been having difficulty sleeping. What is the normal sleep pattern of a person Ms. Brennan's age?
(a) Sleep is consolidated and has a lower percentage of REM sleep.
(b) Sleep is fragmented and typically includes a daytime nap.
(c) Sleep is consolidated, but characterized by sleep latency.
(d) Sleep is fragmented, but characterized by fewer arousals.
Correct answer: (b), see text page 112. Usually, older people experience sleep latency, more arousals and fragmented sleep, and less deep sleep. By age 70, a person's sleep is not consolidated into one block, but usually includes a daytime nap.

21. Which abnormality would the nurse expect to see in Ms. Brennan if she had narcolepsy?
(a) Difficulty falling asleep
(b) Brief attacks of sleep
(c) Difficulty staying asleep
(d) Sleepwalking
Correct answer: (b), see text page 115. Narcolepsy is characterized by brief attacks of sleep that may occur many times a day, during times of physical inactivity or when least expected.

Test bank for Chapter 5, Activities of Daily Living and Sleep Patterns

1. Kate Jones, age 50, comes to the clinic for a follow-up evaluation of her hypertension. The nurse assesses Ms. Jones's health promotion and protection patterns, including ADLs and sleep patterns. Which factor would influence Ms. Jones's ADLs?
(a) Occupation
(b) Environment
(c) Culture
(d) Diet

2. To assess Ms. Jones's personal care ability, the nurse should use which question?
(a) "What are your living arrangements?"
(b) "What do you do when you're not working?"
(c) "What kinds of things do you do when you're alone?"
(d) "Do you have any problems with dressing?"

3. The nurse asks Ms. Jones how she feels about retirement. This question helps assess which ADLs?
(a) Socialization activities
(b) Family responsibility activities
(c) Work and school activities
(d) Recreational activities

4. To improve her cardiovascular status, Ms. Jones has begun an exercise program. What should the nurse tell Ms. Jones about exercise and sleep?
(a) Vigorous exercise before retiring may inhibit sleep.
(b) Sporadic exercise before retiring induces sleep.
(c) Regular exercise inhibits sleep.
(d) Sporadic exercise induces sleep.

5. Ms. Jones also is beginning a weight reduction program. Which effect does diet have on sleep?
(a) A person gaining weight tends to sleep for shorter periods but more deeply than normal.
(b) A person losing weight tends to sleep for shorter periods and may have more fragmented sleep.
(c) A person losing weight tends to sleep longer and deeper than normal.
(d) Diet has little or no effect on sleep-wake patterns.

6. Julie Newman, age 22, is a nurse who works a night shift every 3 weeks. Shift work can disrupt the circadian rhythm. How long is the usual cycle for the circadian rhythm?
(a) 8 hours
(b) 10 hours
(c) 12 hours
(d) 24 hours

7. Maria Palino, age 25, has just given birth to a girl. What should the nurse tell Ms. Palino about her infant's sleeping pattern?
(a) Infants normally have 10 to 14 hours of consolidated sleep daily.
(b) Infants normally have 16 to 20 hours of consolidated sleep daily.
(c) Infants normally have 10 to 14 hours of fragmented sleep daily.
(d) Infants normally have 16 to 20 hours of fragmented sleep daily.

8. Ellen Carver brings her son, Robert, age 3, to the pediatrician for his yearly check-up. When the nurse assesses Robert's sleep and wakefulness patterns, Ms. Carver expresses concern that he still takes an afternoon nap. How should the nurse respond to this statement?
(a) "This is a normal sleep pattern for a 3-year-old."
(b) "He shouldn't need an afternoon nap anymore."
(c) "He probably should take a morning nap as well."
(d) "He must need to sleep longer at night."

9. Ms. Carver also expresses concern that Robert still wets the bed. The nurse should tell her that enuresis is considered abnormal after the child reaches which age?
(a) 2
(b) 3
(c) 4
(d) 5

10. Joe Jarvis, age 40, comes to the physician's office with complaints about sleeping difficulties. What is the average amount of sleep for healthy adults of Mr. Jarvis's age?
(a) 6.5 hours
(b) 7 hours
(c) 7.5 hours
(d) 8 hours

11. At Mr. Jarvis's age, he is most likely to experience which sleeping difficulty?
(a) Difficulty falling asleep
(b) Difficulty staying asleep
(c) Night terrors
(d) Somnambulism

12. Non-rapid eye movement (NREM) sleep usually occurs in how many stages?
(a) One
(b) Two
(c) Four
(d) Five

13. Which stage accounts for the highest percentage of nightly sleep?
(a) Stage 2
(b) Stage 3
(c) Stage 4
(d) Stage 5

14. Which response would be most likely to occur if Mr. Jarvis were awakened during stage 4 sleep?
(a) He would state he felt awake.
(b) He would awaken immediately and be alert.
(c) He would be able to recall his dreams.
(d) He would be difficult to arouse.

15. During which type of sleep does dreaming occur?
(a) REM sleep
(b) NREM sleep
(c) Delta sleep
(d) Transition sleep

16. Mr. Jarvis's health history reveals that he smokes. How may cigarette smoking affect sleep?
(a) It should have no effect on sleep.
(b) It may reduce the amount of time needed to fall asleep.
(c) It may produce a deeper sleep for longer periods.
(d) It may cause lighter sleep with more frequent arousals.

17. Mr. Jarvis also has a high caffeine intake. How may this affect his sleep?
(a) It should have no effect on sleep.
(b) It may increase sleep latency and reduce total sleep time.
(c) It may increase sleep latency and total sleep time.
(d) It may decrease sleep latency and total sleep time.

18. Mr. Jarvis tells the nurse that lately he has tried drinking alcohol before bedtime to help him sleep. The nurse should tell him that alcohol ingestion has which effect on sleep?
(a) It increases deep sleep.
(b) It increases REM activity.
(c) It fragments REM sleep.
(d) It increases sleep latency.

19. Mr. Jarvis tells the nurse that he snores. Which sleep disorder is associated with snoring?
(a) Sleep apnea
(b) Insomnia
(c) Bruxism
(d) Somnambulism

20. Margaret Brennan, age 73, is a recent widow who has been having difficulty sleeping. What is the normal sleep pattern of a person Ms. Brennan's age?
(a) Sleep is consolidated and has a lower percentage of REM sleep.
(b) Sleep is fragmented and typically includes a daytime nap.
(c) Sleep is consolidated, but characterized by sleep latency.
(d) Sleep is fragmented, but characterized by fewer arousals.

21. Which abnormality would the nurse expect to see in Ms. Brennan if she had narcolepsy?
(a) Difficulty falling asleep
(b) Brief attacks of sleep
(c) Difficulty staying asleep
(d) Sleepwalking

6

Nutritional Status

Overview

To help the nurse perform comprehensive nutritional assessments in any setting, Chapter 6 begins by reviewing the physiologic processes related to nutrition. Then it details the components of a nutritional assessment, highlighting developmental considerations for pediatric, pregnant, breast-feeding, and elderly clients. The chapter identifies specific health history questions to assess the client's nutritional status. It also shows how to evaluate nutritional status through physical assessment techniques, such as inspection, palpation, and anthropometric measurements, and laboratory studies. Finally, Chapter 6 describes how to document significant findings and apply the nursing process. It presents the following information:

• Malnutrition can occur as a primary disorder, caused by insufficient nutrient intake, or a secondary disorder, caused by a condition that impairs digestion, absorption, or use of nutrients, or increases nutrient requirements or excretion.

• Ingestion, digestion, absorption, and excretion help maintain adequate nutrition. Cell metabolism, which determines how the body uses nutrients, has two phases: catabolism and anabolism. When anabolism exceeds catabolism, the body gains weight. Carbohydrates, proteins, and fats in the diet supply the energy needed for metabolism.

• Vitamins are essential for metabolism and are water-soluble (B complex and C) or fat-soluble (A, D, E, and K).

• Minerals are essential for many body processes, such as enzyme metabolism and impulse transmission.

• The health history helps identify existing or potential nutrition-related problems. It includes a dietary history, intake record, and psychosocial assessment. When obtaining a health history, the nurse should ask the client about health and illness patterns (including current, past, and family health status), health promotion and protection patterns (such as health beliefs and exercise and activity, nutritional, stress and coping, and socioeconomic patterns), and role and relationship patterns (including self-concept and social support patterns). The nurse should tailor the health history to the client's developmental level. A complete history can help the nurse detect possible malnutrition before signs and symptoms appear.

• To perform a physical assessment, the nurse needs the following equipment: a standing platform scale with height attachment, skinfold calipers, a measuring tape, and a recumbent measuring board. Inspection of the skin, hair, mouth, throat, eyes, nails, posture, muscles, extremities, and thyroid gland can detect abnormalities related to nutritional deficiencies. Palpation may reveal enlarged glands (such as the thyroid and parotid glands) and helps assess the condition of the liver, spleen, teeth, and tongue. Anthropometric measurements help the nurse evaluate the client's height in relation to weight and may reveal inadequate or excess food intake. To determine the client's ideal weight, the nurse first determines body frame size, and then compares the client's height and weight with standard measurement charts.

• Advanced assessment skills include measurements of midarm circumference, triceps skinfold thickness, and midarm muscle circumference. The nurse should use these measurements to determine the amount of skeletal muscle and adipose tissue, which indicate protein and fat reserves.

• Laboratory studies of hemoglobin, hematocrit, red blood cell indices, serum iron, serum albumin, serum transferrin, total iron-binding capacity, total lymphocyte count, and total protein can provide clues to the possible causes of nutritional disorders.

- Documentation of a 24-hour dietary recall, or a 3-, 7-, or 14-day dietary inventory is an important part of nutritional assessment.

Suggested lecture topics

- Review the physiologic processes involved in nutrition.
- Demonstrate how to measure midarm circumference, triceps skinfold thickness, and midarm muscle circumference.
- Have a nutritionist discuss and compare the dietary needs of a well client and an ill client.
- Have a nutritionist describe how dietary needs vary for clients at different growth and developmental levels.

Suggested critical thinking activities

- Have the students plot their own height, weight, and skinfold measurements on standard charts and evaluate the results.
- Pair the students and have them obtain a dietary history—including a 24-hour dietary recall—from each other. Then have the students analyze their findings.
- Have the students develop a nursing care plan based on a case study of a malnourished client.
- Pair the students and have them perform anthropometric arm measurements on each other. Then have the students analyze their findings.

Student study questions and answers

The following study questions are taken from text page 147 of Chapter 6, Nutritional Status. Their answers are based on information in that chapter.

1. A client asks for information on dietary requirements, including the best sources of carbohydrates. What facts do you provide?

Answer
- Experts recommend that 10% to 20% of a person's daily caloric intake comes from protein; about 30% from fat; and 50% to 60% from carbohydrates. Protein-rich foods include poultry, fish, meat, eggs, milk, and cheese (complete proteins) as well as some vegetables and grains (incomplete proteins). Fats are found in vegetable oils and animal fats.
- Carbohydrates, which are ingested as starches (complex carbohydrates) and sugars (simple carbohydrates), are the chief protein-sparing ingredients in a nutritionally sound diet. In general, the diet should include more calories from complex carbohydrates, such as rice, bread, and legumes,

---

Skills laboratory guide: Health history

To collect information about the client's nutritional status, ask questions about health and illness patterns, health promotion and protection patterns, and role and relationship patterns. Sample questions from each category are listed below.

HEALTH AND ILLNESS PATTERNS

- Have you had any recent change in diet?
- Have you experienced any significant weight gain or loss or change in appetite?
- Do you have any food allergies?
- Have you ever had, or been told you have, an eating disorder?
- How much per day do you consume of coffee, tea, cola, and cocoa?
- Do you take any vitamin or mineral supplements? Do you use any "natural" or "health" foods?

HEALTH PROMOTION AND PROTECTION PATTERNS

- Which particular foods do you believe you should eat at this time?
- Which particular foods do you believe you should not eat at this time?
- Where and how is your food prepared?
- Do you have access to adequate storage and refrigeration?
- Do you receive food stamps, Social Security payments, or assistance from WIC?

ROLE AND RELATIONSHIP PATTERNS

- Do you like yourself physically?
- Are you content with your present weight?
- Do you eat alone or with others?
- On a scale of 1 to 10, with 10 being the most important to you, how would you rate mealtimes?

---

than from simple carbohydrates, such as sugar, cookies, and candy. Excessive carbohydrate intake—especially of simple carbohydrates—can cause obesity, predisposing a person to many disorders.

2. Mrs. Adams brings her daughter Kirsten, age 4 months, to the clinic. Kirsten is listless, refuses food and fluid, and appears pale. You weigh Kirsten and find that she is 8 lb, 5 oz. You notice that she sucks weakly on a pacifier. How would you record the following information related to your nursing assessment of Kirsten?
- history (subjective) assessment data
- physical (objective) assessment data
- assessment techniques and equipment
- two appropriate nursing diagnoses
- documentation of findings.

Answer
History (subjective) assessment data
- Mother states child is listless and refuses food and fluids.

Skills laboratory guide: Physical assessment

This chart guides the student during assessment by identifying body areas, special considerations and techniques to be used, and normal findings.

BODY AREA	SPECIAL CONSIDERATIONS	NORMAL FINDINGS
Inspection		
General appearance	• Note size and weight.	• Appropriate size and weight for client's age, sex, and body frame
Skin, hair, and nails	• Note skin color and lesions; hair quality and distribution; thin or split nails.	• Smooth skin, free of lesions and appropriate for client's age • Thick, shiny hair with no alopecia • Smooth nails with no cracks, fissures, thinness, or splitting
Mouth (lips, gingivae, oral mucosa, tongue, teeth)	• Note hydration, cheilosis, redness, inflammation, bleeding gums, or loose teeth.	• Pink, moist lips, free of lesions and cheilosis • Pink oral mucosa, gingivae, and tongue • No redness, swelling, lesions, or bleeding • Teeth in good repair and firmly attached to gingivae
Eyes (eyelids, conjunctiva, cornea)	• Note red or dry conjunctiva, swollen or red lids, or opaque cornea.	• Clear eyes with no dryness, redness, or roughness • Pink, transparent conjunctivae • No eyelid edema or redness • Transparent cornea with no opacities
Musculoskeletal system (posture, extremities, muscles)	• Note the client's posture and the movement of extremities. • Note any gross muscle wasting, atrophy, edema, or hypertrophy.	• Appropriate posture for age • Symmetrical movement of extremities • Symmetrical muscles with no atrophy, hypertrophy, or edema
Palpation		
Mouth	• Note atrophy of papillae or loose teeth.	• Firm tongue with no atrophy of papillae • No loose teeth
Parotid gland	• Note enlargement or tenderness.	• Nontender parotid gland
Thyroid gland	• Note enlargement or tenderness.	• Nontender, nonpalpable thyroid gland
Liver and spleen	• Note enlargement or tenderness.	• Nontender, nonpalpable liver and spleen
Anthropometric measurements	• Measure height and weight, taking serial readings.	• Appropriate height and weight for client's age, sex, and body frame
Height and weight	• Refer clients who are 20% above or below standard for medical evaluation. Keep in mind that height decreases with age in elderly clients. Measure head and chest circumference in infants and small children. In children under age 2, measure length with child supine. Refer clients with values at or below 5th percentile or at or above 95th percentile for medical evaluation.	• Height and weight values correlate on a standard height-weight chart • Height and weight values correlate on standard pediatric growth grids
Advanced assessment skills		
Anthropometric arm measurements	• Measure midarm circumference, triceps skinfold thickness, and midarm muscle circumference. Measure midarm midpoint for accuracy. Apply calipers ⅜″ (1 cm) above midpoint to assess triceps skinfold thickness; take three readings, then compute average. Record all three measurements as percentages of the standard measurements.	• Appropriate arm measurements for client's age and sex

Physical (objective) assessment data
• Weight 8 lb, 5 oz
• Child appears pale.
• Child sucks weakly on pacifier.
Assessment techniques and equipment
• Interview the child's mother about the type and amount of feedings as well as vitamin use. Also find out about recent illnesses, the child's last health care visit, and how long the child has been refusing food and fluid.
• Inspect child's general appearance, especially noting skin and luster of eyes.
• Palpate for skin turgor and bony prominences.
• Measure the child's length with a stature-measuring device.
• Weigh the child nude on an infant scale.
• Plot height and weight on a growth grid.
• Measure the child's head and chest circumference with a measuring tape.
• Compare these measurements to standard growth charts.
Two appropriate nursing diagnoses
• Altered nutrition: less than body requirements, related to inadequate intake of food and fluids
• Fluid volume deficit related to refusal to drink fluids
Documentation of findings
• S—Mother states child is listless and refuses food and fluids.
• O—8 lb, 5 oz, pale, 4-month-old child who sucks weakly on pacifier
• A—Altered nutrition: less than body requirements, related to inadequate intake of food and fluids

3. Karen McNulty, age 18, is pregnant and comes to the prenatal clinic for a checkup. Because of her age and condition, Mrs. McNulty is at nutritional risk. What health history questions would you ask Mrs. McNulty to assess her nutritional status?

Answer
• How have your eating patterns changed since you have become pregnant?
• Are you taking any nutritional supplements, such as vitamins?
• How has your weight changed since you have become pregnant?
• Are you currently breast-feeding another baby?
• What do you eat in a typical day (24 hours)? What snacks and fluids do you consume?
• Do you use any alcohol, drugs, tobacco, caffeine (coffee, tea, cola, or cocoa), or salt? If so, what effects do they produce?
• Do you follow any special diets?

4. What four factors contribute to malnutrition in elderly clients?

Answer
• Poorly fitting dentures, which can decrease nutritional intake and limit variety in diet.
• Physical disabilities that limit mobility and therefore the ability to obtain, prepare, or eat food.
• Nutritionally inadequate diet of soft, refined foods that are low in residue and dietary fiber.
• Social isolation.

5. What assessment techniques are used to determine a client's nutritional status? Correlate the assessment techniques with the body systems involved.

Answer
Inspection and palpation are the assessment techniques used to assess a client's nutritional status. The nurse should inspect the client's skin, hair, and nails (integumentary system) as well as posture, muscles, and extremities (musculoskeletal system). The nurse also should inspect the oral structures, eyes, and thyroid gland; and palpate to detect enlarged glands, such as the thyroid (endocrine system), liver (gastrointestinal system), and spleen (immune system).

Questions, answers, and rationales

1. Raymond Lambert, age 40, is admitted to the critical care unit with a myocardial infarction. The physician orders a lipid profile as well as other tests for Mr. Lambert. Which lipoprotein is associated with the lowest incidence of coronary artery disease (CAD)?
(a) Chylomicrons
(b) Very low-density lipoproteins
(c) Low-density lipoproteins
(d) High-density lipoproteins
Correct answer: (d), see text page 127. Clients with high levels of high-density lipoproteins (HDLs) have a lower incidence of CAD, possibly because HDLs help remove excess cholesterol from the body.

2. Evelyn Granger, age 75, is admitted to the orthopedic unit for fractured hip repair. Because of the stress and immobility associated with this injury, Ms. Granger is at increased risk for developing which metabolic disorder?
(a) Negative nitrogen balance
(b) Hyperlipidemia
(c) Hypoglycemia
(d) Anabolism
Correct answer: (a), see text page 126. Negative nitrogen balance may result from inadequate dietary protein intake, inadequate quality of ingested dietary protein, or excessive tissue breakdown following stress, injury, immobility, or disease.

3. During the health history, the nurse asks basic questions that assess nutritional health. Based on Ms. Granger's developmental status, which additional question should the nurse ask?
(a) "Do you wear dentures?"
(b) "What are your food preferences?"
(c) "Do you have any food allergies?"
(d) "Who prepares your meals?"
Correct answer: (a), see text page 132. The nurse should ask an elderly client about denture wear and fit. Poorly fitted dentures may decrease an elderly client's nutritional intake, contributing to nutritional deficiencies.

4. Ms. Granger reports that she has chronic obstructive pulmonary disease for which she takes bronchodilator, steroid, and diuretic drugs. How may steroid use affect Ms. Granger's nutritional status?
(a) It may cause hypocalcemia.
(b) It may produce hyperkalemia.
(c) It may decrease folic acid absorption.
(d) It may increase vitamin B_{12} excretion.
Correct answer: (a), see text page 130. Steroids can produce adverse effects on nutritional status, causing sodium retention, hypokalemic alkalosis, and hypocalcemia.

5. How may diuretic use affect Ms. Granger's nutritional status?
(a) It may cause hyperglycemia.
(b) It may produce metabolic acidosis.
(c) It may exacerbate osteoporosis.
(d) It may cause fluid and electrolyte imbalances.
Correct answer: (d), see text page 130. Nutrition-related adverse reactions to diuretics may include fluid and electrolyte imbalances, hypokalemia or hyperkalemia, hypocalcemia or hypercalcemia, and metabolic acidosis.

6. The nurse performs a physical assessment of Ms. Granger. Which finding is considered normal for a woman of her age?
(a) Increased weight
(b) Muscle wasting
(c) Decreased height
(d) Increased chest circumference
Correct answer: (c), see text page 144. Height commonly decreases with age because of changes in intervertebral discs, vertebrae, and posture.

7. Martha Small takes her daughter Sandy, age 18, to the physician because she is obsessed about losing weight even though she now appears emaciated from dieting. These findings most likely suggest which eating disorder?
(a) Anorexia nervosa
(b) Bulimia
(c) Kwashiorkor
(d) Pica
Correct answer: (a), see text page 141. Anorexia nervosa usually affects adolescent or young adult females. It is characterized by an emaciated appearance, a morbid fear of being fat, and a compulsion to be thin.

8. During the health history, which question best assesses the effect of role and relationship patterns on Sandy's nutritional status?
(a) "Do you have any food allergies?"
(b) "What is your usual activity pattern?"
(c) "What are your food preferences?"
(d) "Do you like yourself physically?"
Correct answer: (d), see text page 136. Role and relationship patterns focus on body image and relationships with others, which commonly are interrelated with food intake.

9. After obtaining a health history, the nurse assesses Sandy. Which assessment technique is most helpful in detecting nutritional deficiencies?
(a) Inspection
(b) Palpation
(c) Percussion
(d) Auscultation
Correct answer: (a), see text page 137. The nurse obtains information about nutritional deficiencies primarily through inspection. Palpation also provides useful information, but is less important.

10. Which assessment technique helps determine protein and fat reserves?
(a) Height and weight measurements
(b) Anthropometric arm measurements
(c) Chest circumference measurement
(d) Head circumference measurement
Correct answer: (b), see text page 144. Midarm circumference, triceps skinfold thickness, and midarm muscle circumference provide a way to determine the amount of skeletal muscle and adipose tissue, which indicate protein and fat reserves.

11. Sandy's poor nutrition and weight loss place her at risk for negative nitrogen balance. Which laboratory study would best assess for this problem?
(a) Hemoglobin
(b) Total iron-binding capacity
(c) Total protein
(d) Serum transferrin
Correct answer: (c), see text page 126 and 146. Because negative nitrogen balance can result from inadequate protein intake, it could be detected by a total protein test, which is designed to reveals hyperproteinemia and hypoproteinemia.

12. Considering Sandy's excessive weight loss, which term best describes her metabolic state?
(a) Catabolic
(b) Anabolic
(c) Malabsorptive
(d) Hyperexcretory
Correct answer: (a), see text page 125. Catabolism involves the breakdown of complex substances into simpler constituents for energy production or excretion. When catabolism exceeds anabolism, the body loses weight.

13. Rita Blackburn brings her son Andy, age 1, to the pediatrician for his annual check-up. Which measurement is included in Andy's check-up that would not be included in an adult's check-up?
(a) Head and chest circumference
(b) Midarm circumference
(c) Triceps skinfold thickness
(d) Thigh circumference
Correct answer: (a), see text page 142. Head and chest circumference are anthropometric measurements that are included in the physical assessment of infants and children.

14. At the same time, Ms. Blackburn brings her daughter Becky, age 4, for her annual check-up. The nurse plots Becky's height and weight on a pediatric growth grid. Normal growth is represented by which range of percentiles?
(a) 50th to 100th percentile
(b) 25th to 75th percentile
(c) 10th to 100th percentile
(d) 5th to 95th percentile
Correct answer: (d), see text page 144. Measurements that fall between the 5th and 95th percentiles represent normal growth for most clients.

15. The physician prescribes a vitamin supplement for Andy. What is the main purpose of vitamins?
(a) To promote normal metabolism
(b) To maintain acid-base balance
(c) To maintain fluid and electrolyte balance
(d) To remove excess cholesterol
Correct answer: (a), see text page 128. Vitamins are active organic compounds that are essential for normal metabolism; they contribute to enzyme reactions that facilitate the metabolism of amino acids, fats, and carbohydrates.

16. Joseph Greenspan, age 52, has hypertension and is 40 pounds overweight. As part of Mr. Greenspan's treatment, the physician prescribes a weight reduction program. Which history question best assesses the effect of health promotion and protection patterns on Mr. Greenspan's nutritional status?
(a) "Have you had any significant weight gain or loss?"
(b) "Do you eat alone or with others?"
(c) "Are you content with your present weight?"
(d) "Where and how is your food prepared?"
Correct answer: (d), see text page 136. All of these questions help assess nutritional status. However, questions about health beliefs and exercise and activity, nutritional, stress and coping, and socioeconomic patterns can best assess health promotion and protection patterns.

17. The nurse should use which assessment tool to evaluate Mr. Greenspan's nutritional patterns?
(a) Anthropometric measurements
(b) Height and weight measurements
(c) 24-hour diet recall
(d) Lipid profile
Correct answer: (c), see text page 133. To assess nutritional patterns, the nurse obtains a dietary history, using a 24-hour diet recall, 3-day or 7- to 14-day dietary inventory, food frequency form, or similar tool.

18. Maureen Keller, age 30, has Crohn's disease, which has produced severe weight loss, dry skin, muscle wasting, and frequent diarrhea. As a result, Ms. Keller has developed marasmus. This disorder is a deficiency of which nutrients?
(a) Calories
(b) Vitamins
(c) Minerals
(d) Fluids
Correct answer: (a), see text page 141. Maramus is a caloric deficiency that causes depletion of body fat and lean body mass.

19. Kwashiorkor is similar to marasmus. How do these nutritional deficiencies differ?
(a) Kwashiorkor produces more severe weight loss.
(b) Kwashiorkor causes more extensive muscle wasting.
(c) Kwashiorkor is marked by normal body weight; marasmus, by weight loss.
(d) Kawshiorkor causes decreased body fat; marasmus does not.
Correct answer: (c), see text page 144. In kwashiorkor, depleted visceral protein, normal to excessive body fat, and normal body weight are characteristic. In marasmus, body fat and lean body mass are depleted.

20. Ms. Keller undergoes several laboratory tests. Which test detects visceral protein depletion?
(a) Hemoglobin
(b) Hematocrit
(c) Serum iron
(d) Serum albumin
Correct answer: (d), see text page 145. Also known as hypoalbuminemic malnutrition, depleted visceral protein decreases the serum albumin level.

Test bank for Chapter 6, Nutritional Status

1. Raymond Lambert, age 40, is admitted to the critical care unit with a myocardial infarction. The physician orders a lipid profile as well as other tests for Mr. Lambert. Which lipoprotein is associated with the lowest incidence of coronary artery disease (CAD)?
(a) Chylomicrons
(b) Very low-density lipoproteins
(c) Low-density lipoproteins
(d) High-density lipoproteins

2. Evelyn Granger, age 75, is admitted to the orthopedic unit for fractured hip repair. Because of the stress and immobility associated with this injury, Ms. Granger is at increased risk for developing which metabolic disorder?
(a) Negative nitrogen balance
(b) Hyperlipidemia
(c) Hypoglycemia
(d) Anabolism

3. During the health history, the nurse asks basic questions that assess nutritional health. Based on Ms. Granger's developmental status, which additional question should the nurse ask?
(a) "Do you wear dentures?"
(b) "What are your food preferences?"
(c) "Do you have any food allergies?"
(d) "Who prepares your meals?"

4. Ms. Granger reports that she has chronic obstructive pulmonary disease for which she takes bronchodilator, steroid, and diuretic drugs. How may steroid use affect Ms. Granger's nutritional status?
(a) It may cause hypocalcemia.
(b) It may produce hyperkalemia.
(c) It may decrease folic acid absorption.
(d) It may increase vitamin B_{12} excretion.

5. How may diuretic use affect Ms. Granger's nutritional status?
(a) It may cause hyperglycemia.
(b) It may produce metabolic acidosis.
(c) It may exacerbate osteoporosis.
(d) It may cause fluid and electrolyte imbalances.

6. The nurse performs a physical assessment of Ms. Granger. Which finding is considered normal for a woman of her age?
(a) Increased weight
(b) Muscle wasting
(c) Decreased height
(d) Increased chest circumference

7. Martha Small takes her daughter Sandy, age 18, to the physician because she is obsessed about losing weight even though she now appears emaciated from dieting. These findings most likely suggest which eating disorder?
(a) Anorexia nervosa
(b) Bulimia
(c) Kwashiorkor
(d) Pica

8. During the health history, which question best assesses the effect of role and relationship patterns on Sandy's nutritional status?
(a) "Do you have any food allergies?"
(b) "What is your usual activity pattern?"
(c) "What are your food preferences?"
(d) "Do you like yourself physically?"

9. After obtaining a health history, the nurse assesses Sandy. Which assessment technique is most helpful in detecting nutritional deficiencies?
(a) Inspection
(b) Palpation
(c) Percussion
(d) Auscultation

10. Which assessment technique helps determine protein and fat reserves?
(a) Height and weight measurements
(b) Anthropometric arm measurements
(c) Chest circumference measurement
(d) Head circumference measurement

11. Sandy's poor nutrition and weight loss place her at risk for negative nitrogen balance. Which laboratory study would best assess for this problem?
(a) Hemoglobin
(b) Total iron-binding capacity
(c) Total protein
(d) Serum transferrin

12. Considering Sandy's excessive weight loss, which term best describes her metabolic state?
(a) Catabolic
(b) Anabolic
(c) Malabsorptive
(d) Hyperexcretory

13. Rita Blackburn brings her son Andy, age 1, to the pediatrician for his annual check-up. Which measurement is included in Andy's check-up that would not be included in an adult's check-up?
(a) Head and chest circumference
(b) Midarm circumference
(c) Triceps skinfold thickness
(d) Thigh circumference

14. At the same time, Ms. Blackburn brings her daughter Becky, age 4, for her annual check-up. The nurse plots Becky's height and weight on a pediatric growth grid. Normal growth is represented by which range of percentiles?
(a) 50th to 100th percentile
(b) 25th to 75th percentile
(c) 10th to 100th percentile
(d) 5th to 95th percentile

15. The physician prescribes a vitamin supplement for Andy. What is the main purpose of vitamins?
(a) To promote normal metabolism
(b) To maintain acid-base balance
(c) To maintain fluid and electrolyte balance
(d) To remove excess cholesterol

16. Joseph Greenspan, age 52, has hypertension and is 40 pounds overweight. As part of Mr. Greenspan's treatment, the physician prescribes a weight reduction program. Which history question best assesses the effect of health promotion and protection patterns on Mr. Greenspan's nutritional status?
(a) "Have you had any significant weight gain or loss?"
(b) "Do you eat alone or with others?"
(c) "Are you content with your present weight?"
(d) "Where and how is your food prepared?"

17. The nurse should use which assessment tool to evaluate Mr. Greenspan's nutritional patterns?
(a) Anthropometric measurements
(b) Height and weight measurements
(c) 24-hour diet recall
(d) Lipid profile

18. Maureen Keller, age 30, has Crohn's disease, which has produced severe weight loss, dry skin, muscle wasting, and frequent diarrhea. As a result, Ms. Keller has developed marasmus. This disorder is a deficiency of which nutrients?
(a) Calories
(b) Vitamins
(c) Minerals
(d) Fluids

19. Kwashiorkor is similar to marasmus. How do these nutritional deficiencies differ?
(a) Kwashiorkor produces more severe weight loss.
(b) Kwashiorkor causes more extensive muscle wasting.
(c) Kwashiorkor is marked by normal body weight; marasmus, by weight loss.
(d) Kawshiorkor causes decreased body fat; marasmus does not.

20. Ms. Keller undergoes several laboratory tests. Which test detects visceral protein depletion?
(a) Hemoglobin
(b) Hematocrit
(c) Serum iron
(d) Serum albumin

7

Skin, Hair, and Nails

Overview

To prepare the nurse to assess the skin, hair, and nails, Chapter 7 reviews the anatomy and physiology of these structures. Then it presents the health history and physical assessment for these structures, highlighting developmental and cultural variations and the significance of abnormal findings. The chapter covers the following points:

- The skin has two distinct layers, the epidermis and the dermis, overlying a layer of subcutaneous fat. Epidermal appendages include the hair, nails, and sebaceous, apocrine, and eccrine glands.

- The surface skin layer, the epidermis, has two layers: a superficial keratinized layer of cells that are shed continuously or worn away, and a deeper germinal layer that produces new cells to replace the superficial ones.

- The dermis also has two layers: superficial papillary dermis and reticular dermis. A collagenous membrane (the basement membrane) anchors the epidermis to the papillary dermis. The subcutaneous fat layer beneath the dermis acts as a mechanical and thermal insulator.

- Numerous appendages occur throughout the skin: hair, nails, and sebaceous, apocrine, and eccrine glands. Hair and hair follicles cover the body except the palms, soles, and mucocutaneous junctions. Sebaceous glands, which appear throughout the body except for the palms and soles, secrete sebum (a lipid substance) into the hair follicles. Nails, which serve a protective function, are situated over the dorsal surface of the distal end of each digit. The underlying vascular nail bed gives the nail plate its pink color. The apocrine and eccrine glands are sweat glands.

The apocrine glands are found in the axilla and groin near hair follicles; the eccrine glands are located over most of the body except the lips.

- Because the skin can affect and be affected by every body system, skin problems can result from disorders in other areas of the body. Therefore, skin assessment can provide important information for the evaluation of most illnesses, not just for primary skin disorders.

- Skin assessment includes a thorough health history followed by careful inspection and palpation.

- When conducting the health history, the nurse can establish trust by providing a comfortable environment and using terms that are familiar to the client. Without such rapport, the client may be embarrassed to discuss or reveal lesions on private parts of the body.

- During the physical assessment, the nurse first evaluates the client's body weight, fluid status, general appearance, and vital signs. Then the nurse inspects and palpates all skin areas and appendages, including the mucous membranes of the mouth and eyes.

- The nurse assesses the skin for color, texture, consistency, temperature, turgor, and lesions, comparing similar body areas.

- When assessing primary skin lesions, the nurse notes the morphology, distribution, location, and configuration, as well as any secondary changes that may have occurred.

- During the physical assessment, the nurse should document skin lesions by their descriptive characteristics as well as their nomenclature.

- The nurse should document all assessment findings and use them in the nursing process to plan, implement, and evaluate the client's nursing care.

Skills laboratory guide: Health history

To collect information about the client's skin, hair, and nails, ask questions about health and illness patterns, health promotion and protection patterns, and role and relationship patterns. Sample questions from each category are listed below.

HEALTH AND ILLNESS PATTERNS

- What aspect of your skin problem bothers you the most?
- Where on your body did the skin problem begin?
- When did you first notice these changes?
- How does your skin feel?
- Have you noticed skin changes in other areas?
- Does anything make the problem worse?
- Does anything make the problem better?
- Have you used any home remedies or prescription or over-the-counter drugs to try to resolve your problem?
- Have you recently had any other illnesses?
- Have you noticed any unusual overall or patchy hair loss?
- Have you noticed any changes in your nails?
- Have you had any allergic reactions?
- Has anyone in your family had a skin problem?

HEALTH PROMOTION AND PROTECTION PATTERNS

- What do you do to try to keep your skin healthy? What things would you like to do for your skin but feel unable to do?
- What type of soap, skin creams, lotions, and other skin and hair products do you use?
- Have you recently experienced any stress or emotional problems? If so, how have you handled these problems?

ROLE AND RELATIONSHIP PATTERNS

- How has your skin problem affected your daily activities?
- How does the affected area look to you?
- How does the problem make you feel?

- For more information about skin, hair, and nail assessment, see pages 1PG through 9PG of the Photo Gallery in the text.

Suggested lecture topics

- Review the anatomy and physiology of the skin, hair, and nails, using overhead projections or other visual aids. (For visual aids, see the transparency master, *Anatomy of the skin,* as well as page 1PG in the text.)
- Discuss health history questions that are important to skin, hair, and nail assessment, and explain the rationales behind these questions.
- Using a live model and the proper equipment, demonstrate how to inspect and palpate the skin, hair, and nails.
- Using audiovisual aids, discuss normal and abnormal findings of a skin, hair, and nail assessment. Include typical developmental and cultural variations in your discussion. (For visual aids, see pages 2PG through 9PG in the text.)

Suggested critical thinking activities

- Pair the students according to sex, and have them perform a skin, hair, and nail assessment—including a history and physical assessment—on each other.
- Have the students document their assessment findings on the Skills Laboratory Assessment Guide.
- Have the entire class critique these assessment findings.
- Using a case history of a client with a skin disorder, have the students develop a nursing care plan.

Student study questions and answers

The following study questions are taken from text pages 180 and 181 of Chapter 7, Skin, Hair, and Nails. Their answers are based on information in that chapter.

1. How would you compare the location, secretions, and function of the apocrine, eccrine, and sebaceous glands of the skin?

Answer
- Located primarily in the axillary and anogenital areas, the apocrine glands have no known biological function, but produce a fluid. Bacteria decompose this fluid when it reaches the skin surface, causing adult body odor.
- Eccrine glands are distributed widely over the entire body. They secrete sweat—a watery, odorless fluid with a sodium concentration equal to that of plasma. Sweat is vital to body temperature regulation.
- Sebaceous glands occur in all parts of the skin except on the palms and soles; they are most prominent on the scalp, face, upper torso, and anogenital region. These glands secrete sebum, a lipid substance, into hair follicles and directly onto the skin surface. Sebum may help waterproof the hair and skin, promote absorption of fat-soluble substances into the dermis, play a role in vitamin D_3 production, and serve some antibacterial function.

2. You have been assigned to the newborn nursery. What are three normal skin variations of the newborn about which parents may express concern?

Answer
A normal physiologic jaundice, related to destruction of excess red blood cells and marked by a yellow skin tone, may occur within 2 to 3 days after birth and usually resolves within a week. Capillary hemangioma (stork bites)—small, reddened areas on the upper eyelids, bridge of the nose, and nape of the neck—result from localized vascular congestion and disappear as the skin thickens. Milia—small, white papules primarily over the nose, chin, and forehead—result from plugged sebaceous glands and usually disappear spontaneously a few weeks after birth.

Skills laboratory guide: Physical assessment

This chart guides the student during assessment by identifying body areas, special considerations and techniques to be used, and normal findings.

BODY AREA	SPECIAL CONSIDERATIONS	NORMAL FINDINGS
Inspection		
General assessment	• Note body weight, age, general appearance, signs of fluid balance, and effects of systemic disorders. • Weigh the client daily at the same time with the same scale. • Weight changes within 48 hrs usually reflect fluid changes.	• Appropriate body weight for age, sex, and body frame • Appropriate general appearance for stated age • No signs of fluid imbalance or systemic disorders
Skin	• Observe color, particularly noting jaundice, pallor, erythema, or cyanosis. Also note any areas of hyperpigmentation, hygiene, and odor. Sun-exposed skin areas usually are darker than nonexposed areas. • Note any vascular changes. If detected, assess for color, location, blanching, and pulsation. • Note any skin lesions. If detected, assess for morphology, distribution, location, configuration, and individual characteristics. • Make side-to-side comparisons. • Transilluminate, if indicated. • Be aware of the following cultural and ethnic considerations: Hygiene and grooming may vary with culture; Futcher's line—pigmented line running diagonally from shoulder to elbow—and deep pigmentation lines on palms and soles normally occur in dark-skinned clients; dark-skinned infants commonly appear lighter until age 2 to 3 months. • Be aware of the following developmental considerations: In neonates, physiologic jaundice may occur 2 to 3 days after birth; it should resolve in about 1 week; normal newborn skin lesions may include port-wine stains, hemangiomas, and Mongolian spots; infants with less subcutaneous fat appear redder; adolescents commonly have acne and body odor; pregnant clients may exhibit chloasma, linea nigra, spider angiomas, varicose veins, and striae.	• Uniform skin color with slightly darker exposed areas • No jaundice, pallor, erythema, cyanosis, or hyperpigmentation • Good skin hygiene; no offensive odors • No vascular lesions • No skin lesions
Hair and scalp	• Note color, quantity, texture, distribution, lesions, alopecia, and pediculosis. Hair color, quantity, texture, and distribution may be affected by race and ethnic origin. Neonates born with hair shed it within the first 3 months. At puberty, male and female adolescents develop hair growth in the axillae and pubic area. Male adolescents develop facial hair and often profusion, darkening, and thickening of body hair. Pregnant clients may experience hair straightening, increased oiliness, and partial hair loss. Elderly clients typically develop gray hair and hair loss.	• Appropriate hair color, quantity, texture, and distribution for client's age, race, and ethnic origin • No scalp lesions, alopecia, or pediculosis
Nails	• Note color, consistency, smoothness, symmetry, ridges, cracks, length, bitten edges, cleanliness, angle of attachment, and clubbing. In elderly clients, the toenails may appear yellowed, thickened, and more fragile.	• Pink, smooth, symmetrical, well-groomed nails without ridges, cracks, or bitten edges • 160-degree angle of attachment, no clubbing.

continued

Skills laboratory guide: Physical assessment *continued*

BODY AREA	SPECIAL CONSIDERATIONS	NORMAL FINDINGS
Palpation		
Skin	• Note texture, coarseness, or thinning. Texture varies with age: unlike an adult's skin, an infant's or an elderly client's skin is thin and fragile. • Note temperature, excessively hot or cold areas, and asymmetry. • Note excessive dryness or moistness, turgor, and mobility. • Pregnancy increases perspiration. Elderly clients may have drier skin and decreased turgor and mobility. • Note skin lesions, tenderness, induration, consistency, and pulsations. • Wear gloves when palpating lesions. • Use dorsal part of hand to assess moisture and temperature changes.	• Smooth, soft skin that is warm and dry bilaterally • No excessive dryness or diaphoresis • Good skin turgor and mobility • No lesions
Hair and scalp	• Note texture and consistency of hair; and mobility, tenderness, and lesions of scalp.	• Medium texture hair • Mobile scalp with no tenderness or lesions
Nails	• Note firmness, adherence to nail beds, and sponginess. Pregnant clients may have brittle nails. • Check capillary refill time.	• Firm nails that adhere well to nail bed and exhibit no sponginess • Rapid capillary refill

3. What effects do each of the following conditions have on the skin?
• anemia
• decreased oxygenation
• fever
• liver disease
• pregnancy

Answer
• Anemia can cause skin and mucous membrane pallor.
• Decreased blood oxygenation commonly produces cyanosis (a bluish tinge) of the skin and mucous membranes.
• Fever may cause the skin to become warm and flushed.
• Liver disease, such as viral hepatitis, commonly produces jaundice with a characteristic yellow coloration of the sclera and skin.
• Pregnancy can cause several skin changes, including hyperpigmentation (generalized or localized to the face [chloasma], moles, or areolae), linea nigra (a brownish black streak on the midline of the abdomen), striae (stretch marks), and varicose veins.

4. What harmful effects on the skin, hair, and nails can the following behaviors produce?
• taking excessively hot showers and baths
• long-term braiding or corn-rowing of hair
• exposing unprotected skin to cleaning solvents
• sunbathing or using a tanning booth

Answer
• Repeated washing in excessively hot water can cause skin dryness.
• Traction produced by regular hair braiding can result in scalp hair loss (traction alopecia).
• Skin exposure to cleaning solvents may result in localized irritation, allergic responses, and, with certain solvents, an increased risk of skin cancer.
• Excessive exposure to sunlight or overuse of tanning booths may produce skin dryness and wrinkling, as well as an increased risk of skin cancer.

5. John Peterson, age 44, has been admitted with a fever of 102° F (38.9° C); red, puffy eyes; and a generalized red, raised rash with a few small blisters of 2 days' duration. He also reports discomfort from superficial, eroded lesions in his mouth. During the interview, Mr. Peterson asks you to dim the lights because they bother his eyes. He says he has had a seizure disorder for the past 5 years, which until recently was well controlled. He began taking phenytoin sodium (Dilantin) a few days ago. How would you relate the following information in an assessment of Mr. Peterson?
• history (subjective) assessment data
• physical (objective) assessment data
• assessment techniques and equipment
• two appropriate nursing diagnoses
• documentation of your findings.

Answer

History (subjective) assessment data
• Complaints of pruritus and painful mouth sores
• Complaints of photosensitivity
• Five-year history of seizure disorder
• Phenytoin sodium (Dilantin) regimen begun several days ago

Physical (objective) assessment data
• Male, age 44
• Fever of 102° F
• Red, puffy eyes
• Generalized erythematous rash with several small blisters

Assessment techniques and equipment
• Interview client regarding past health history, current medications, allergies, ability to consume food and fluids (because of oral lesions), and exposure to infectious diseases.
• Inspect skin and mucous membranes of the eyes and mouth for color, vascular changes, and lesions.
• Palpate skin for texture, temperature, moisture, turgor, and lesions.
• Use the following equipment: good overhead lighting, tongue depressor, penlight, and gloves for oral examination.

Two appropriate nursing diagnoses
• Impaired skin integrity related to adverse drug reaction (Dilantin)
• Pain related to pruritus

Documentation of findings
• S—Client complains of pruritus, painful mouth sores, and photosensitivity. Client has a 5-year history of seizure disorder. Has been taking phenytoin sodium (Dilantin) for several days.
• O—T 102° F, eyes red and swollen, generalized erythematous rash with small blisters
• A—Impaired skin integrity related to adverse drug reaction (Dilantin)

Questions, answers, and rationales

1. Mary Dwyer, age 62, seeks care for a skin lesion on her arm. The nurse could use which question to assess Ms. Dwyer's health promotion and protection patterns related to skin?
(a) "How does your skin feel?"
(b) "Have you noticed skin changes in other areas?"
(c) "How does the affected area look to you?"
(d) "How would you describe your usual skin exposure to the sun?"
Correct answer: (d), see text pages 163 and 164. Health promotion and protection patterns include environmental factors that may cause or aggravate skin disorders. Excessive, unprotected sun exposure increases the risk of skin cancer.

2. After determining that Ms. Dwyer's skin lesion is cancerous, the physician removes it surgically. The nurse provides postoperative instruction about skin care and protection, including the use of sunscreens. Which structure normally protects the skin from ultraviolet light?
(a) Langerhans' cells
(b) Melanocytes
(c) Eccrine glands
(d) Basal cells
Correct answer: (b), see text page 155. Melanocytes protect the skin by producing melanin to help filter ultraviolet light (irradiation).

3. The skin normally uses ultraviolet light to synthesize which vitamin?
(a) A
(b) B_6
(c) C
(d) D_3
Correct answer: (d), see text page 155. In response to ultraviolet light, the skin forms vitamin D_3 (cholecalciferol), which plays a role in preventing rickets.

4. Margaret Whiting, age 75, is admitted to the orthopedic unit for fractured hip repair. Because Ms. Whiting is at high risk for developing skin problems, the nurse performs a thorough skin assessment. Which finding may be a normal result of aging?
(a) Increased skin temperature
(b) Increased moisture
(c) Decreased turgor
(d) Decreased texture
Correct answer: (c), see text pages 173 and 177. With age, the dermis becomes less elastic from loss of collagen and elastin fibers. This causes decreased turgor (elasticity).

5. The nurse also may detect which other normal, developmental change in Ms. Whiting?
(a) Increased growth of pubic hair
(b) Increased oiliness of hair
(c) Increased growth of facial hair
(d) Increased thickness of hair
Correct answer: (c), see text page 177. The decreased ratio of estrogen to androgen in the elderly female client may cause changes in hair distribution, including baldness, increased growth of coarse facial hair, and loss of axillary and pubic hair.

6. The nurse checks Ms. Whiting's skin temperature. When doing this, the nurse should use which part of the hand?
(a) Dorsal surface
(b) Ventral surface
(c) Fingertips
(d) Finger pads
Correct answer: (a), see text page 171. The nurse should assess temperature with the dorsal surface of the fingers or hands, which are most sensitive to temperature perception.

7. What else might the nurse assess to evaluate Ms. Whiting's vascular status?
(a) Skin turgor
(b) Capillary refill
(c) Skin moisture
(d) Skin texture
Correct answer: (b), see text page 173. Assessment of capillary refill evaluates central and peripheral cyanosis related to reduced peripheral blood supply.

8. Janet Canfield, age 28, is 8½ months pregnant. She is most likely to display which normal skin color variation?
(a) Vitiligo
(b) Erythema
(c) Cyanosis
(d) Chloasma
Correct answer: (d), see text pages 170 and 177. Chloasma, the mask of pregnancy, causes tan to brown patches on the face. This hyperpigmentation results from hormonal changes.

9. Ms. Canfield also may have striae. This lesion falls into which classification?
(a) Primary
(b) Annular
(c) Arciform
(d) Secondary
Correct answer: (d), see text page 172. Striae is an example of a secondary lesion; it is marked by atrophy, or thinning of the skin surface.

10. After giving birth, Ms. Canfield expresses concern that her baby daughter has stork bites (reddened areas at the nape of the neck). What should the nurse tell her about these skin lesions?
(a) They are normal and disappear as the skin thickens.
(b) They are a sign of a common congenital anomaly.
(c) They result from trauma during delivery.
(d) They result from blocked apocrine glands.
Correct answer: (a), see text page 176. Capillary hemangioma (stork bites) may affect the upper eyelids, bridge of the nose, or nape of the neck in a neonate. They result from vascular congestion and disappear as the skin thickens.

11. Ms. Canfield's daughter develops milia (small, white raised lesions over the nose, chin, and forehead). Milia are an example of which type of primary lesion?
(a) Macule
(b) Papule
(c) Patch
(d) Keloid
Correct answer: (b), see text page 172 and 176. A papule is a firm, inflammatory, raised lesion up to 0.5 cm (¼″) diameter.

12. The physician informs Ms. Canfield that her daughter has physiologic jaundice. How long does this disorder usually last?
(a) 24 hours
(b) 2 to 3 days
(c) 1 week
(d) 2 weeks
Correct answer: (c), see text page 175. Normal physiologic jaundice (related to the destruction of excess red blood cells) may occur 2 to 3 days after birth, but should resolve in about a week.

13. JoAnn Stoll, age 3, is admitted to the hospital with nausea, vomiting, and diarrhea that have persisted for 4 days. The suspected cause is gastroenteritis. During the initial assessment, the nurse detects tenting. What does this finding indicate?
(a) Dehydration
(b) Polycythemia vera
(c) Peripheral cyanosis
(d) Clubbing
Correct answer: (a), see text page 173. Tenting (decreased skin turgor) normally may occur in elderly clients because of decreased elastin content, but it more commonly results from dehydration.

14. The nurse is likely to detect which other assessment finding?
(a) Dry mucous membranes
(b) Decreased bowel sounds
(c) Pale mucous membranes
(d) Severe edema
Correct answer: (a), see text page 166. Dry mucous membranes suggest dehydration; this finding would be consistent with the client's probable diagnosis.

15. Barbara Brown, age 45, has pernicious anemia. This disorder is likely to produce which sign?
(a) Longitudinal nail ridges
(b) Beau's lines
(c) Paronychia
(d) Clubbing
Correct answer: (b), see text page 171. Beau's lines (transverse depressions in all nails) may result from severe, acute illness; malnutrition; or anemia.

16. Helen McCullen, age 70, has shingles, a disorder that produces lesions along the course of cutaneous nerves. Which term best describes this lesion configuration?
(a) Annular
(b) Confluent
(c) Arciform
(d) Herpetiform
Correct answer: (d), see text page 167. Herpetiform lesions, which run along the course of cutaneous nerves, commonly accompany some herpes virus infections.

17. While assessing Ms. McCullen, the nurse notes that her skin is dry, which may be normal in an elderly client. What accounts for this developmental skin change?
(a) Decreased sebum production
(b) Impaired peripheral circulation
(c) Arteriosclerosis
(d) Decreased apocrine gland production
Correct answer: (a), see text pages 155, 157, and 177. Decreased numbers of functioning sebaceous and sweat glands cause dry skin and impaired thermoregulation in the elderly client.

18. Sean Armstrong, age 14, receives minocycline hydrochloride (Micocin) to treat severe acne accompanied by scarring—a type of secondary lesion. What causes secondary lesions?
(a) Trauma
(b) Primary lesion changes
(c) Infection
(d) External irritation
Correct answer: (b), see text page 172. Secondary lesions result from changes in primary lesions.

19. Because minocycline hydrochloride is a tetracycline, the nurse should instruct Sean to be alert for which possible adverse skin reaction?
(a) Dry skin
(b) Photosensitivity
(c) Chloasma
(d) Purpura
Correct answer: (b), see text page 163. Many drugs affect the skin. Various tetracyclines can produce photosensitivity as an adverse reaction.

20. Sean is experiencing characteristic changes for his age, such as increased body hair and adult body odor. Which glands are responsible for adult body odor?
(a) Apocrine
(b) Eccrine
(c) Sebaceous
(d) Sweat
Correct answer: (a), see text page 158 and 175. Bacterial decomposition of the fluid produced by the apocrine glands results in body odor.

Test bank for Chapter 7, Skin, Hair, and Nails

1. Mary Dwyer, age 62, seeks care for a skin lesion on her arm. The nurse could use which question to assess Ms. Dwyer's health promotion and protection patterns related to skin?
(a) "How does your skin feel?"
(b) "Have you noticed skin changes in other areas?"
(c) "How does the affected area look to you?"
(d) "How would you describe your usual skin exposure to the sun?"

2. After determining that Ms. Dwyer's skin lesion is cancerous, the physician removes it surgically. The nurse provides postoperative instruction about skin care and protection, including the use of sunscreens. Which structure normally protects the skin from ultraviolet light?
(a) Langerhans' cells
(b) Melanocytes
(c) Eccrine glands
(d) Basal cells

3. The skin normally uses ultraviolet light to synthesize which vitamin?
(a) A
(b) B_6
(c) C
(d) D_3

4. Margaret Whiting, age 75, is admitted to the orthopedic unit for fractured hip repair. Because Ms. Whiting is at high risk for developing skin problems, the nurse performs a thorough skin assessment. Which finding may be a normal result of aging?
(a) Increased skin temperature
(b) Increased moisture
(c) Decreased turgor
(d) Decreased texture

5. The nurse also may detect which other normal, developmental change in Ms. Whiting?
(a) Increased growth of pubic hair
(b) Increased oiliness of hair
(c) Increased growth of facial hair
(d) Increased thickness of hair

6. The nurse checks Ms. Whiting's skin temperature. When doing this, the nurse should use which part of the hand?
(a) Dorsal surface
(b) Ventral surface
(c) Fingertips
(d) Finger pads

7. What else might the nurse assess to evaluate Ms. Whiting's vascular status?
(a) Skin turgor
(b) Capillary refill
(c) Skin moisture
(d) Skin texture

8. Janet Canfield, age 28, is 8½ months pregnant. She is most likely to display which normal skin color variation?
(a) Vitiligo
(b) Erythema
(c) Cyanosis
(d) Chloasma

9. Ms. Canfield also may have striae. This lesion falls into which classification?
(a) Primary
(b) Annular
(c) Arciform
(d) Secondary

10. After giving birth, Ms. Canfield expresses concern that her baby daughter has stork bites (reddened areas at the nape of the neck). What should the nurse tell her about these skin lesions?
(a) They are normal and disappear as the skin thickens.
(b) They are a sign of a common congenital anomaly.
(c) They result from trauma during delivery.
(d) They result from blocked apocrine glands.

11. Ms. Canfield's daughter develops milia (small, white raised lesions over the nose, chin, and forehead). Milia are an example of which type of primary lesion?
(a) Macule
(b) Papule
(c) Patch
(d) Keloid

12. The physician informs Ms. Canfield that her daughter has physiologic jaundice. How long does this disorder usually last?
(a) 24 hours
(b) 2 to 3 days
(c) 1 week
(d) 2 weeks

13. JoAnn Stoll, age 3, is admitted to the hospital with nausea, vomiting, and diarrhea that have persisted for 4 days. The suspected cause is gastroenteritis. During the initial assessment, the nurse detects tenting. What does this finding indicate?
(a) Dehydration
(b) Polycythemia vera
(c) Peripheral cyanosis
(d) Clubbing

14. The nurse is likely to detect which other assessment finding?
(a) Dry mucous membranes
(b) Decreased bowel sounds
(c) Pale mucous membranes
(d) Severe edema

15. Barbara Brown, age 45, has pernicious anemia. This disorder is likely to produce which sign?
(a) Longitudinal nail ridges
(b) Beau's lines
(c) Paronychia
(d) Clubbing

16. Helen McCullen, age 70, has shingles, a disorder that produces lesions along the course of cutaneous nerves. Which term best describes this lesion configuration?
(a) Annular
(b) Confluent
(c) Arciform
(d) Herpetiform

17. While assessing Ms. McCullen, the nurse notes that her skin is dry, which may be normal in an elderly client. What accounts for this developmental skin change?
(a) Decreased sebum production
(b) Impaired peripheral circulation
(c) Arteriosclerosis
(d) Decreased apocrine gland production

18. Sean Armstrong, age 14, receives minocycline hydrochloride (Micocin) to treat severe acne accompanied by scarring—a type of secondary lesion. What causes secondary lesions?
(a) Trauma
(b) Primary lesion changes
(c) Infection
(d) External irritation

19. Because minocycline hydrochloride is a tetracycline, the nurse should instruct Sean to be alert for which possible adverse skin reaction?
(a) Dry skin
(b) Photosensitivity
(c) Chloasma
(d) Purpura

20. Sean is experiencing characteristic changes for his age, such as increased body hair and adult body odor. Which glands are responsible for adult body odor?
(a) Apocrine
(b) Eccrine
(c) Sebaceous
(d) Sweat

8

Head and Neck

Overview

Chapter 8 describes how to assess the head, neck, and related structures, including the face, nose, paranasal sinuses, mouth, and oropharynx. It also provides the necessary information to analyze assessment findings and use them in the nursing process. The chapter includes the following information:

- The eight bones of the cranium are joined by immobile joints called sutures. These bones, together with the 14 bones of the face, protect and support the brain, eyes, and other structures. The sinuses are hollow structures within the facial bones. The nose is composed of bone and cartilage. The mouth includes the lips, tongue, mucosa, gingivae, teeth, and salivary glands.

- The neck is held erect by the sternocleidomastoid and trapezius muscles, ligaments, and the cervical vertebrae. These structures form the anterior and posterior triangles, important assessment landmarks.

- When assessing the head and neck, the nurse asks health history questions that evaluate the client's health and illness patterns. These questions focus on head and neck injuries, fractures, surgery, swelling, infections, range of motion, nasal discharge, mouth lesions, swallowing, chewing, voice changes, nosebleeds, and allergies.

- To assess health promotion and protection patterns, the nurse asks questions that uncover information about smoking, headache relief, neck tightness relief, occupational stresses, risk of head injury, and mouth-care patterns.

- To assess role and relationship patterns, the nurse asks questions that uncover the effects of a head or neck problem on the client's self-perception, family relationships, and activities of daily living.

- A basic physical assessment includes inspection and palpation of the head and face; auscultation of the vessels in the head; inspection and palpation of the nose; inspection, palpation, and percussion of the frontal and maxillary sinuses; inspection of the mouth (including the lips, tongue, mucosa, gingivae, teeth, and salivary glands) and oropharynx; palpation of the lips and tongue; inspection and palpation of the neck; and auscultation of the carotid arteries.

- To perform a basic head and neck assessment in a pediatric client, the nurse also palpates the fontanels and measures head circumference. Normal assessment findings can vary greatly between adults and children, especially in dentition, tonsil size, and breathing patterns. Pregnant and elderly clients also may exhibit differences in normal findings.

- The nurse applies advanced assessment skills, as needed. These include direct inspection of the nostrils (nares) by flashlight and nasal speculum or by ophthalmoscope handle with nasal attachment; illumination of the septum; and transillumination of the sinuses by flashlight or by ophthalmoscope handle with nasal attachment.

- The nurse documents all assessment findings and uses them in the nursing process to plan and evaluate the client's care.

- For more information about head and neck assessment, see pages 10PG through 15PG of the Photo Gallery in the text.

Suggested lecture topics

- Using audiovisual aids, review the anatomic structures of the head and neck. (For visual aids, see the transparency

masters, *Anatomy of the head and neck* and *Structures of the mouth,* as well as pages 10PG through 11PG in the text.)
• Discuss and explain the rationales for health history questions that assess the head and neck.
• Demonstrate how to inspect, palpate, percuss, and auscultate the head and neck structures. (For visual aids, see pages 12PG through 14PG in the text.)
• Demonstrate advanced assessment skills, including transillumination of the sinuses and direct inspection of the nostrils. (For a visual aid, see page 12PG in the text.)

Suggested critical thinking activities

• Pair the students and have them perform a head and neck assessment, including history and physical assessment, on each other.
• Have the students document their assessment findings on the Skills Laboratory Assessment Guide.
• Have the entire class critique these assessment findings.
• Using a case study of a client with a head or neck problem, have the students develop a nursing care plan.

Student study questions and answers

The following study questions are taken from text pages 204 and 205 of Chapter 8, Head and Neck. Their answers are based on information in that chapter.

1. The head and neck contain various anatomic structures. What are these structures and which techniques can you use to assess them?

Answer
• Major cranial bones include the frontal bone, the right and left temporal bones, the right and left parietal bones, and the ethmoid, sphenoid, and occipital bones. In infants, the anterior and posterior fontanels and palpable suture lines join the cranial bones. Major facial structures include the maxilla; the mandible; frontal, sphenoid, nasal, zygomatic, occipital, temporal, and parietal bones; the frontal and maxillary sinuses; and facial muscles and nerves. Nasal structures include the nasal septum, the nostrils, the turbinates, and the mucous membranes; mouth structures include the lips, tongue, gingivae, teeth, salivary ducts, uvula, hard and soft palates, palatine tonsils, and mucous membranes. Neck structures include the cervical vertebrae, ligaments, and neck and shoulder muscles, such as the trapezius, sternocleidomastoid, and omohyoid muscles. The neck also houses the internal and external jugular veins and the carotid arteries; cervical spinal nerves; cervical lymph nodes; and the thyroid gland.
• Physical assessment of the head and neck involves inspecting and palpating the head and face; auscultating the vessels in the head; inspecting and palpating the nose;

inspecting, palpating, and percussing the frontal and maxillary sinuses; inspecting the mouth (including the lips, tongue, mucosa, gingivae, teeth, and salivary glands) and oropharynx; palpating the lips and tongue; inspecting and palpating the neck; and auscultating the carotid arteries.

2. For a client with a head or neck problem, which health history questions are the most important to ask? Why?

Answer
• The most important questions about the head and neck are those related to pain—headache, neck stiffness or pain, and sore throat. Other important questions assess head and neck injuries, fractures, surgery, swelling, infections, range of motion, nasal discharge, mouth lesions, swallowing, chewing, voice changes, nosebleeds, and allergies.
• Headaches often result from a minor problem, such as muscle tension, but sometimes may point to a serious condition, such as intracranial tumor or hemorrhage. Neck

Skills laboratory guide: Health history

To collect information about a client's head and neck, ask questions about health and illness patterns, health promotion and protection patterns, and role and relationship patterns. Sample questions from each category are listed below.

HEALTH AND ILLNESS PATTERNS

• Have you ever had head trauma, skull surgery, or jaw or facial fractures?
• Do you have frequent headaches? If so, how often do they occur? What precedes them and what relieves them?
• Have you ever had any swelling over your face, jaws, or mastoid process?
• Do you have a history of sinus infections or tenderness?
• Do you have any nasal discharge or postnasal drip?
• Do you have frequent or prolonged nosebleeds?
• Have you had any mouth lesions, ulcers, or cold sores? If so, how would you describe them? How long have you had them? Do they recur?
• Do you have any difficulty swallowing or chewing?
• Have you experienced any hoarseness or noticed any changes in the sound of your voice?

HEALTH PROMOTION AND PROTECTION PATTERNS

• Do you smoke a pipe?
• Do you chew tobacco or use snuff?
• If you suffer from headaches or tightness in the neck or jaw, what do you do for relief?
• What are your mouth-care habits?

ROLE AND RELATIONSHIP PATTERNS

• Does your head or neck problem affect the way you feel about yourself or the way you relate to your family?
• Has your head or neck problem interfered with your activities of daily living or normal sexual activity?

Skills laboratory guide: Physical assessment

This chart guides the student during assessment by identifying the body areas, special considerations and techniques to be used, and normal findings.

BODY AREA	SPECIAL CONSIDERATIONS	NORMAL FINDINGS
Inspection		
Head	• Note size, shape, symmetry, and position; scalp condition; and hair distribution. • In neonates, head asymmetry may result from molding during vaginal delivery.	• Normocephalic, erect, midline head • No scalp lesions • Evenly distributed hair
Face	• Note facial expression, skin color and condition, edema, and lesions; and abnormal movements, such as tics. • Assess symmetry of facial features by inspecting nasolabial folds and palpebral fissures. • Note hair distribution.	• Appropriate facial expression • No pallor, cyanosis, jaundice, tics, lesions, or periorbital edema • Symmetrical nasolabial folds and palpebral fissures • Normal hair distribution
Nose	• Note position, symmetry, and contour; any areas of deformity, swelling, or discoloration; and any nasal discharge or flaring. • Inspect the nose using a nasal speculum and flashlight or an ophthalmoscope with a nasal attachment, if needed.	• Midline, intact, symmetrical nose; septum aligned with bridge of nose • No deformity, swelling, discoloration, or nasal discharge; mild nasal flaring
Frontal and maxillary sinuses	• Note inflammation and edema. The frontal sinuses are located just above the eyes near the midline; the maxillary sinuses, on each side of the nose and just below the zygomatic bone. • Transilluminate the sinuses using an ophthalmoscope with a nasal attachment, if needed.	• No inflammation or edema
Lips	• Note color, condition, symmetry, and lesions.	• Pink, moist, symmetrical lips • No lesions
Oral mucosa	• Note color, patency, hydration, lesions, and any unusual breath odors. Fordyce's spots—small, yellowish white raised lesions—are the normal sebaceous glands of the buccal mucosa.	• Pink, smooth, moist oral mucosa with no lesions • No unusual odors • Bluish or patchily pigmented mucosa in dark-skinned clients
Gingivae	• Note color and condition of gingivae and any bleeding, retraction, and lesions.	• Pink, moist, slightly irregular gingivae with no spongy or edematous areas • No bleeding, retraction, or lesions
Teeth	• Note number, color, condition, and any missing or loose teeth, and occlusion of upper and lower jaws.	• 32 teeth in an adult; up to 20 teeth in a child • White to ivory teeth in good repair with smooth edges and no visible caries • Good occlusion: upper teeth extend slighly beyond and over lower teeth
Tongue	• Note position, color, mobility, and lesions.	• Midline, moist, smooth, pink tongue with no lesions • Geographic tongue (normal variant)
Stensen's and Wharton's ducts	• Note color and signs of inflammation. Stensen's ducts open at the level of the second molar on the buccal mucosa. Wharton's ducts open under the tongue. • Saliva production normally decreases with aging.	• Pink, moist ducts with no inflammation
Hard and soft palates	• Note color, symmetry, deformities, lesions, or areas of tenderness or inflammation.	• Intact pink to light red palates with symmetrical lines • No deformities, lesions, tenderness, or inflammation
Oropharynx	• Note color, lesions, swelling, exudate, and enlargement of uvula or tonsils. • Assess tonsil size as +1, normal; +2, tonsils between pillars and uvula; +3, tonsils touching uvula; +4, tonsils midline.	• Pink, moist oropharynx with no inflammation or exudates • Pink, nonhypertrophied (+1) tonsils and uvula with no exudates

Skills laboratory guide: Physical assessment *continued*

BODY AREA	SPECIAL CONSIDERATIONS	NORMAL FINDINGS
Inspection *continued*		
Neck	• Note size, condition of skin, symmetry, range of motion, pulsations, venous distention, and lymph node or thyroid enlargement. Many elderly clients experience decreased neck range of motion. • Locate the anterior and posterior triangles of the neck to assess for symmetry. • Inspect the neck as the client swallows.	• Proportionate size neck with intact skin • Symmetrical muscles with full range of motion • No visible pulsations, masses, swelling, venous distention, or lymph node or thyroid enlargement • Rising larynx, trachea, and thyroid with swallowing
Palpation		
Head	• Note symmetry, contour, masses, tenderness, scalp mobility and condition, and hair texture. • In children under age 2, measure head circumference and palpate fontanels.	• Symmetrical head with no masses, tenderness, or lesions • Freely movable scalp with no dryness, lesions, or scars • Medium texture hair with no oiliness or brittleness
Face	• Note skin condition, muscle tone and movements, temporal artery pulses, and temporomandibular joint (TMJ) function.	• Smooth, nontender facial skin • Good muscle tone and symmetrical movement • Equal temporal artery pulses • No crepitation on palpation of TMJ
Nose	• Note areas of pain, tenderness, swelling, or deformity. • Assess nostril patency by occluding each one separately.	• No pain, tenderness, swelling, or deformities • Patent nostrils
Frontal and maxillary sinuses	• Note tenderness on palpation. For frontal sinuses, apply light pressure under the ridges of the upper orbits. For maxillary sinuses, apply pressure over the cheek bones.	• Nontender sinuses
Lips and tongue	• Assess muscle tone and surface characteristics. • Wear gloves when palpating the lips and tongue.	• Soft, pink to red, symmetrical lips with good muscle tone and no lesions, lumps, ulcers, or edema • Slightly rough, freely movable tongue with good muscle tone
Oropharynx	• Assess gag reflex. The presence of the gag reflex and symmetrical rise of the uvula reflect intact cranial nerves IX and X.	• Gag reflex present
Neck	• Assess position of trachea. • Note symmetry, masses, cervical lymphadenopathy, and pulsations.	• Midline trachea • Symmetrical neck structures with no masses or cervical lymphadenopathy or tenderness • Equal carotid pulses
Percussion		
Frontal and maxillary sinuses	• Note any tenderness or dullness. • Use direct percussion for the sinuses.	• Nontender, resonant sinuses
Auscultation		
Temporal, periorbital, occipital, and carotid arteries	• Use the bell of the stethoscope. • Note any bruits.	• No bruits

stiffness or pain can result from such disorders as muscle spasm, trauma, osteoporosis, arthritis, or cervical lymphadenopathy. Throat pain and voice changes may result from bacterial or viral infections of the oropharynx or tonsils, such as strep throat. Difficult swallowing and chewing may be caused by dental or neuromuscular prob-lems. The nurse also should ask about recent head, neck, or nose injuries or surgery and about any limitations in moving the head and neck caused by past fractures, muscle spasms, or bruises. Movement limitations could indicate cervical vertebral problems, alerting the nurse to use caution when palpating and assessing range of motion in the neck. Swelling and nasal discharge may accompany recurrent infections or allergies. Nosebleeds may result from various causes, ranging from hypertension to irritation caused by excessively dry heat. Mouth lesions may result from various causes, such as poor-fitting dentures or mouth cancer.

3. A child's head and neck differ greatly from those of an elderly client. What differences in physical assessment findings can you expect to see?

Answer

• To assess the head and neck of a child under age 2, the nurse must perform these additional techniques: measurement of head circumference and inspection and palpation of the fontanels. The nurse also should keep in mind that a neonate's head shape may have been altered by vaginal delivery and that the bridge of an infant's nose may appear slightly flattened. These findings usually change as the child ages. Normal assessment findings can vary greatly between adults and children, especially in dentition, tonsil size, and breathing patterns.

• To assess the head and neck of an elderly client, the nurse should use the same techniques as for a younger adult. However, the normal findings may be slightly different. Palpation of an elderly client's head and face may reveal skin wrinkling and some loss of skin elasticity. An elderly client also may exhibit gingival recession and inflammation and may have loose teeth, dry mucous membranes from decreased salivary output, and longitudinal or latitudinal fissures in the tongue. Because many elderly clients have decreased range of motion or neck pain from osteoporosis, arthritis, or other disorders, the nurse should instruct the client to move slowly and carefully to avoid pain during assessment of range of motion.

4. Janet Gray, age 68, comes to the outpatient clinic complaining of chronic neck pain that she has had for 2 months. She has no history of fever or recent injury. How would you report the following information related to your nursing assessment of Ms. Gray?
• history (subjective) assessment data
• physical (objective) assessment data
• assessment techniques and equipment
• two nursing diagnoses
• documentation of findings.

Answer

History (subjective) assessment data
• Client reports neck pain that has persisted for 2 months.
• Client reports no history of neck injury.

Physical (objective) assessment data
• Female, age 68
• Temperature 98.4° F (36.9° C)

Assessment techniques and equipment
• Interview client about current and past health history and current medication use.
• Inspect and palpate the neck.
• Assess neck range of motion.
• No special equipment is needed.

Two nursing diagnoses
• Chronic pain related to neck muscle spasms
• Impaired physical mobility related to neck pain

Documentation of findings
• S—Client complains of chronic neck pain that has persisted for 2 months.
• O—T 98.4° F, P 82, R 20, BP 118/70. Client can move neck only 20 degrees to left and right. Client experiences moderate muscle spasm and pain on lateral movement, extension, and flexion. Cervical X-ray reveals osteoporotic degeneration of cervical spine.
• A—Chronic pain related to neck muscle spasms

5. Lisa Nelson, age 5, is brought to the emergency department by her mother. Lisa complains of a sore throat, and her mother says she has had a fever of 102° to 103° F (38.9° to 39.4° C) for the past 24 hours. Lisa has been reluctant to eat or drink because of her sore throat. How would you report the following information related to your nursing assessment of Lisa?
• history (subjective) assessment data
• physical (objective) assessment data
• assessment techniques and equipment
• two nursing diagnoses
• documentation of findings.

Answer

History (subjective) assessment data
• Client complains of sore throat.
• Client's mother reports client has had fever of 102° to 103° F for past 24 hours.
• Client's mother reports that client has not been eating or drinking well because of her sore throat.

Physical (objective) assessment data
• Female, age 5
• Fever of 102.4° F

Assessment techniques and equipment
• Interview client and mother regarding client's current and past health history, current medication use, and history of allergies.
• Inspect the mouth and oropharynx with a tongue depressor and a flashlight (if necessary).
• Inspect the internal ear with an otoscope.
• Palpate the neck.
• Monitor fluid intake and output.

Two nursing diagnoses
• Pain related to throat inflammation
• Potential fluid volume deficit related to decreased fluid intake and fever

Documentation of findings
• S—Client complaining of sore throat, fever, and inability to eat or drink.
• O—T 102.4° F, P 110, R 32, BP 90/60. Bilateral cervical lymphadenopathy noted, with 2 cm movable nodes palpated. Neck ROM normal, with no pain elicited on movement. Tympanic membranes pearly gray with good mobility. Mucous membranes slightly dry. Throat bright red with yellow and white exudate on oropharynx and +3 tonsillar hypertrophy.
• A—Pain related to throat inflammation

Questions, answers, and rationales

1. Upon admission to the hospital with right-side weakness, Terence Lambert, age 70, undergoes a comprehensive assessment to help confirm or rule out cerebrovascular accident (CVA). To assess the symmetry of his facial features, the nurse should inspect which area?
(a) Ears
(b) Uvula
(c) Bulbar fissures
(d) Nasolabial folds
Correct answer: (d), see text page 191. To determine facial symmetry, the nurse should inspect the palpebral fissures (openings between the eyelids) and nasolabial folds (creases extending from the angle of the nose to the corner of the mouth).

2. The nurse also auscultates Mr. Lambert's temporal artery. Which sounds may be detected here?
(a) S_1 and S_2
(b) Murmurs
(c) Bruits
(d) Thrills
Correct answer: (c), see text page 193. The nurse should auscultate the periorbital, temporal, and occipital arteries with the bell of the stethoscope. Auscultation normally reveals no sounds in these arteries; however, bruits may be detected.

3. Before allowing Mr. Lambert to eat, the nurse assesses his gag reflex. What is the correct technique for evaluating this reflex?
(a) Place a tongue blade on the anterior aspect of the tongue and have the client say "ah."
(b) Place a tongue blade on the middle of the tongue and have the client cough.
(c) Place a tongue blade lightly on the posterior aspect of the tongue.
(d) Place a tongue blade on the client's uvula.
Correct answer: (c), see text pages 198 and 199. To assess the gag reflex, the nurse gently touches the posterior aspect of the tongue with a tongue depressor. This action normally elicits gagging.

4. This gag reflex test assesses which cranial nerves?
(a) IX and X
(b) V and VII
(c) IX and XII
(d) V and X
Correct answer: (a), see text page 199. Gagging during the gag reflex test indicates that cranial nerves IX and X (the glossopharyngeal and vagus nerves) are intact.

5. When assessing Mr. Lambert's oral structures, the nurse can expect to see which normal finding associated with his developmental status?
(a) Gingival hypertrophy
(b) Dry mucous membranes
(c) Tonsillar hypertrophy
(d) Glossal atrophy
Correct answer: (b), see text page 201. With aging, salivary output decreases. This may cause dryness of the mucous membranes, which may interfere with chewing and make the membranes more susceptible to breakdown.

6. Maureen Albertson, age 22, seeks care for recurrent headaches. During the health history interview, the nurse asks Ms. Albertson to describe the headaches. Which description typically characterizes vascular headaches?
(a) Intermittent, deep-seated pain that is relieved by analgesics
(b) Tight sensation in the occipital or temporal area that is relieved by analgesics
(c) Pain that is most intense in the morning and relieved by analgesics
(d) Throbbing, unilateral pain that is not relieved by analgesics
Correct answer: (d), see text page 187. Vascular headaches produce a throbbing, typically unilateral pain that is not relieved by analgesics.

7. During the physical assessment, the nurse palpates Ms. Albertson's temporomandibular joints. Which assessment finding is normal?
(a) Crepitus
(b) Tenderness
(c) Smooth movement
(d) Slight clicking
Correct answer: (c), see text page 192. The nurse evaluates the temporomandibular joints for movability, approximation, and discomfort. Normally, palpation reveals smooth movement, good approximation, and no pain.

8. For many years, Jane Schultz, age 53, has taken a steroid drug as prescribed to treat chronic obstructive pulmonary disease (COPD). Prolonged use of steroid drugs may cause which facial change?
(a) Mask-like expression
(b) Moon-shaped face
(c) Dull expression
(d) Exophthalmos
Correct answer: (b), see text page 193. Prolonged use or high doses of steroids may cause the face to assume a rounded "moon" shape, with red cheeks, increased facial hair, and possibly edema.

9. Ms. Schultz has smoked cigarettes for more than 30 years. Assessment of her oral mucosa may reveal which abnormal finding that may be a precursor to cancer?
(a) Leukoplakia
(b) Pale membranes
(c) Cheilitis
(d) Cheilosis
Correct answer: (a), see text page 199. Leukoplakia, a thickened, white patch on the buccal membrane, may be precancerous.

10. Sue Lee, a 25-year-old Asian woman, has just given birth to a healthy boy. The nurse inspects the Asian newborn's head and neck. Which finding is considered normal?
(a) Decreased palpebral fissures
(b) Prominent epicanthal folds
(c) Increased nasolabial folds
(d) Low-set ears
Correct answer: (b), see text page 192. Prominent epicanthal folds (vertical folds of skin over the inner canthus of the eye) are normal facial features in Asians.

11. The nurse also assesses the newborn's fontanels. How should the newborn be positioned for this assessment?
(a) Supine
(b) Prone
(c) Seated upright
(d) Left lateral
Correct answer: (c), see text page 200. The fontanels should be assessed with the infant quiet and seated upright. Pressure from postural changes or intense crying can cause the fontanels to bulge or seem abnormally tense.

12. Because the child is under age 2, the nurse should assess which additional area?
(a) Sinus patency
(b) Neck range of motion
(c) Head circumference
(d) Gag reflex
Correct answer: (c), see text page 200. To assess a child under age 2, the nurse should measure the head circumference and assess the fontanels.

13. Lucy Bowes brings her son Johnny, age 5, to the pediatrician's office because he has had a fever of 102° F (38.9° C) and a persistent cough for 48 hours. As part of the assessment, the nurse inspects Johnny's tonsils. Where do the tonsils normally lie?
(a) Behind the pillars
(b) In front of the pillars
(c) Between the pillars and uvula
(d) Next to the uvula
Correct answer: (a), see text pages 196 and 198. Normally, the tonsils are behind the pillars (the supporting structures of the soft palate).

14. How many temporary teeth should the nurse expect to find in Johnny's mouth?
(a) Up to 10
(b) Up to 15
(c) Up to 20
(d) Up to 32
Correct answer: (c), see text page 197. A child may have up to 20 temporary (deciduous or baby) teeth. The first tooth usually erupts by age 6 months; the last, by age 30 months. All temporary teeth usually are shed between age 6 and 13.

15. The pediatrician prescribes an antibiotic for Johnny. Which antibiotic would be avoided because it may discolor the teeth?
(a) Penicillin
(b) Amoxicillin
(c) Erythromycin
(d) Tetracycline
Correct answer: (d), see text page 190. Tetracycline can produce enamel hypoplasia and permanent yellow-gray to brown tooth discoloration in children under age 8.

16. Pam Dawson, age 36, seeks care for sinusitis. To assess the maxillary sinuses, where should the nurse palpate?
(a) Below the eyebrows
(b) On the bridge of the nose
(c) Below the cheekbones
(d) Over the temporal areas
Correct answer: (c), see text page 194. To assess the maxillary sinuses, the nurse should palpate on either side of the nose below the zygomatic bone (cheekbone).

17. The nurse should use which type of percussion to assess the sinuses?
(a) Direct
(b) Indirect
(c) Fist
(d) Blunt
Correct answer: (a), see text page 194. The nurse percusses by gently tapping the index or middle finger directly over the sinuses.

18. Which other assessment technique may the nurse use to assess the sinuses?
(a) Ballottement
(b) Auscultation
(c) Transillumination
(d) Ophthalmoscopy
Correct answer: (c), see text page 196. If sinus palpation and percussion cause tenderness, transillumination may help the nurse fully evaluate the frontal and maxillary sinuses.

19. The nurse also assesses Ms. Dawson's oral structures. To assess Stensen's duct openings, the nurse should inspect which area?
(a) Floor of the mouth
(b) Buccal mucosa
(c) Hard palate
(d) Soft palate
Correct answer: (b), see text page 195. Stensen's duct openings appear as small, white rimmed openings at the level of the second molar in each cheek.

20. The nurse uses the anterior and posterior triangles as landmarks when assessing Ms. Dawson's glands and cervical lymph nodes. Which muscles form these triangles?
(a) Sternocleidomastoid and trapezius
(b) Omohyoid and cervical
(c) Sternocleidomastoid and scalene
(d) Scalene and trapezius
Correct answer: (a), see text page 185. The sternocleidomastoid and trapezius muscles and adjoining bones create the two anatomical landmarks of the neck, the anterior and posterior triangles.

Test bank for Chapter 8, Head and Neck

1. Upon admission to the hospital with right-side weakness, Terence Lambert, age 70, undergoes a comprehensive assessment to help confirm or rule out cerebrovascular accident (CVA). To assess the symmetry of his facial features, the nurse should inspect which area?
(a) Ears
(b) Uvula
(c) Bulbar fissures
(d) Nasolabial folds

2. The nurse also auscultates Mr. Lambert's temporal artery. Which sounds may be detected here?
(a) S_1 and S_2
(b) Murmurs
(c) Bruits
(d) Thrills

3. Before allowing Mr. Lambert to eat, the nurse assesses his gag reflex. What is the correct technique for evaluating this reflex?
(a) Place a tongue blade on the anterior aspect of the tongue and have the client say "ah."
(b) Place a tongue blade on the middle of the tongue and have the client cough.
(c) Place a tongue blade lightly on the posterior aspect of the tongue.
(d) Place a tongue blade on the client's uvula.

4. This gag reflex test assesses which cranial nerves?
(a) IX and X
(b) V and VII
(c) IX and XII
(d) V and X

5. When assessing Mr. Lambert's oral structures, the nurse can expect to see which normal finding associated with his developmental status?
(a) Gingival hypertrophy
(b) Dry mucous membranes
(c) Tonsillar hypertrophy
(d) Glossal atrophy

6. Maureen Albertson, age 22, seeks care for recurrent headaches. During the health history interview, the nurse asks Ms. Albertson to describe the headaches. Which description typically characterizes vascular headaches?
(a) Intermittent, deep-seated pain that is relieved by analgesics
(b) Tight sensation in the occipital or temporal area that is relieved by analgesics
(c) Pain that is most intense in the morning and relieved by analgesics
(d) Throbbing, unilateral pain that is not relieved by analgesics

7. During the physical assessment, the nurse palpates Ms. Albertson's temporomandibular joints. Which assessment finding is normal?
(a) Crepitus
(b) Tenderness
(c) Smooth movement
(d) Slight clicking

8. For many years, Jane Schultz, age 53, has taken a steroid drug as prescribed to treat chronic obstructive pulmonary disease (COPD). Prolonged use of steroid drugs may cause which facial change?
(a) Mask-like expression
(b) Moon-shaped face
(c) Dull expression
(d) Exophthalmos

9. Ms. Schultz has smoked cigarettes for more than 30 years. Assessment of her oral mucosa may reveal which abnormal finding that may be a precursor to cancer?
(a) Leukoplakia
(b) Pale membranes
(c) Cheilitis
(d) Cheilosis

10. Sue Lee, a 25-year-old Asian woman, has just given birth to a healthy boy. The nurse inspects the Asian newborn's head and neck. Which finding is considered normal?
(a) Decreased palpebral fissures
(b) Prominent epicanthal folds
(c) Increased nasolabial folds
(d) Low-set ears

11. The nurse also assesses the newborn's fontanels. How should the newborn be positioned for this assessment?
(a) Supine
(b) Prone
(c) Seated upright
(d) Left lateral

12. Because the child is under age 2, the nurse should assess which additional area?
(a) Sinus patency
(b) Neck range of motion
(c) Head circumference
(d) Gag reflex

13. Lucy Bowes brings her son Johnny, age 5, to the pediatrician's office because he has had a fever of 102° F (38.9° C) and a persistent cough for 48 hours. As part of the assessment, the nurse inspects Johnny's tonsils. Where do the tonsils normally lie?
(a) Behind the pillars
(b) In front of the pillars
(c) Between the pillars and uvula
(d) Next to the uvula

14. How many temporary teeth should the nurse expect to find in Johnny's mouth?
(a) Up to 10
(b) Up to 15
(c) Up to 20
(d) Up to 32

15. The pediatrician prescribes an antibiotic for Johnny. Which antibiotic would be avoided because it may discolor the teeth?
(a) Penicillin
(b) Amoxicillin
(c) Erythromycin
(d) Tetracycline

16. Pam Dawson, age 36, seeks care for sinusitis. To assess the maxillary sinuses, where should the nurse palpate?
(a) Below the eyebrows
(b) On the bridge of the nose
(c) Below the cheekbones
(d) Over the temporal areas

17. The nurse should use which type of percussion to assess the sinuses?
(a) Direct
(b) Indirect
(c) Fist
(d) Blunt

18. Which other assessment technique may the nurse use to assess the sinuses?
(a) Ballottement
(b) Auscultation
(c) Transillumination
(d) Ophthalmoscopy

19. The nurse also assesses Ms. Dawson's oral structures. To assess Stensen's duct openings, the nurse should inspect which area?
(a) Floor of the mouth
(b) Buccal mucosa
(c) Hard palate
(d) Soft palate

20. The nurse uses the anterior and posterior triangles as landmarks when assessing Ms. Dawson's glands and cervical lymph nodes. Which muscles form these triangles?
(a) Sternocleidomastoid and trapezius
(b) Omohyoid and cervical
(c) Sternocleidomastoid and scalene
(d) Scalene and trapezius

9

Eyes and Ears

Overview

Although the eyes and ears differ in structure and function, they have several similarities. They are both sources of perception (sight and hearing), usually are assessed sequentially, and are evaluated with similar techniques: screening tests (for vision and hearing), inspection, palpation, and advanced assessment skills using an ophthalmoscope or an otoscope. After exploring the structures and functions of the eyes and ears, Chapter 9 describes their nursing assessments in detail. Here are the chapter highlights:

• The eyelids, conjunctiva, and lacrimal apparatus form the extraocular structures of the eye. During the physical assessment, the nurse inspects and palpates these structures.

• Six muscles—four rectus and two oblique—control eye movement. To assess the functioning of these extraocular muscles, the nurse uses the six cardinal positions of gaze test, the cover-uncover test, and the corneal light reflex test.

• Retinal structures include the optic disk, four sets of retinal blood vessels, the macula, and the fovea centralis. To view these structures, the nurse uses an ophthalmoscope.

• When obtaining a health history, the nurse should ask for the date of the client's last eye examination. The answer provides information about how well the client takes care of health needs and serves as a basis for health teaching.

• The nurse also should ask what medications the client takes. The answer may reveal self-treatment of an eye condition or use of medications that can cause vision disorders.

• To assess the client's vision, the nurse performs visual acuity tests for near vision and distance vision and assesses extraocular muscle function.

• When performing an eye assessment on a child, the nurse uses the appropriate tools—for example, the Snellen E chart or the Stycar cards instead of the Snellen alphabet chart—when testing visual acuity.

• The nurse documents all eye assessment findings and uses them in the nursing process to plan, implement, and evaluate the client's care.

• The auricle and the external auditory canal compose the external ear. The tympanic membrane separates the external ear from the middle ear, which contains the three ossicles—the malleus, incus, and stapes. The inner ear contains the bony labyrinth, which houses the vestibule, the cochlea, and the semicircular canals.

• To view the tympanic membrane and the bulge of the handle of the malleus, the nurse uses an otoscope. The other middle and inner ear structures are not visible.

• When obtaining a health history, the nurse should ask for the date of the client's last ear examination. The answer provides information about how well the client takes care of health needs and serves as a basis for health teaching.

• During the health history, the nurse also should ask the client about medication use, particularly noting any drugs that may be used to self-treat an ear condition or that can cause hearing problems.

• Basic ear assessment techniques include inspection, palpation, and auditory screening. Advanced assessment calls for an otoscopic examination.

• To conduct an auditory screening, the nurse uses the voice, a watch, and a tuning fork. The voice and watch tick tests

Skills laboratory guide: Health history

To collect information about the client's eyes and ears, ask questions about health and illness patterns, health promotion and protection patterns, and role and relationship patterns. Sample questions from each category are listed below.

EYES	EARS
Health and illness patterns	**Health and illness patterns**
• Do you have any problems with your eyes? • Do you wear or have you ever worn corrective lenses? If so, for how long? Are they glasses or hard or soft contact lenses? • For what eye condition do you wear corrective lenses? • When did you last have your lenses changed? • Have you ever had blurred vision? • Have you ever seen spots, floaters, or halos around lights? If yes, is the change sudden or has it occurred for a while? • Do you suffer from frequent eye infections or inflammation? • Have you ever had eye surgery or an eye injury? • What medications are you taking, including prescription or over-the-counter medications and home remedies? • Has anyone in your family ever been treated for cataracts, glaucoma, or blindness?	• Have you recently noticed any difference in your hearing in one or both ears? • Do you have ear pain? • Do you ever have trouble with ear wax? If so, what do you do for it? • Have you had an ear injury? If so, describe the injury and treatment. • Have you experienced ringing or crackling in your ears? • Have you recently had a foreign body in your ear? • Do you suffer from frequent ear infections? • Have you had drainage from your ears? If so, when and how was it treated? • Have you had problems with balance, dizziness, or vertigo? • Have you been taking any prescription or over-the-counter medications or home remedies for your ears or for any conditions? • Has anyone in your family had hearing problems?
Health promotion and protection patterns	**Health promotion and protection patterns**
• When was your last eye examination? • Does your health insurance cover eye examinations and lenses? • Does your occupation require close use of your eyes, such as long-term reading or prolonged use of a video display terminal? • Does the air where you work or live contain anything that causes you eye problems? • Do you wear goggles when working with power tools, chain saws, or table saws or when engaging in sports that might irritate or endanger the eye, such as swimming, fencing, or playing racquetball?	• When was your last ear examination or hearing test? • Do you work around loud equipment, such as heavy machinery, air guns, or airplanes? If so, do you wear ear protectors? • Do you have any concerns about your ears or other symptoms that you would like to discuss?
Role and relationship patterns	**Role and relationship patterns**
• If you wear glasses, are they a problem for you? • If you are visually impaired, do you have difficulty fulfilling home or work obligations? • If you are visually impaired, are your social activities curtailed? If so, to what extent?	• Does your hearing difficulty interfere with your activities of daily living? • Does your hearing difficulty affect your relationships with other people? If so, how?

are gross screenings. The Weber's and Rinne tests—performed with a tuning fork—evaluate air and bone conduction and are more conclusive.

• The nurse documents all ear assessment findings and uses them in the nursing process to plan, implement, and evaluate the client's care.
• For more information about eye and ear assessment, see pages 16PG through 33PG of the Photo Gallery in the text.

Suggested lecture topics

Eyes
• Using audiovisual aids, review the anatomy and physiology of the eyes, discussing developmental variations in pediatric and elderly clients. (For visual aids, see the transparency master, *Extraocular and intraocular structures,* as well as page 16PG in the text.)
• Discuss health history questions important to eye assessment, explaining the rationales for asking them.
• Demonstrate the proper use of equipment in physical assessment of the eye, including eye charts and the ophthalmoscope.

Skills laboratory guide: Physical assessment

This chart guides the student during assessment by identifying body areas, special considerations and techniques to be used, and normal findings.

BODY AREA	SPECIAL CONSIDERATIONS	NORMAL FINDINGS
Eye function testing		
Far vision	• Use the Snellen eye chart for a literate adult or the Snellen E chart or Stycar chart for a child or an illiterate client. A child's far vision does not reach 20/20 until age 7.	• Test each eye separately and together. If client wears corrective lenses, test visual acuity with and without lenses. • 20/20 far vision right eye (OD), left eye (OS), and both eyes (OU) with no more than two mistakes
Near vision	• Note the client's ability to read newsprint held 12" to 14" (30.5 to 35.6 cm) from the eyes. • Use different size symbols instead of newsprint for a child or an illiterate client. • Test each eye separately and together.	• Intact near vision OD, OS, OU
Color vision	• Note client's ability to identify patterns of colored dots on color plates.	• Intact color vision
Extraocular muscle (EOM) function	• Perform the six cardinal positions of gaze test, noting any nystagmus or deviation of one eye. • Perform the cover-uncover test, noting any movement or wandering of one eye. • Perform the corneal light reflex test, noting light reflection on the cornea. • Refer to an ophthalmologist a child who fails one test or an adult who fails more than one test.	• Intact EOM OU; parallel, yoked eye movement • Steady eyes; no movement or wandering • Symmetrical corneal light reflex OU
Peripheral vision	• Note the client's ability to identify a moving object from peripheral (superior, temporal, inferior, and nasal) visual fields. This test is subjective because it compares the client's peripheral vision to the nurse's.	• Field of vision about 50 degrees from the top, 60 degrees medially, 70 degrees downward, and 110 degrees laterally
Eye inspection		
Eyelids	• Note color, general appearance, and edema.	• Color consistent with client's complexion • Complete closure over sclera • No edema, scaling, or lesions • Symmetrical palpebral folds; no lid lag
Eyelashes	• Note position and distribution of lashes.	• Equally distributed eyelashes that curve outward along the eyelids
Eyeball	• Note color and clarity.	• Bright, clear eyes
Lacrimal apparatus	• Note excessive tearing or dryness. Elderly clients may have decreased tear production. • Note inflammation and swelling of puncta.	• No inflammation, swelling, excessive tearing, or excessive dryness
Conjunctiva	• Note color and condition of conjunctiva. • Pull down lower eyelid to examine bulbar conjunctiva; evert eyelid to inspect palpebral conjunctiva.	• Clear, pink conjunctiva free from engorged blood vessels and drainage
Sclera	• Note color and condition of sclera. Small, dark-pigmented spots on the sclera are normal in dark-skinned clients.	• White sclera

Skills laboratory guide: Physical assessment *continued*

BODY AREA	SPECIAL CONSIDERATIONS	NORMAL FINDINGS
Eye inspection *continued*		
Cornea	• Note color, abrasions, and opacities. • Inspect cornea by shining light tangentially. Whitish ring around the edge of the cornea (arcus senilis) is a normal finding in elderly clients.	• Clear, transparent cornea • No opacities or abrasions
Anterior chamber	• Note color, size, shape, and any abnormalities. • Calculate the depth of the anterior chamber from the client's side.	• Clear, transparent anterior chamber • No bleeding, bulging, or other abnormalities
Iris	• Note size, shape, color, and the presence of any bulging. • Inspect iris from the side.	• Equal irises in size, shape, and color • Flat irises when viewed from the side
Pupils	• Note size, shape, reaction to light, and accommodation. Pupil size varies with age. Elderly clients may exhibit decreased accommodation. • Note mydriasis or miosis.	• Pupils equal, round, reactive to light, and accommodation (PERRLA); direct and consensual reaction (Direct reaction refers to pupil constriction in response to direct stimulation by light; consensual reaction, to pupil constriction in response to stimulation of the opposite eye.) • No mydriasis or miosis
Eye palpation		
Eyelids	• Note edema, tenderness, and excessive tearing.	• No edema, tenderness, or tearing on palpation
Eyeball	• Palpate with the tips of both index fingers on the eyelids over the sclera while the client looks down.	• Equally firm eyeballs
Lacrimal apparatus	• Palpate below eyebrow near the client's nose. • Observe the punctum for regurgitation of purulent material or excessive tears, which may indicate nasolacrimal duct blockage.	• No tenderness, swelling, regurgitation of purulent material, or excessive tears
Advanced eye assessment: Ophthalmoscopic examination		
Red reflex	• Note presence of red reflex, color, opacities, or dark spots. • Red reflex assessment is the only part of the ophthalmoscopic examination that is performed on an infant. • Examine from an oblique angle.	• Positive orange-red red reflex OU • No opacities or spots
Retinal vessels	• Note vessel color, the size ratio of arterioles to veins, the arteriole light reflex, and the arteriovenous (AV) crossings.	• Vessels free of exudate, bleeding, and narrowing • 2:3 or 4:5 AV ratio • Smooth AV crossings without nicking or narrowing
Retina	• Note color, consistency, hemorrhages, and exudates.	• Light yellow to orange retina with a background free from hemorrhages, aneurysms, and exudates
Optic disk	• Note color, margins, papilledema, or disk atrophy. • Look for the optic disk on the nasal side of the retina.	• Orange-red optic disk with distinct margins • No papilledema or disk atrophy
Macula	• Note color, hemorrhages, exudates, or lesions. • Always examine the macula last because it is very sensitive to light. • Look for the macula temporal to the optic disk.	• Darker macula than retinal background • No hemorrhages, exudates, or lesions
Ear function tests		
Gross hearing screening	• Use the whispered voice test to assess low-pitched sound; the watch tick test for high-pitched sounds.	• Whispered phrase heard bilaterally at a distance of 1' to 2' (30 to 60 cm) and repeated correctly • Watch tick heard bilaterally at a distance of 5" (13 cm)

continued

Skills laboratory guide: Physical assessment   *continued*

BODY AREA	SPECIAL CONSIDERATIONS	NORMAL FINDINGS
Ear function tests *continued*		
Weber's test	• Place vibrating tuning fork on top of client's head or in the middle of the forehead.	• Sound perceived equally in both ears
Rinne test	• Place vibrating tuning fork on mastoid process until the sound cannot be heard (for bone conduction test), then in front of the ear canal until the sound cannot be heard (for air conduction test). Compare the time for air conduction and bone conduction.	• Sound from air conduction heard twice as long as sound from bone conduction (2:1 ratio) bilaterally
Ear inspection		
External ear	• Note position, symmetry, angle of attachment, color, size, drainage, nodules, and lesions. • Align top of the helix with outer canthus of eye to assess position.	• Vertical ear position with not more than a 10-degree lateral-posterior slant • Similarly shaped ears, colored the same as the face, and sized in proportion to the head • No redness, drainage, nodules, or lesions • Small amount of yellow-orange cerumen
Ear palpation		
External ear	• Note tenderness, swelling, nodules, or lesions in the external ear and mastoid process. • Check for pain or tenderness by pulling the helix backward.	• Firm pinna • No pain, tenderness, swelling, nodules, or lesions
Advanced ear assessment: Otoscopic examination		
External canal	• Note inflammation, lesions, drainage, and cerumen. Use the largest speculum that fits comfortably in the client's external ear canal. • Straighten the canal by pulling the auricle up and back in adults; down and back in children.	• Varying amounts of hair and dry, gray-brown cerumen • No inflammation, scaling, lesions, or drainage
Tympanic membrane	• Note color, condition, and position of landmarks. • Look for bulging, retraction, perforation, bleeding, mobility, and lesions.	• Pearly gray, intact tympanic membrane with appropriately placed landmarks: light reflex at 7 o'clock in left ear; 5 o'clock in right ear • No bulging, retraction, perforation, bleeding, or lesions
Malleus	• Note color and position of malleus and malleolar folds.	• Dense whitish streak (malleus) originating from the superior hemisphere of the tympanic membrane • Folds in the small white projection of the short process of the malleus

• Describe normal eye assessment findings, including cultural and developmental variations. (For visual aids, see the transparency master, *Inspecting the conjunctivae,* as well as pages 17PG through 25 PG in the text.)

• Discuss abnormal findings and their implications. (For visual aids, see pages 26PG through 29PG in the text.)

Ears

• Using audiovisual aids, review the anatomy and physiology of the ears, discussing developmental variations in pediatric and elderly clients. (For visual aids, see the transparency master, *Structures of the ear,* as well as page 30PG in the text.)

• Discuss health history questions important to ear assessment, explaining the rationales for asking them.

• Demonstrate how to perform the Weber's and Rinne tests and how to use an otoscope. Describe how to modify assessment techniques for a child. (For visual aids, see the transparency master, *Otoscopic view of the tympanic membrane,* as well as pages 32PG through 33PG in the text.)

• Describe normal ear assessment findings, including cultural and developmental variations. (For visual aids, see pages 31PG through 33PG in the text.)

• Discuss abnormal findings and their implications. (For visual aids, see page 33PG in the text.)

Suggested critical thinking activities

Eyes
- Pair the students and have them perform a complete eye assessment on each other, including history and physical assessment.
- Have the students document their assessment findings on the Skills Laboratory Assessment Guide.
- Have the entire class critique these assessment findings.
- Have the students demonstrate the techniques used to assess a child's and an infant's eyes and compare them to the techniques used to assess an adult's eyes.
- Using a case study of a client with a vision problem, have the students develop a nursing care plan.

Ears
- Pair the students and have them perform a complete ear assessment on each other, including history and physical assessment.
- Have the students document their assessment findings on the Skills Laboratory Assessment Guide.
- Have the entire class critique these assessment findings.
- Have the students demonstrate the techniques used to assess a child's and an infant's ears and compare them to the techniques used to assess an adult's ears.
- Using a case study of a client with a hearing problem, have the students develop a nursing care plan.

Student study questions and answers

The following study questions are taken from text page 241 of Chapter 9, Eyes and Ears. Their answers are based on information in that chapter.

1. When your eyes see an object, such as a red rose, how do they transmit its image to the brain? (Describe this process in terms of the anatomy and physiology of the eye.)

Answer
Normally, the cornea, aqueous humor, lens, and vitreous humor refract light rays from an object and focus these rays on the fovea of the retina, where an inverted and reversed image forms clearly. Within the retina, rods and cones turn the projected image into an impulse and transmit it to the optic nerves. The impulse travels to the optic chiasma, where the two optic nerves unite and then split again into two optic tracts that continue to the optic section of the cerebral cortex in the brain. There, the inverted and reversed image on the retina changes back to its original form.

2. When a client reports an eye problem, such as blurred vision, what techniques should you use to collect physical assessment data about the eye?

Answer
To collect physical assessment data about the eye, the nurse should:
- test distance vision and near vision
- assess extraocular muscle function using the six cardinal positions of gaze test, the cover-uncover test, and the corneal light reflex test
- test peripheral vision
- inspect and palpate external ocular structures
- test the pupillary response to light
- perform an ophthalmoscopic examination.

3. When your ears hear a sound, such as a musical note, how do they transmit its perception to the brain? (Describe this process in terms of the anatomy and physiology of the ear.)

Answer
Sound waves travel through the ear by two pathways: air conduction and bone conduction. In air conduction, sound waves travel in the air through the external and middle ear to the inner ear. In bone conduction, sound waves travel through bone to the inner ear. Vibrations transmitted through air and bone stimulate nerve impulses in the inner ear. The cochlear branch of the acoustic nerve (cranial nerve VIII) transmits these vibrations to the auditory area of the cerebral cortex, where the temporal lobe of the brain interprets the sound.

4. When inspecting the right ear canal and tympanic membrane, what normal findings should you expect to see? What three common abnormal findings might you see? What could cause these abnormal findings?

Answer
- The ear canal normally has varying amounts of hair and dry, grayish brown cerumen. It should be free from inflammation and scaling. The right tympanic membrane should appear pearly gray and glistening. The annulus should appear white and denser than the rest of the membrane. The light reflex, which usually appears as a bright cone of light with its point directed at the umbo and its base at the periphery of the membrane, should be in the 5 o'clock position in the right tympanic membrane (the 7 o'clock position in the left membrane). The handle of the malleus should look like a dense whitish streak in the middle of the membrane.
- Common abnormalities noted on otoscopic examination include tympanic membrane inflammation, altered light reflex, and tympanic membrane retraction. An inflamed membrane, along with a decreased or absent light reflex, may indicate otitis media. These findings accompanied by a retracted membrane may point to serous otitis media.

5. Mrs. Traynor brings her son Tim, age 6 months, to the outpatient clinic because he has had a fever of 101° to 102° F (38.3° to 38.9° C) for the past 24 hours. She reports that he was fussy yesterday, awoke three times last night, and has been fussy today. He is drinking well but has a decreased appetite. Mrs. Traynor noticed him pulling on his ears. How would you document the following information related to your nursing assessment of Tim?
• history (subjective) assessment data
• physical (objective) assessment data
• assessment techniques and equipment
• nursing diagnoses
• documentation of your findings.

Answer
History (subjective) assessment data
• Mother reports that child has had a fever of 101° to 102° F for the past 24 hours.
• Mother reports that the child has been fussy, is sleeping and eating poorly, and is pulling on his ears.
Physical (objective) assessment data
• Male, age 6 months
• Temperature 101.4° F
Assessment techniques and equipment
Interview mother about her child's current and past health history, current medication use, and ear care practices.
• Inspect the external ear structures.
• Palpate the external ear and the mastoid process.
• Perform gross hearing tests, using a ticking watch and the voice.
• Inspect the ear canal and tympanic membrane, using an otoscope.
Two appropriate nursing diagnoses
• Pain related to ear inflammation and fever
• Sensory or perceptual alteration: auditory, related to inflamed tympanic membrane and pain
Documentation of findings
• S—Client has had a fever of 101° to 102° F for the past 24 hours and is fussy, sleeping and eating poorly, and pulling on his ears.
• O—T 101.4° F. Right and left tympanic membranes inflamed with diminished light reflexes and landmarks
• A—Pain related to ear inflammation and fever

Questions, answers, and rationales

Eyes

1. Eleanor Barrett, age 57, seeks care because she has been having difficulty focusing while reading. The nurse begins by taking Ms. Barrett's health history, obtaining a detailed description of her eye problems. Which symptom may suggest glaucoma?
(a) Halos
(b) Styes
(c) Pain
(d) Diplopia
Correct answer: (a), see text page 213. The sudden appearance of spots, floaters, or halos may indicate a retinal detachment or glaucoma.

2. The nurse also obtains Ms. Barrett's medical history. Which disorder can affect her vision adversely?
(a) Arthritis
(b) Pulmonary disease
(c) Diabetes
(d) Colitis
Correct answer: (c), see text page 213. Diabetes causes noninflammatory changes in the retina (retinopathy) that can lead to blindness.

3. To assess Ms. Barrett's distance vision, the nurse is most likely to use which tool?
(a) Stycar chart
(b) Ishihara test
(c) Ophthalmoscope
(d) Snellen eye chart
Correct answer: (d), see text page 216. All of these tools may be used to assess the eyes. However, the Snellen eye chart is used to assess distance vision.

4. If Ms. Barrett's distance vision is 20/30, which of the following statements is true?
(a) The client can read from 20′ what a person with normal vision can read at 30′.
(b) The client can read from 30′ what a person with normal vision can read at 20′.
(c) The client can read the entire chart from 30′.
(d) The client can read the chart from 20′ with the left eye, and from 30′ with the right eye.
Correct answer: (a), see text page 216. The numerator, which is always 20, is the distance in feet between the chart and the client. The denominator, which ranges from 10 to 200, indicates from what distance a normal eye can read the chart.

5. The nurse may use which test to assess Ms. Barrett's extraocular muscle function?
(a) Superior field test
(b) Pupillary reaction test
(c) Denver Eye Screening Examination
(d) Six cardinal positions of gaze test
Correct answer: (d), see text page 217. The six cardinal positions of gaze test evaluates the function of each of the six extraocular muscles.

6. The extraocular muscle function test also assesses which cranial nerves?
(a) I, II, and III
(b) II, III, and VII
(c) III, IV, and VI
(d) VI, VII, and VIII
Correct answer: (c), see text page 217. Besides testing the function of the extraocular muscles, the six cardinal positions of gaze test evaluates the cranial nerves responsible for their movement (cranial nerves III, IV, and VI).

7. Madeline Lithgow brings her son Joey, age 6, to the pediatrician's office for his annual physical examination. During the health history, which question is most appropriate for Joey's vision assessment?
(a) "Do you have difficulty seeing at night?"
(b) "Do you have any problems discerning colors?"
(c) "Do you have problems with glare?"
(d) "How are you doing in school?"
Correct answer: (d), see text page 215. Poor progress in school could indicate a visual disturbance in a child. The other questions are more appropriate for an elderly client.

8. The eye examination reveals that Joey has a lazy eye. Which test best detects this eye disorder?
(a) Cover-uncover test
(b) Snellen test
(c) Near vision test
(d) Peripheral vision test
Correct answer: (a), see text pages 217 and 219. The cover-uncover test assesses the fusion reflex, which makes binocular vision possible. During this test, the lazy eye exhibits wandering.

9. Anna Bryon, age 68, has obstructive jaundice. This could be detected by inspecting which structure of the eye?
(a) Iris
(b) Sclera
(c) Cornea
(d) Anterior chamber
Correct answer: (b), see text page 222. Jaundice from liver disease manifests itself first in the sclera, which becomes yellow (scleral icterus).

10. James Thomas, age 31, is admitted to the emergency department with head trauma caused by an automobile accident. While assessing Mr. Thomas's eyes, the nurse notes that the left pupil constricts simultaneously when the right pupil receives direct light. His left pupil exhibits which reaction?
(a) Direct pupillary reaction
(b) Consensual pupillary reaction
(c) Convergence reaction
(d) Corneal light reflex reaction
Correct answer: (b), see text pages 221 and 222. The pupil receiving the direct light constricts directly, while the other pupil constricts simultaneously and consensually.

11. The nurse also tests Mr. Thomas's pupils for accommodation. What is the normal pupillary response to this test?
(a) Constriction and convergence
(b) Constriction and divergence
(c) Dilation and convergence
(d) Dilation and divergence
Correct answer: (a), see text page 222. As the client's eyes focus on an object across the room and then about 2′ away, the pupils should constrict and converge equally on the object.

12. Using an ophthalmoscope, the nurse continues to assess Mr. Thomas's eyes. Which finding may indicate increased intracranial pressure?
(a) Papilledema
(b) Lens opacities
(c) Optic disc atrophy
(d) Hordeolum
Correct answer: (a), see text page 225. Blurred optic disk borders are the major diagnostic sign of papilledema, which usually occurs with increased intracranial pressure.

13. When assessing Mr. Thomas's fundus, the nurse should assess which structure last?
(a) Arteriovenous crossing
(b) Physiologic cup
(c) Optic disk
(d) Macula
Correct answer: (d), see text page 227. The nurse should examine the macula last because it is very light-sensitive. The client will become uncomfortable if the light shines too long on it.

14. Joan Blocker, age 72, is undergoing her annual eye examination. Because of her age, which assessment finding is considered normal?
(a) Arcus senilis
(b) Xanthelasma
(c) Hordeolum
(d) Nystagmus
Correct answer: (a), see text page 225. An elderly client's cornea normally may exhibit arcus senilis, a thin, gray-white surrounding ring caused by lipid deposits.

15. Ms. Blocker's assessment includes an ophthalmoscopic examination. How do the retinal vessels normally appear?
(a) Arterioles are smaller and brighter than veins.
(b) Arterioles are larger and darker than veins.
(c) Arterioles are smaller and darker than veins.
(d) Arterioles are larger and brighter than arterioles.
Correct answer: (a), see text page 211. The arterioles normally are 25% smaller than the veins and brighter in color.

Ears

16. Carol Burke has brought her daughter Katie, age 3, to the clinic. Ms. Burke reports that Katie has had a fever of 101.4° F (38.5° C), nasal congestion, and irritability for the past 2 days. She also states that Katie has had two ear infections in the past year. During the health history, the nurse asks Ms. Burke questions to assess Katie's ear problem. Which question is likely to provide the most useful information?
(a) "Does Katie's ear hurt?"
(b) "Does Katie have any problems hearing?"
(c) "Does Katie tug at either ear?"
(d) "Does anyone in the family have hearing problems?"
Correct answer: (c), see text page 233. All of these questions may be useful in an ear assessment. However, because a young child usually cannot describe symptoms accurately, questions about the child's behavior provide the most useful information in a pediatric health history.

17. Before inserting the otoscope into Katie's ears, the nurse should palpate which areas for tenderness?
(a) Tragus, mastoid process, and helix
(b) Tragus, cochlea, and lobule
(c) Mastoid process, incus, and malleus
(d) Helix, umbo, and tragus
Correct answer: (a), see text pages 235 and 238. Before inserting the otoscope, the nurse should palpate the external ear (especially the tragus) and mastoid process and should pull the helix backward to determine the presence of pain or tenderness.

18. During the otoscopic examination, the nurse inspects the tympanic membrane. What is its normal color?
(a) Light pink
(b) Deep red
(c) Pearly gray
(d) Yellow-white
Correct answer: (c), see text page 232. The tympanic membrane normally appears pearly gray, shiny, and translucent.

19. The physician prescribes a drug to treat Katie's ear infection. Which drugs must be administered cautiously because of their ototoxic effects?
(a) Carbapenems
(b) Penicillins
(c) Aminoglycosides
(d) Cephalosporins
Correct answer: (c), see text page 234. All aminoglycosides are ototoxic and may cause tinnitus, vertigo, and hearing loss.

20. Joe Larkin, age 45, is having difficulty hearing with his left ear. To assess the problem, the nurse performs various hearing tests. Which test evaluates air and bone conduction?
(a) Whispered voice test
(b) Watch tick test
(c) Weber's test
(d) Rinne test
Correct answer: (d), see text page 236. The Rinne test compares air conduction and bone conduction in both ears.

21. When performing Weber's test, where should the nurse place the tuning fork?
(a) On the mastoid process
(b) In front of the ear
(c) On the forehead
(d) On the tragus
Correct answer: (c), see text page 236. In the Weber's test, which evaluates bone conduction, the nurse should place the tuning fork on the top of the client's head at midline or in the middle of client's forehead.

22. During the otoscopic examination, how should the nurse hold Mr. Larkin's ear?
(a) Pull the helix up and back.
(b) Pull the lobule down and forward.
(c) Pull the lobule down and back.
(d) Pull the helix up and forward.
Correct answer: (a), see text page 238. To straighten the ear canal of an adult, the nurse should grasp the helix of the auricle between the thumb and index finger and pull it up and back.

23. The otoscopic examination reveals cerumen build-up. Which type of hearing loss may this cause?
(a) Sensorineural
(b) Perceptive
(c) Conductive
(d) Central
Correct answer: (c), see text page 235. Conductive hearing loss occurs from interference with the functioning of the external and middle ear structures. It may result from such causes as a cerumen plug in the canal or otitis media.

Test bank for Chapter 9, Eyes and Ears

Eyes

1. Eleanor Barrett, age 57, seeks care because she has been having difficulty focusing while reading. The nurse begins by taking Ms. Barrett's health history, obtaining a detailed description of her eye problems. Which symptom may suggest glaucoma?
(a) Halos
(b) Styes
(c) Pain
(d) Diplopia

2. The nurse also obtains Ms. Barrett's medical history. Which disorder can affect her vision adversely?
(a) Arthritis
(b) Pulmonary disease
(c) Diabetes
(d) Colitis

3. To assess Ms. Barrett's distance vision, the nurse is most likely to use which tool?
(a) Stycar chart
(b) Ishihara test
(c) Ophthalmoscope
(d) Snellen eye chart

4. If Ms. Barrett's distance vision is 20/30, which of the following statements is true?
(a) The client can read from 20′ what a person with normal vision can read at 30′.
(b) The client can read from 30′ what a person with normal vision can read at 20′.
(c) The client can read the entire chart from 30′.
(d) The client can read the chart from 20′ with the left eye, and from 30′ with the right eye.

5. The nurse may use which test to assess Ms. Barrett's extraocular muscle function?
(a) Superior field test
(b) Pupillary reaction test
(c) Denver Eye Screening Examination
(d) Six cardinal positions of gaze test

6. The extraocular muscle function test also assesses which cranial nerves?
(a) I, II, and III
(b) II, III, and VII
(c) III, IV, and VI
(d) VI, VII, and VIII

7. Madeline Lithgow brings her son Joey, age 6, to the pediatrician's office for his annual physical examination. During the health history, which question is most appropriate for Joey's vision assessment?
(a) "Do you have difficulty seeing at night?"
(b) "Do you have any problems discerning colors?"
(c) "Do you have problems with glare?"
(d) "How are you doing in school?"

8. The eye examination reveals that Joey has a lazy eye. Which test best detects this eye disorder?
(a) Cover-uncover test
(b) Snellen test
(c) Near vision test
(d) Peripheral vision test

9. Anna Bryon, age 68, has obstructive jaundice. This could be detected by inspecting which structure of the eye?
(a) Iris
(b) Sclera
(c) Cornea
(d) Anterior chamber

10. James Thomas, age 31, is admitted to the emergency department with head trauma caused by an automobile accident. While assessing Mr. Thomas's eyes, the nurse notes that the left pupil constricts simultaneously when the right pupil receives direct light. His left pupil exhibits which reaction?
(a) Direct pupillary reaction
(b) Consensual pupillary reaction
(c) Convergence reaction
(d) Corneal light reflex reaction

11. The nurse also tests Mr. Thomas's pupils for accommodation. What is the normal pupillary response to this test?
(a) Constriction and convergence
(b) Constriction and divergence
(c) Dilation and convergence
(d) Dilation and divergence

12. Using an ophthalmoscope, the nurse continues to assess Mr. Thomas's eyes. Which finding may indicate increased intracranial pressure?
(a) Papilledema
(b) Lens opacities
(c) Optic disc atrophy
(d) Hordeolum

13. When assessing Mr. Thomas's fundus, the nurse should assess which structure last?
(a) Arteriovenous crossing
(b) Physiologic cup
(c) Optic disk
(d) Macula

14. Joan Blocker, age 72, is undergoing her annual eye examination. Because of her age, which assessment finding is considered normal?
(a) Arcus senilis
(b) Xanthelasma
(c) Hordeolum
(d) Nystagmus

15. Ms. Blocker's assessment includes an ophthalmoscopic examination. How do the retinal vessels normally appear?
(a) Arterioles are smaller and brighter than veins.
(b) Arterioles are larger and darker than veins.
(c) Arterioles are smaller and darker than veins.
(d) Arterioles are larger and brighter than arterioles.

Ears

16. Carol Burke has brought her daughter Katie, age 3, to the clinic. Ms. Burke reports that Katie has had a fever of 101.4° F (38.5° C), nasal congestion, and irritability for the past 2 days. She also states that Katie has had two ear infections in the past year. During the health history, the nurse asks Ms. Burke questions to assess Katie's ear problem. Which question is likely to provide the most useful information?
(a) "Does Katie's ear hurt?"
(b) "Does Katie have any problems hearing?"
(c) "Does Katie tug at either ear?"
(d) "Does anyone in the family have hearing problems?"

17. Before inserting the otoscope into Katie's ears, the nurse should palpate which areas for tenderness?
(a) Tragus, mastoid process, and helix
(b) Tragus, cochlea, and lobule
(c) Mastoid process, incus, and malleus
(d) Helix, umbo, and tragus

18. During the otoscopic examination, the nurse inspects the tympanic membrane. What is its normal color?
(a) Light pink
(b) Deep red
(c) Pearly gray
(d) Yellow-white

19. The physician prescribes a drug to treat Katie's ear infection. Which drugs must be administered cautiously because of their ototoxic effects?
(a) Carbapenems
(b) Penicillins
(c) Aminoglycosides
(d) Cephalosporins

20. Joe Larkin, age 45, is having difficulty hearing with his left ear. To assess the problem, the nurse performs various hearing tests. Which test evaluates air and bone conduction?
(a) Whispered voice test
(b) Watch tick test
(c) Weber's test
(d) Rinne test

21. When performing Weber's test, where should the nurse place the tuning fork?
(a) On the mastoid process
(b) In front of the ear
(c) On the forehead
(d) On the tragus

22. During the otoscopic examination, how should the nurse hold Mr. Larkin's ear?
(a) Pull the helix up and back.
(b) Pull the lobule down and forward.
(c) Pull the lobule down and back.
(d) Pull the helix up and forward.

23. The otoscopic examination reveals cerumen build-up. Which type of hearing loss may this cause?
(a) Sensorineural
(b) Perceptive
(c) Conductive
(d) Central

10

Respiratory System

Overview

Because the body depends on the respiratory system to survive, respiratory assessment constitutes a critical aspect of a client's health evaluation. Chapter 10 prepares the nurse to perform a thorough respiratory assessment. After a brief discussion of respiratory system anatomy and physiology, the chapter focuses on pertinent questions to ask and areas to discuss during the health history. Then it explores physical assessment of the upper and lower airways. The chapter also identifies developmental considerations, respiratory disorders, and proper documentation of assesment findings, including laboratory results. It covers the following information:

- The respiratory system basically functions to exchange oxygen and carbon dioxide in the lungs and tissues, and to maintain acid-base balance.
- The respiratory system includes the upper airways, the lower airways, and the thoracic cage, which protects the lungs. The nose, mouth, nasopharynx, oropharynx, laryngopharynx, and larynx compose the upper airways. The trachea, bronchi, and lungs compose the lower airways.
- The external intercostal muscles and the diaphragm—the major muscles of respiration—work to provide normal respiration. The pulmonary artery from the right ventricle and the pulmonary veins to the left atrium provide pulmonary circulation.
- External respiration refers to air exchange in the lungs and occurs through ventilation, pulmonary perfusion, and diffusion. Internal respiration refers to air exchange in the tissues and occurs through diffusion only.

- The nervous system affects ventilation by controlling breathing from the respiratory center in the medulla and pons. The medulla stimulates contraction of the diaphragm and external intercostal muscles. The musculoskeletal system and pulmonary system also affect ventilation.
- Pulmonary perfusion promotes external respiration by allowing gas exchange to occur at alveolar levels. Diffusion occurs when oxygen and carbon dioxide travel between the alveoli and capillaries.
- Developmental factors affect the respiratory system. For example, a pediatric client may have small airways, which may increase the risk of respiratory problems; a pregnant client may have an increased tidal volume and respiratory rate; an elderly client may exhibit musculoskeletal changes (such as cartilage calcification) that may affect respiration.
- Respiratory system assessment begins with the health history, which should investigate the chief complaint in detail. The most common respiratory complaints include dyspnea, cough, sputum production, and chest pain or discomfort. The health history also should investigate the client's past health status, physiologic system status, developmental status, health promotion and protection patterns, and role and relationship patterns.
- The client should be seated during the assessment to allow access to the anterior and posterior thorax. Assessment equipment should include a stethoscope, felt-tipped pen, ruler, and tape measure.
- To assess the client's oxygenation, the nurse should inspect for cyanosis and finger clubbing. Inspection should continue with an assessment of the rate, rhythm, and quality of respirations. The nurse should note the type and

depth of breathing. Inspection of the thorax evaluates chest shape, symmetry, expansion, and the use of accessory muscles of respiration.

- Using palpation, the nurse should check the position of the trachea, note the presence of aortic pulsations in the suprasternal notch, and assess anterior and posterior respiratory excursion. Costal angle palpation can detect tenderness and changes in size.
- Percussion helps determine how much gas, liquid, or solid exists in the lungs. Mediate percussion over bones elicits dullness; over healthy lung tissue, resonance.
- Using the diaphragm of the stethoscope, the nurse should auscultate the anterior, lateral, and posterior thorax. To auscultate properly, the nurse begins at a point on one side of the chest, then moves to the same point on the other side of the chest. Normal breath sounds include tracheal, bronchial, bronchovesicular, and vesicular sounds. Tracheal sounds normally occur over the trachea; bronchial sounds, over the manubrium; bronchovesicular sounds, over the upper third of the sternum anteriorly and in the interscapular area posteriorly; vesicular sounds, in the lung periphery.
- The nurse should classify breath sounds according to location, intensity, characteristic sound, pitch, and duration during the inspiratory and expiratory phases. Adventitious (abnormal) breath sounds include crackles, wheezes, rhonchi, and pleural friction rubs.
- Advanced assessment skills include palpation for tactile fremitus, measurement of diaphragmatic excursion, and auscultation of voice resonance.
- The nurse should document respiratory assessment findings, including the results of any laboratory tests, using the nursing process.
- For more information about respiratory system assessment, see pages 34PG through 43PG of the Photo Gallery in the text.

Suggested lecture topics

- Review respiratory system anatomy and physiology, using overhead projections or other audiovisual aids. (For visual aids, see the transparency master, *Respiratory system structures,* as well as pages 34PG through 37PG in the text.)
- Discuss variations in respiratory system anatomy and physiology in pediatric, pregnant, and elderly clients.
- Identify appropriate questions to ask during the health history and provide rationales for asking them.
- Demonstrate how to inspect, palpate, percuss, and auscultate the respiratory system. (For visual aids, see the transparency masters, *Thorax palpation* and *Thorax percussion,* as well as pages 37PG through 43PG in the text.)
- Using audiovisual aids, identify normal and abnormal breath sounds.

Skills laboratory guide: Health history

To collect information about the client's respiratory system, ask questions about health and illness patterns, health promotion and protection patterns, and role and relationship patterns. Sample questions from each category are listed below.

HEALTH AND ILLNESS PATTERNS

- Do you have shortness of breath? Does position, medication, or relaxation relieve it?
- Do you have a cough? Does it sound dry, hacking, barking, or congested?
- Do you cough up sputum?
- Do you have chest pain? Is it constant or intermittent? Is it localized? Does any activity produce pain? Does pain occur when you breathe normally or when you breathe deeply?
- Have you had any lung problems, such as asthma or tuberculosis?
- How many pillows do you sleep on? Does this number represent a change from your previous number?
- Do you have allergies that flare up in different seasons?
- Do you smoke tobacco? If so, for how long have you been smoking? How much do you smoke?
- Do you use a nebulizer or other breathing aid?

HEALTH PROMOTION AND PROTECTION PATTERNS

- When was your last chest X-ray? Tuberculosis test?
- Which home remedies do you use for respiratory problems?
- Does your breathing problem affect your daily activities?
- Do you have any hobbies that expose you to respiratory irritants, such as glues, paints, and sprays?
- Do you have any breathing difficulty when eating?
- Does stress at home or work affect your breathing?
- What is your current occupation? Are you exposed to any known respiratory irritants at work?

ROLE AND RELATIONSHIP PATTERNS

- How supportive has your family been during your respiratory illness?
- How has your breathing problem affected your sexual activity? Have you found ways to decrease the effect of breathing problems on sexual activity? Would you care to discuss them?

- Compare normal assessment findings for an adult client with those of pediatric, pregnant, and elderly clients.
- Identify abnormal respiratory assessment findings and the common disorders that they may reveal.

Suggested critical thinking activities

- Pair the students and have them perform a respiratory assessment, including history and physical assessment, on each other.
- Have the students document their findings on the Skills Laboratory Assessment Guide.
- Have the entire class critique these assessment findings.

Skills laboratory guide: Physical assessment

This chart guides the student during assessment by identifying body areas, special considerations and techniques to be used, and normal findings.

BODY AREA	SPECIAL CONSIDERATIONS	NORMAL FINDINGS
Inspection		
Skin	• Note skin color. In a dark-skinned client, inspect mucous membranes for color changes.	• No cyanosis or pallor
Fingertips and toes	• Note clubbing and nail thinning.	• 160-degree angle between the nail and the point where it enters the skin
Respirations	• Assess respiratory rate, pattern, quality, and depth; describe the respiratory pattern rather than label it. • Note position of comfort.	• Appropriate respiratory rate for the client's age • Eupneic respirations with moderate chest wall expansion • Ability to assume a supine position
Anterior and posterior thorax	• Note structural deformities, thoracic cage shape, degree of costal angle, chest movement symmetry, accessory muscle use, and skin condition. • In pediatric and elderly clients, the ratio of anteroposterior to lateral diameter of the thorax is close to 1:1. Women tend to use thoracic muscles for breathing; men and small children, abdominal muscles.	• No structural deformities • 1:2 ratio of anteroposterior to lateral diameter of thorax • Costal angle < 90 degrees • Symmetrical chest movement • No retractions or use of accessory muscles; no pursed-lip breathing or nasal flaring • Intact skin with no unusual color, lumps, or lesions
Palpation		
Trachea	• Palpate the trachea for position.	• Midline trachea
Suprasternal notch	• Use your fingertips to evaluate the strength and regularity of the client's aortic pulsations.	• Regular pulsations
Anterior and posterior thorax	• Use your fingertips and palms of one or both hands. Assess systematically, alternating palpation from one side of the thorax to the other. Palpate the costal angle gently to avoid causing pain. • Note pain, masses, crepitus, and skin irregularities. • Assess respiratory excursion at the second, fifth, and tenth intercostal spaces (ICS) anteriorly, and at the infrascapular and interscapular areas posteriorly.	• No pain, masses, crepitus, or skin irregularities • Costal angle < 90 degrees • Symmetrical respiratory excursion with no lag
Percussion		
Anterior, lateral, and posterior thorax	• Use mediate percussion and avoid percussing over bones. • Percuss systematically, comparing sound variations from one side to the other. • Note areas of hyperresonance and dullness.	• Anterior thorax resonance from below the clavicle to the fifth ICS on the right and to the third ICS on the left • Lateral thorax resonance from the sixth to the eighth ICS • Posterior thorax resonance to the level of T10 bilaterally
Auscultation		
Anterior, lateral, and posterior thorax	• Use stethoscope diaphragm to listen systematically, beginning at the upper lobes and moving from side to side and down. • Note normal breath sounds (tracheal, bronchial, bronchovesicular, and vesicular sounds) and adventitious breath sounds (crackles, wheezes, rhonchi, and rubs). If adventitious sounds are present, ask the client to cough. Then listen again. In children, breath sounds are normally more bronchovesicular.	• Clear lungs • Tracheal sounds over trachea; bronchial sounds over the manubrium; bronchovesicular sounds over the upper third of the sternum anteriorly and between the scapula posteriorly; vesicular sounds in the lung periphery • No adventitious sounds

Skills laboratory guide: Physical assessment *continued*

BODY AREA	SPECIAL CONSIDERATIONS	NORMAL FINDINGS
Advanced assessment skills		
Tactile fremitus	• Use open palms to palpate the client's chest for tactile fremitus, comparing side to side. • Palpate systematically from central airways to lung periphery and back. • Note areas of increased or decreased fremitus.	• Bilaterally equal vibrations • Vibrations in the upper chest close to the bronchi that decrease and then disappear toward the lung periphery
Diaphragmatic excursion	• Percuss down the posterior thorax on the right and left sides from the lower border of the scapula to the point where the percussion note changes from resonance to dullness while the client holds a deep breath, then exhales fully and pauses before inhaling.	• Excursion of 1¼" to 2¼" (3 to 6 cm)
Voice resonance	• Assess for bronchophony by auscultating while the client says "ninety-nine." Note clear sound transmission (bronchophony). • Assess for egophony by auscultating while the client says "e." Note an "a" sound and nasal or bleating voice sounds (egophony). • Assess for whispered pectoriloquy by auscultating while the client whispers "one-two-three." Note clear sound transmission (whispered pectoriloquy).	• Muffled, indistinct, or barely audible sounds • No bronchophony, egophony, or whispered pectoriloquy

• Using a case study of a client with a respiratory disorder, have the students develop a nursing care plan.

• Using audiovisual aids, have the students differentiate normal and abnormal breath sounds.

Student study questions and answers

The following study questions are taken from text page 281 of Chapter 10, Respiratory System. Their answers are based on information in that chapter.

1. What are the four most common signs and symptoms of respiratory dysfunction and why must they be thoroughly explored during assessment?

Answer

• Dyspnea. Shortness of breath, or dyspnea, occurs when breathing cannot meet the body's metabolic needs for oxygen. It usually increases the work of breathing. In the early stages of pulmonary disease, a decrease in physical activity decreases the body's metabolic needs, which easily relieves dyspnea. A client unconsciously may control exertional dyspnea (shortness of breath alleviated by rest) by limiting activity.

• Cough. This respiratory defense mechanism usually occurs in response to irritation in the tracheobronchial system and may begin in the pharynx, larynx, or trachea. Dust, debris, secretions, or foreign objects may trigger the cough reflex, which forcefully expels substances from the airway. A cough may be effective or ineffective, productive or nonproductive, or intermittent or constant.

• Sputum production. The body produces sputum as a respiratory defense mechanism. Normal sputum is clear to white, tasteless, odorless, and scant. Changes in the color, taste, smell, or amount of sputum may indicate pulmonary infection.

• Chest pain. Clients with respiratory disorders frequently report this symptom. Chest pain may have a pulmonary, cardiac, or musculoskeletal origin. Because the lungs themselves have no pain-sensitive nerve endings, pulmonary chest pain usually is a late sign of lung disease (except when it results from trauma).

2. You may need to assess for respiratory excursion, diaphragmatic excursion, tactile fremitus, and egophony in a client with a respiratory disorder. How would you describe the step-by-step procedure to perform each assessment?

Answer

• To evaluate respiratory excursion, plan to assess three areas on the client's anterior thorax and two areas on the client's posterior thorax.

• For all three areas on the anterior thorax, stand in front of the client, who may either sit or stand. To assess the first area, place your hands on the anterior chest wall, thumbs equidistant from the sternum, with the rest of your fingers spread over the thorax. As the client takes a deep breath, observe your thumbs, which should separate simultaneously and equally to a distance several centimeters from the sternum. To assess the second area, place your thumbs at the fifth intercostal space and repeat the procedure. To assess the third area, place your thumbs at the tenth intercostal space and repeat the procedure.

- For the posterior thorax areas, stand behind the client and place your thumbs in the infrascapular area on either side of the spine at the level of the tenth rib. Grasp the lateral rib cage and rest your palms gently over the lateroposterior surface. As the client inhales, the posterior chest should move upward and outward and your thumbs should move apart. When the client exhales, your thumbs should return to the midline and again touch. Repeat the procedure after placing your thumbs equally lateral to the vertebral column in the interscapular area, with your fingers extending into the axillary area.

- To assess diaphragmatic excursion—the distance that the diaphragm travels between inhalation and exhalation—instruct the client to take a deep breath and hold it while you percuss down the right side of the posterior thorax. Begin at the lower border of the scapula and continue until the percussion note changes from resonance to dullness, which identifies the location of the diaphragm. Using a washable, felt-tipped pen, mark this point with a small line. Ask the client to take a few normal breaths, then to exhale completely and hold it while you percuss again to locate the point where the resonant sound becomes dull. Mark this point with a small line. Repeat this procedure on the left side of the posterior thorax. Then, using a tape measure or ruler, measure the distance between the two marks on each side of the chest. The distance between them reflects diaphragmatic excursion. Normally, the distance is 1¼″ to 2¼″ (3 to 6 cm).

- To assess tactile fremitus, place the ulnar surface of your hand against the client's chest. Have the client repeat a resonant phrase as you move your hands over the client's chest from the central airways to the lung periphery and back. Repeat this procedure on the posterior thorax. You should feel vibrations of equal intensity on either side of the chest. The fremitus normally occurs in the upper chest. Little or no fremitus should occur in the lower chest.

- To assess for egophony, ask the client to repeat the letter "e" as you auscultate the lungs. Normally, the letter sounds muffled and nondistinct. If the letter sounds like "a" and the voice sounds nasal or bleating, you have heard egophony caused by lung tissue consolidation.

3. Mr. Egars, age 72, comes to the clinic complaining of shortness of breath, an inability to catch his breath after climbing a flight of stairs, and the need to sleep on more pillows than usual. What health history questions would you ask Mr. Egars to assess his respiratory problem?

Answer
- Is your shortness of breath constant or intermittent?
- Does a position change, medication, or relaxation relieve it? Does anything aggravate it?
- How many stairs can you climb before you begin to feel short of breath?
- Do you have a cough? Does it produce sputum?

4. Mrs. Miner, age 26, brings her son Timmy, age 4, to the office for a well-family visit. As you assess their respiratory systems, how would you modify your auscultation technique, and what differences in normal breath sounds would you expect to find?

Answer
For Mrs. Miner, use the diaphragm of an adult stethoscope, auscultating at numerous sites. For Timmy, use a smaller pediatric stethoscope on fewer sites. Because a child's chest is more resonant than an adult's, expect Timmy's breath sounds to be harsher and more bronchial than his mother's. Also expect differentiation of sounds to be more difficult with Timmy.

5. Mrs. Lund, age 62, is admitted to the hospital from the emergency department. She reports having shortness of breath, a productive cough, fever, and chest pain that worsens with deep breathing and coughing. When you assess Mrs. Lund's vital signs, you find that her temperature is 102.4° F (39° C) (rectally), her blood pressure is 160/92 mm Hg, her pulse is 120 and regular, and her respiratory rate is 32 with deep, regular respirations. How would you report the following information related to your nursing assessment of Mrs. Lund?
- history (subjective) assessment data
- physical (objective) assessment data
- two appropriate nursing diagnoses
- assessment techniques and equipment
- documentation of your findings.

Answer
History (subjective) assessment data
- Complaining of shortness of breath
- Complaining of productive cough
- Complaining of chest pain that worsens with deep breathing and coughing
Physical (objective) assessment data
- Female, age 62
- Fever of 102.4° F (rectally)
- Blood pressure 160/92 mm Hg
- Pulse 120 and regular
- Respirations 32, regular and deep
Two appropriate nursing diagnoses
- Ineffective airway clearance related to lung congestion
- Hyperthermia related to lung congestion

Assessment techniques and equipment
- Interview the client regarding her current symptoms (using the PQRST method), past health history, and medications use.
- Inspect the client's skin color, use of accessory muscles of respiration, inspiration and expiration, and symmetry of chest expansion.
- Palpate the chest to detect pain and assess respiratory excursion and tactile fremitus.
- Percuss the left lung and lower right lobe.
- Auscultate the lungs using a stethoscope.

Documentation of findings
- S—Client complains of shortness of breath, productive cough, and chest pain that worsens with deep breathing and coughing.
- O—T 102.4° F (rectally); P 120 and regular; R 32, regular and deep; B/P 160/92
- A—Ineffective airway clearance related to lung congestion

Questions, answers, and rationales

1. Jeffrey Greenaway, age 53, is admitted to the hospital with acute exacerbation of chronic obstructive pulmonary disease (COPD). Upon inspection, the nurse notes that Mr. Greenaway has a barrel chest. What is the normal ratio of the anteroposterior to lateral diameter of the chest?
(a) 1:1
(b) 1:2
(c) 1:3
(d) 1:4
Correct answer: (b), see text page 253. In the adult, the lateral diameter of the chest is broader by up to twice the anteroposterior diameter (1:2 ratio).

2. COPD may affect which anatomical angle?
(a) Angle of Louis
(b) Sternal angle
(c) Costal angle
(d) Scapular angle
Correct answer: (c), see text page 262. The costal angle (angle between the ribs and sternum above the xiphoid process) normally is less than 90 degrees. It widens if the chest wall is expanded chronically as in COPD.

3. The nurse observes that Mr. Greenaway is using his intercostal muscles for breathing. Adult males normally use which muscles for breathing?
(a) Intercostal
(b) Abdominal
(c) Thoracic
(d) Cervical
Correct answer: (b), see text pages 261 and 262. Infants, adult males, and sleeping clients usually exhibit abdominal breathing, using the abdominal muscles.

4. While inspecting Mr. Greenaway, the nurse remains alert for signs of cyanosis. How is central cyanosis different from peripheral cyanosis?
(a) Central cyanosis affects the ears; peripheral cyanosis does not.
(b) Central cyanosis affects the nail beds; peripheral cyanosis does not.
(c) Central cyanosis affects the mucous membranes; peripheral cyanosis does not.
(d) Central cyanosis affects the tip of the nose; peripheral cyanosis does not.
Correct answer: (c), see text page 260. Central and peripheral cyanosis may affect the extremities and ears; only central cyanosis affects the mucous membranes.

5. The nurse also inspects Mr. Greenaway's fingers for clubbing. Which angle of nail attachment is the minimum that indicates clubbing?
(a) 90 degrees
(b) 120 degrees
(c) 160 degrees
(d) 180 degrees
Correct answer: (d), see text page 261. Normally, the angle of nail attachment is 160 degrees. Clubbing occurs when that angle increases to 180 degrees or more.

6. While palpating Mr. Greenaway's thorax, the nurse assesses respiratory excursion. What does this technique assess?
(a) Chest movement
(b) Breath sounds
(c) Lung vibration
(d) Voice sounds
Correct answer: (a), see text page 264. Respiratory excursion assesses chest wall expansion during inspiration and chest contraction during expiration.

7. During palpation, the nurse should use which part of the hand to assess tactile fremitus?
(a) Palm
(b) Fingerpads
(c) Fingertips
(d) Dorsal surface
Correct answer: (a), see text page 275. To assess tactile fremitus, the nurse should place the open palm flat against the client's chest without touching the chest with the fingers.

8. Mr. Greenaway is likely to display which type of tactile fremitus?
(a) Normal
(b) Increased
(c) Decreased
(d) Absent
Correct answer: (c), see text page 275. Conditions that cause more air than normal to be blocked or trapped in the lungs, such as COPD, result in decreased tactile fremitus.

9. While assessing Mr. Greenaway's thorax, the nurse should use which type of percussion?
(a) Blunt
(b) Immediate
(c) Mediate
(d) Fist
Correct answer: (c), see text page 268. To percuss a client's thorax, the nurse should use mediate percussion and follow the same sequence, comparing sound variations from one side to the other.

10. Percussion over a healthy lung normally elicits which sound?
(a) Tympany
(b) Dullness
(c) Resonance
(d) Hyperresonance
Correct answer: (c), see text page 267. Percussion over a healthy lung elicits a resonant sound—hollow and loud, with a low pitch and long duration.

11. Percussion over Mr. Greenaway's lungs is likely to produce which sound?
(a) Tympany
(b) Dullness
(d) Resonance
(d) Hyperresonance
Correct answer: (d), see text page 269. Hyperresonance may result from overinflation of the lung, such as occurs with COPD.

12. The nurse auscultates Mr. Greenaway's breath sounds. Which sounds normally are heard over the peripheral lung fields?
(a) Tracheal
(b) Bronchial
(c) Bronchovesicular
(d) Vesicular
Correct answer: (d), see text page 270. Vesicular sounds result from laminar airflow moving through the alveolar ducts and alveoli at low flow rates. They are heard best in the periphery of the lungs.

13. Which physical assessment technique should the nurse use to assess for diaphragmatic excursion?
(a) Inspection
(b) Palpation
(c) Percussion
(d) Auscultation
Correct answer: (c), see text page 278. The nurse assesses diaphragmatic excursion by marking the place where percussion notes change during deep inspiration and during expiration and then measuring the distance between them.

14. What is the normal range of diaphragmatic excursion?
(a) 1 to 2 cm
(b) 2 to 4 cm
(c) 3 to 6 cm
(d) 4 to 8 cm
Correct answer: (c), see text page 275. Normal diaphragmatic excursion is 1¼″ to 2¼″ (3 to 6 cm).

15. Roberta Howard, age 67, seeks care for a respiratory disorder. Which health history question would be most helpful in detecting pleuritis?
(a) "Does pain occur when you breathe deeply?"
(b) "Do you have allergies that flare up?"
(c) "How many pillows do you sleep on?"
(d) "Do you cough up sputum?"
Correct answer: (a), see text page 255. All of these questions are appropriate for a respiratory history. However, pain that increases with deep breathing suggests a pulmonary (pleuritic) disorder.

16. Auscultation of Ms. Howard's thorax reveals a pleural friction rub. How can the nurse differentiate this sound from other abnormal breath sounds?
(a) Rubs occur during inspiration only and clear with coughing.
(b) Rubs occur during expiration only and produce a light popping, nonmusical sound.
(c) Rubs occur during inspiration only and may be heard anywhere.
(d) Rubs occur during inspiration and expiration and produce a squeaking or grating sound.
Correct answer: (d), see text page 271. Pleural friction rubs, which produce a squeaking or grating sound, are heard in the lateral lung fields during inspiration and expiration.

17. Stanley Walters, age 74, is admitted to the hospital with aspiration pneumonia of the right middle lung lobe. To assess this lobe, the nurse should use which approach?
(a) Posterior
(b) Dorsal
(c) Lateral
(d) Oblique
Correct answer: (c), see text page 269. Because of its location, the right middle lung lobe should be assessed using a lateral auscultation and percussion sequence.

18. Which age-related factor may have contributed to the development of aspiration pneumonia in Mr. Walters?
(a) Decreased cough reflex
(b) Decreased activity level
(c) Decreased ventilatory effort
(d) Decreased distensibility of lung tissue
Correct answer: (a), see text page 275. A decreased cough reflex increases the risk of aspiration in elderly clients.

19. When auscultating Mr. Walters's breath sounds, the nurse detect crackles. Which statement accurately characterizes crackles?
(a) Crackles usually occur during inspiration.
(b) Crackles are unaffected by coughing.
(c) Crackles are heard only in central airways.
(d) Crackles occur during inspiration and expiration.
Correct answer: (a), see text page 271. Crackles usually occur during inspiration, may be heard anywhere, and may clear with coughing.

20. Because Mr. Walters has pneumonia, the nurse also assesses voice resonance. When he says "e," it sounds like "a" on auscultation over the affected area. This is an example of which type of resonance?
(a) Bronchophony
(b) Whsphered pectoriloquy
(c) Egophony
(d) Stridor
Correct answer: (c), see text page 278. Egophony is present when a spoken "e" sounds like "a" and the voice sounds nasal or bleating during auscultation.

21. Which laboratory test is likely to be ordered to assess Mr. Walters for hypoxia?
(a) Sputum culture and sensitivity
(b) Arterial blood gas analysis
(c) Red blood cell count
(d) Total hemoglobin
Correct answer: (b), see text page 279. Although all of these tests may be used in a respiratory assessment, arterial blood gas analysis evaluates gas exchange in the lungs, providing an objective measurement of the client's oxygenation.

Test bank for Chapter 10, Respiratory System

1. Jeffrey Greenaway, age 53, is admitted to the hospital with acute exacerbation of chronic obstructive pulmonary disease (COPD). Upon inspection, the nurse notes that Mr. Greenaway has a barrel chest. What is the normal ratio of the anteroposterior to lateral diameter of the chest?
(a) 1:1
(b) 1:2
(c) 1:3
(d) 1:4

2. COPD may affect which anatomical angle?
(a) Angle of Louis
(b) Sternal angle
(c) Costal angle
(d) Scapular angle

3. The nurse observes that Mr. Greenaway is using his intercostal muscles for breathing. Adult males normally use which muscles for breathing?
(a) Intercostal
(b) Abdominal
(c) Thoracic
(d) Cervical

4. While inspecting Mr. Greenaway, the nurse remains alert for signs of cyanosis. How is central cyanosis different from peripheral cyanosis?
(a) Central cyanosis affects the ears; peripheral cyanosis does not.
(b) Central cyanosis affects the nail beds; peripheral cyanosis does not.
(c) Central cyanosis affects the mucous membranes; peripheral cyanosis does not.
(d) Central cyanosis affects the tip of the nose; peripheral cyanosis does not.

5. The nurse also inspects Mr. Greenaway's fingers for clubbing. Which angle of nail attachment is the minimum that indicates clubbing?
(a) 90 degrees
(b) 120 degrees
(c) 160 degrees
(d) 180 degrees

6. While palpating Mr. Greenaway's thorax, the nurse assesses respiratory excursion. What does this technique assess?
(a) Chest movement
(b) Breath sounds
(c) Lung vibration
(d) Voice sounds

7. During palpation, the nurse should use which part of the hand to assess tactile fremitus?
(a) Palm
(b) Fingerpads
(c) Fingertips
(d) Dorsal surface

8. Mr. Greenaway is likely to display which type of tactile fremitus?
(a) Normal
(b) Increased
(c) Decreased
(d) Absent

9. While assessing Mr. Greenaway's thorax, the nurse should use which type of percussion?
(a) Blunt
(b) Immediate
(c) Mediate
(d) Fist

10. Percussion over a healthy lung normally elicits which sound?
(a) Tympany
(b) Dullness
(c) Resonance
(d) Hyperresonance

11. Percussion over Mr. Greenaway's lungs is likely to produce which sound?
(a) Tympany
(b) Dullness
(d) Resonance
(d) Hyperresonance

12. The nurse auscultates Mr. Greenaway's breath sounds. Which sounds normally are heard over the peripheral lung fields?
(a) Tracheal
(b) Bronchial
(c) Bronchovesicular
(d) Vesicular

13. Which physical assessment technique should the nurse use to assess for diaphragmatic excursion?
(a) Inspection
(b) Palpation
(c) Percussion
(d) Auscultation

14. What is the normal range of diaphragmatic excursion?
(a) 1 to 2 cm
(b) 2 to 4 cm
(c) 3 to 6 cm
(d) 4 to 8 cm

15. Roberta Howard, age 67, seeks care for a respiratory disorder. Which health history question would be most helpful in detecting pleuritis?
(a) "Does pain occur when you breathe deeply?"
(b) "Do you have allergies that flare up?"
(c) "How many pillows do you sleep on?"
(d) "Do you cough up sputum?"

16. Auscultation of Ms. Howard's thorax reveals a pleural friction rub. How can the nurse differentiate this sound from other abnormal breath sounds?
(a) Rubs occur during inspiration only and clear with coughing.
(b) Rubs occur during expiration only and produce a light popping, nonmusical sound.
(c) Rubs occur during inspiration only and may be heard anywhere.
(d) Rubs occur during inspiration and expiration and produce a squeaking or grating sound.

17. Stanley Walters, age 74, is admitted to the hospital with aspiration pneumonia of the right middle lung lobe. To assess this lobe, the nurse should use which approach?
(a) Posterior
(b) Dorsal
(c) Lateral
(d) Oblique

18. Which age-related factor may have contributed to the development of aspiration pneumonia in Mr. Walters?
(a) Decreased cough reflex
(b) Decreased activity level
(c) Decreased ventilatory effort
(d) Decreased distensibility of lung tissue

19. When auscultating Mr. Walters's breath sounds, the nurse detect crackles. Which statement accurately characterizes crackles?
(a) Crackles usually occur during inspiration.
(b) Crackles are unaffected by coughing.
(c) Crackles are heard only in central airways.
(d) Crackles occur during inspiration and expiration.

20. Because Mr. Walters has pneumonia, the nurse also assesses voice resonance. When he says "e," it sounds like "a" on auscultation over the affected area. This is an example of which type of resonance?
(a) Bronchophony
(b) Whispered pectoriloquy
(c) Egophony
(d) Stridor

21. Which laboratory test is likely to be ordered to assess Mr. Walters for hypoxia?
(a) Sputum culture and sensitivity
(b) Arterial blood gas analysis
(c) Red blood cell count
(d) Total hemoglobin

11

Cardiovascular System

Overview

Because of the prevalence of congenital and acquired cardiovascular disorders, the nurse must be able to assess cardiac health and to evaluate a sick client's response to therapy and ability to resume activities of daily living. Chapter 11 prepares the student for these responsibilities by presenting the following information:

- The cardiovascular system includes the heart and blood vessels. Its main function is to deliver oxygenated blood to body tissues and remove waste products. The heart consists of four chambers (the left and right atria and the left and right ventricles) and four valves (two atrioventricular [AV] valves and two semilunar [SL] valves).

- Pulmonary circulation is the network of blood vessels that travels through the lungs to pick up oxygen and release carbon dioxide. The systemic circulation takes oxygen and nutrients to the cells and removes waste products. The coronary circulation supplies nutrients to and removes waste from the heart cells.

- The extrinsic and intrinsic conduction systems control myocardial contraction. The extrinsic system includes the autonomic nervous system. The intrinsic system includes the sinoatrial node, atrioventricular nodes, the bundle of His, right and left bundle branches, and Purkinje fibers.

- The cardiac cycle has two phases: systole (ventricular contraction) and diastole (ventricular relaxation). The first heart sound (S_1) results from AV valve closing, which marks the beginning of systole. The second heart sound (S_2) results from SL valve closing, which marks the start of diastole.

- The cardiovascular health history should include questions about the client's health and illness patterns, risk factors of cardiac disease, and signs and symptoms of cardiac disease, such as chest pain, dyspnea, syncope, edema, palpitations, fatigue, and cyanosis.

- The nurse also should ask questions about the client's health promotion and protection patterns and role and relationship patterns.

- After measuring the client's height, weight, and vital signs, the nurse should inspect related structures, including the skin, hair, nails, and eyes.

- Cardiovascular inspection includes jugular vein assessment to detect distention and estimate central venous pressure, and precordium evaluation to identify pulsations, heaves, and lifts.

- The nurse palpates the central and peripheral pulses to assess their rate, rhythm, symmetry, contour, and strength. The nurse palpates the precordium for cardiac impulses over the sternoclavicular, aortic, pulmonic, right and left ventricular, and epigastric areas, noting the size and location of each impulse.

- Percussion can be used to assess the size of the heart, but the more accurate X-ray usually is used.

- Using the stethoscope diaphragm, the nurse auscultates for high-pitched S_1 and S_2. With the stethoscope bell, the nurse auscultates for low-pitched murmurs and gallops. S_1 sounds loudest over the mitral and tricuspid areas, and S_2 is loudest over the aortic and pulmonic areas. Heart sound assessment should identify the pitch, intensity, duration, timing in the cardiac cycle, quality, location, and radiation of any sound. The nurse also should auscultate for bruits in the abdominal aorta and carotid, femoral, and popliteal arteries.

- Advanced assessment skills include identification of the jugular venous pulse wave form and auscultation of extra heart sounds, murmurs, and other abnormal heart sounds. S_3 and S_4, the extra heart sounds, are heard best over the mitral and tricuspid areas and occur early or late in diastole. These low-pitched sounds are heard best with the stethoscope bell. They can be normal or abnormal. Murmurs can be innocent or pathologic. If a murmur is present, the nurse should note its location, timing in the cardiac cycle, pitch, pattern, quality, and intensity. Clicks and snaps are high-pitched abnormal sounds. Rubs are harsh, scratchy, or creaking sounds.

- After documenting and reviewing all assessment data, the nurse should formulate nursing diagnoses and plan, implement, and evaluate the client's care.
- For more information about cardiovascular system assessment, see pages 44PG through 54PG of the Photo Gallery in the text.

Suggested lecture topics

- Review the anatomy and physiology of the heart and blood vessels. (For visual aids, see the transparency master, *Cardiovascular structures*, as well as pages 44PG through 45PG in the text.)
- Discuss health history questions important to cardiovascular assessment of various age groups.
- Demonstrate how to inspect, palpate, percuss, and auscultate the cardiovascular system. (For visual aids, see transparency masters, *Precordium inspection and palpation* and *Cardiac auscultation*, as well as pages 45PG through 52PG in the text.)
- Discuss normal assessment findings and normal variations in pediatric, pregnant, and elderly clients.
- Compare normal and abnormal heart sounds, using appropriate audio aids.
- Discuss common abnormalities that may be found during cardiovascular assessment of an adult and a child. (For visual aids, see pages 53PG through 54PG in the text.)
- Explain the relationship between heart sounds and cardiac events.

Suggested critical thinking activities

- Pair the students and have them perform a cardiovascular assessment on each other.
- Have the students document their assessment findings on the Skills Laboratory Assessment Guide. Then have them critique each other's assessment findings.
- Using audio aids, have the students identify various normal and abnormal heart sounds.
- Using a case study of a client with a cardiovascular complaint, have the students develop a nursing care plan.

Skills laboratory guide: Health history

To collect information about the client's cardiovascular system, ask questions about health and illness patterns, health promotion and protection patterns, and role and relationship patterns. Sample questions from each category are listed below.

HEALTH AND ILLNESS PATTERNS

- Do you ever have chest pain or discomfort? (Perform a symptom analysis.)
- Do you ever experience shortness of breath? If so, is it accompanied by coughing?
- Do you ever feel dizzy when you change positions?
- Does your heart ever feel like it is pounding, racing, or skipping beats?
- Do you have any ulcers or sores on your legs?
- Were you born with a heart problem?
- Have you had rheumatic fever? If so, when?
- Do you have high blood pressure, high cholesterol, or diabetes mellitus?
- Has anyone in your family been treated for heart disease or high blood pressure?

HEALTH PROMOTION AND PROTECTION PATTERNS

- Do you smoke or drink? If so, how much?
- Do you experience episodes of shortness of breath or coughing during the night?
- Do you exercise routinely? Has your pattern of exercise changed?
- When you walk or exercise, do you experience leg pain?
- Do you follow any special diet? Do you eat at fast-food restaurants?
- Do you feel pressured to complete tasks in a short time?
- What causes you to feel stressed? How often does this occur?
- How do you cope with stress in your life?

ROLE AND RELATIONSHIP PATTERNS

- Do you think of yourself as a healthy or sick person?
- What are your typical responsibilities at home?
- Have they changed since you developed a health problem?
- Has your usual pattern of sexual activity changed in any way?

Student study questions and answers

The following study questions are taken from text page 332 of Chapter 11, Cardiovascular System. Their answers are based on information in that chapter.

1. Mr. Jenkins, age 56, comes to the ambulatory care center complaining of two 3-minute episodes of chest pain that were accompanied by shortness of breath and sweating. He says that he has felt more tired than usual for the past 2 months. His risk factors of cardiac disease include family history (father died of a heart attack at age 60), cigarette smoking (1 pack per day for 40 years), hypertension, and inactivity.

Skills laboratory guide: Physical assessment

This chart guides the student during assessment by identifying body areas, special considerations and techniques to be used, and normal findings.

BODY AREA	SPECIAL CONSIDERATIONS	NORMAL FINDINGS
Inspection		
General appearance	• Note apparent and chronological age as well as other aspects of general appearance.	• Appearance consistent with client's chronological age • Well-nourished, well-developed appearance • Alert and energetic
Body weight	• Note any weight change, especially a sudden weight gain (possibly due to fluid retention). • Observe for cardiac cachexia (muscle weakness and wasting).	• Weight appropriate for age and height • No recent weight gain • No cardiac cachexia
Vital signs	• Note temperature, pulse, respirations, and blood pressure. • Compare blood pressure in all extremities. • Check for orthostatic (postural) hypotension, pulse pressure, and auscultatory gaps during blood pressure measurement.	• Vital signs within normal limits for client's age • No orthostatic hypotension • No auscultatory gap • Pulse pressure of 30 to 50 mmHg
Skin, hair, and nails	• Note skin color, temperature, turgor, lesions, and edema. (If edema is present, check and grade any pitting.) • Differentiate central from peripheral cyanosis. • In a dark-skinned client, inspect the buccal mucosa for cyanotic changes. • Note hair distribution on extremities and the proportion of the extremities to the trunk. • Check nails for color, capillary refill, clubbing, shape, and splinter hemorrhages.	• No cyanosis, flushing, or pallor • Warm, dry skin with good turgor • No lesions • No periorbital, sacral, peripheral, or pedal edema • Even, symmetrical hair distribution • Extremities in proportion to trunk • Pink nails with no cyanosis, clubbing, or splinter hemorrhages • Rapid capillary refill • Smooth, rounded nails
Eyes	• Note xanthelasma, yellowish sclera, and arcus senilis. • During the ophthalmoscopic examination, note arteriovenous (AV) nicking, exudates, and hemorrhages. • Check for Musset's sign (rhythmic head bobbing in time to the heartbeat). • Arcus senilis is normal in elderly clients, but may indicate hyperlipidemia in clients under age 65.	• Clear, bright eyes • No xanthelasma or yellowish sclera • Smooth AV crossings; no retinal exudates or hemorrhages • No Musset's sign
Jugular veins	• Inspect for neck vein distention. • Estimate venous pressure. • Check for neck vein distention with client in supine position and at a 45-degree angle.	• No neck vein distention • Internal jugular vein pulsation 2 cm above the angle of Louis with the client at a 45-degree angle
Precordium	• Inspect the sternoclavicular, aortic, pulmonic, right ventricular, left ventricular (apical), and epigastric areas. • Use tangential lighting to cast shadows across the precordium. • Note pulsations, lifts, or heaves in all areas. • Have an obese client or one with pendulous breasts sit up, rather than lie supine, to make pulsations easier to see.	• No lifts or heaves in any area • No sternoclavicular pulsation • Slight aortic, pulmonic, right ventricular, and epigastric pulsations • Point of maximum impulse (PMI) in left ventricular area; no pulsation displacement
Palpation		
Central and peripheral pulses	• Palpate the carotid, brachial, radial, femoral, popliteal, dorsalis pedis, and posterior tibialis pulses. Note the pulse rate, rhythm, symmetry, contour, and strength at each site. • Palpate right and left carotids separately. Weak pulses (+1) are common in elderly clients. Bounding pulses (+3) are common when cardiac output increases, as in pregnancy or exercise.	• 60 to 100 beats/minute • Regular rhythm • Symmetrical, smooth upstroke and rapid descent • +2 amplitude bilaterally

Skills laboratory guide: Physical assessment *continued*

BODY AREA	SPECIAL CONSIDERATIONS	NORMAL FINDINGS
Palpation *continued*		
Precordium	• Palpate the sternoclavicular, aortic, pulmonic, right ventricular, left ventricular (apical), and epigastric areas, using your fingerpads. • Note size and duration of impulses, thrills, lifts, or heaves. • Note size, duration, and diffusion of PMI as well as any displacement, lifts, or heaves. If PMI is not palpable, roll the supine client to the left-lateral recumbent position.	• No thrills, lifts, or heaves in any area • Slight sternoclavicular pulsation possible • No palpable aortic, pulmonic, or right ventricular pulsations • Palpable PMI roughly 2 cm in diameter in left ventricular area; no displacement or diffusion • Slight epigastric pulsations possible; no diffusion
Percussion		
Precordium	• Note change in percussion note from resonance to dullness to identify the cardiac borders and estimate the heart size.	• Left border of heart at midclavicular line in fifth intercostal space
Auscultation		
Precordium	• Auscultate the aortic, pulmonic, tricuspid, and mitral (apical) areas, in sequence, with the diaphragm and then the bell of the stethoscope. • Note rate, rhythm, pitch, intensity, duration, timing in cardiac cycle, quality, location, and radiation of S_1 and S_2. • Note and characterize any splits or abnormal sounds, such as murmurs, S_3, and S_4. • To differentiate systole from diastole, remember that the carotid pulse occurs simultaneously with S_1, that S_1 is louder than S_2 in the apical area, that S_2 is louder than S_1 at the base, and that S_1 occurs simultaneously with a palpable PMI. • To facilitate auscultation in an obese client or a client with COPD, have the client assume the left-lateral recumbent position or the seated, forward-leaning position. • Split S_2 is easier to detect because of respiratory variation. S_3 and S_4 are best heard at the apex and may be normal in young adults. • Innocent systolic murmurs may occur in pregnant and pediatric clients.	• Heart rate normal for client's age. In a heart rate less than 100 beats/minute, systole is shorter than diastole. In a heart rate greater than 100 beats/minute, diastole is shorter. • Normal splits occur over site of second valve closure. • In the aortic area: regular rate and rhythm; 2/6 intensity; high pitch; short duration; no radiation, splitting, or murmurs; S_2 greater than S_1. • In the pulmonic area: regular rate and rhythm; 2/6 intensity; high pitch; systolic short duration; no radiation or murmurs; split S_2 during inspiration; S_2 greater than S_1. • In the tricuspid area: regular rate and rhythm; 3/6 intensity; high pitch; systolic short duration; no radiation, murmurs, rubs, clicks, or opening snaps; split S_1 possible; S_1 greater than S_2. • In the apical area: regular rate and rhythm; 3/6 intensity; high pitch; systolic short duration; no radiation, splitting, murmurs, clicks, or opening snaps; S_1 greater than S_2.
Central and peripheral arteries	• Auscultate the carotid, femoral, and popliteal arteries as well as the abdominal aorta. • Use stethoscope bell to listen for bruits.	• No bruits in central or peripheral arteries
Advanced assessment skills		
Jugular vein	• Observe the right internal jugular vein. • Plot the jugular venous pulse as a wave form.	• Three ascending waves (a, c, and v) separated by two descending waves (x and y)

His pulse is 92 and irregular; blood pressure, 156/94; temperature, 98° F; and respirations, 16 and unlabored. He is 5′ 8″ tall and weighs 205 lb. His color appears normal, and his skin feels warm and dry. His neck veins exhibit no distention while he is seated. All pulses are palpable, equal, and +2. During auscultation, his lungs sound clear and his first and second heart sounds are normal with no gallops, murmurs, or rubs.

Just as you are about to leave the room, Mr. Jenkins develops substernal chest pain that radiates down his left arm. Auscultation reveals a third heart sound, and Mr. Jenkins develops dyspnea and diaphoresis. His chest pain subsides after 3 minutes.

How would you describe the following information related to your nursing assessment of Mr. Jenkins?
• history (subjective) assessment data
• physical (objective) assessment data
• assessment techniques and equipment
• two appropriate nursing diagnoses
• documentation of your findings.

Answer

History (subjective) assessment data
- Client complains of two episodes of substernal chest pain radiating down the left arm associated with shortness of breath and diaphoresis.
- Client complains of unusual tiredness.
- Client risk factors include family history, cigarette smoking, hypertension, and inactivity.

Physical (objective) assessment data
- Male, age 56
- Pulse 92 and irregular
- Blood pressure 156/94
- Temperature 98° F
- Respirations 16 and unlabored
- Height: 5' 8"
- Weight: 205 lb
- No neck vein distention
- S_1 and S_2 normal with no murmurs, gallops, or rubs
- S_3 during episode of pain
- Warm, dry skin with normal color. All pulses palpable, equal, and +2 (on a scale of 0 to +3).

Assessment techniques and equipment
- Interview the client about his past and family health status as well as health promotion and protection patterns.
- Observe the client at rest and during activity.
- Obtain the blood pressure with the proper size cuff and the bell of the stethoscope.
- Inspect the neck veins.
- Palpate all pulses.
- Auscultate heart sounds with the bell and diaphragm of the stethoscope in all four listening areas.

Two appropriate nursing diagnoses
- Pain related to myocardial ischemia
- Knowledge deficit related to cardiac risk factors and life-style changes

Documentation of findings
- S—Client complains of chest pain with dyspnea and diaphoresis, and unusual tiredness. Client has a family history of cardiac disease, smokes, has hypertension, and is inactive.
- O—T 98° F, P 92 and irregular, R 16 and unlabored, BP 156/94. No neck vein distention. S_1 and S_2 normal; S_3 auscultated during episode of pain. Warm, dry skin with normal color. All pulses palpable, equal, and +2.
- A—Pain related to myocardial ischemia

2. What are the usual differences in physical assessment findings for a client with arterial peripheral vascular disease and a client with venous peripheral vascular disease?

Answer

Arterial peripheral vascular disease typically causes the following assessment findings: pallor, cool skin, weak pulses, lack of hair growth, and dry, open lesions on the lower extremities. Venous peripheral vascular disease typ- ically produces these assessment findings: purplish discoloration of feet, edema of feet and lower extremities, and wet, open lesions with red or purplish edges on the lower extremities.

3. Mr. Young, age 55, was admitted to the hospital with a diagnosis of myocardial infarction. While caring for Mr. Young, you perform a physical assessment. What areas will you focus on to provide information about his cardiovascular status?

Answer

Assessment areas for such a client should include auscultation of heart sounds (especially for an S_4, which occurs with an MI) and blood pressure and pulse measurements. Assessment also should include skin color evaluation to check tissue perfusion.

4. Mrs. Schaeffer, age 73, has a history of congestive heart failure. As a public health nurse, you see her every week to assess her cardiovascular status. During the assessment, which areas should you focus on and why?

Answer

When assessing Mrs. Schaefer, you would focus on the following assessment areas:
- Activity tolerance. Decreased activity may indicate worsening congestive heart failure (CHF) or the need for medication changes.
- Weight gain. This may be an early sign of fluid retention.
- Edema. This may be a later sign of fluid retention and worsening CHF.
- Dyspnea. This symptom indicates increased pulmonary congestion.
- Heart rate and rhythm. Increased heart rate or irregular rhythm may indicate worsening CHF.
- Palpation of the pulses. Pulse pressure weakens as cardiac output decreases.
- Color changes. Pale or cyanotic skin may reflect decreased tissue perfusion or low cardiac output.
- Heart sounds. A new third or fourth heart sound or a new murmur may indicate worsening CHF.
- Lung sounds. New crackles at the bases may indicate increased pulmonary congestion.

5. Whether you work in a hospital or outpatient setting, all clients require heart sound auscultation. What are the four cardiac auscultatory sites? Where are they located? What mechanical events occur during the two normal heart sounds?

Answer
- Auscultatory sites: The four cardiac auscultatory sites include the aortic area, located in the second intercostal space along the right sternal border; the pulmonic area,

located in the second intercostal space at the left sternal border; the tricuspid area, located in the fifth intercostal space along the left sternal border; and the mitral area, located in the fifth intercostal space near the left midclavicular line.

- S_1 mechanical events: The first heart sound coincides with the mitral and tricuspid valve closure and marks the beginning of systole. Ventricular pressure increases with contraction, forcing open the aortic and pulmonic valves. Blood then is ejected from the ventricles into the arteries.
- S_2 mechanical events: The second heart sound coincides with the closing of the aortic and pulmonic valves and marks the beginning of diastole. Ventricular filling occurs when the mitral and tricuspid valves open.

Questions, answers, and rationales

1. Leonard Brown, age 70, is admitted to the critical care unit with uncontrolled hypertension. As part of the complete cardiovascular assessment, the nurse palpates Mr. Brown's point of maximum impulse (PMI) at the apex. What is the normal size of the left ventricular impulse?
(a) Less than 1 cm
(b) About 2 cm
(c) 3 to 4 cm
(d) More than 4 cm
Correct answer: (b), see text page 311. At the PMI, light palpation normally reveals a tap with each heartbeat over a space that is roughly ¾ ″ (2 cm) in diameter.

2. The nurse continues the cardiovascular assessment by auscultating Mr. Brown's heart sounds. Which of the following actions produces the first heart sound (S_1)?
(a) Opening of the mitral and tricuspid valves
(b) Closing of the mitral and tricuspid valves
(c) Opening of the aortic and pulmonic valves
(d) Closing of the aortic and pulmonic valves
Correct answer: (b), see text page 317. Mitral and tricuspid valve closing produces S_1, marking the beginning of systole or ventricular contraction.

3. Which of the following actions produce the second heart sound (S_2)?
(a) Opening of the mitral and tricuspid valves
(b) Closing of the mitral and tricuspid valves
(c) Opening of the aortic and pulmonic valves
(d) Closing of the aortic and pulmonic valves
Correct answer: (d), see text page 318. Aortic and pulmonic valve closing produces S_2, marking the end of systole.

4. When auscultating Mr. Brown's heart sounds, the nurse should hear S_1 best at which auscultatory site?
(a) Pulmonic area
(b) Aortic area
(c) Erb's point
(d) Mitral area
Correct answer: (d), see text page 317. Because S_1 results from mitral and tricuspid valve closure, it is heard best at the mitral or apical area.

5. The nurse should hear S_2 best at which auscultatory site?
(a) Mitral area
(b) Tricuspid area
(c) Erb's point
(d) Aortic area
Correct answer: (d), see text page 318. Because S_2 results from aortic and pulmonic valve closure, it is heard best at the aortic area.

6. When auscultating the tricuspid area, the nurse may hear which normal heart sound?
(a) Split first heart sound
(b) Split second heart sound
(c) Third heart sound
(d) Fourth heart sound
Correct answer: (a), see text page 317. The best location to listen for a split S_1 is over the tricuspid area at the lower left sternal border.

7. Because Mr. Brown has hypertension, the nurse can expect to hear which extra heart sound?
(a) Third heart sound
(b) Fourth heart sound
(c) Opening snap
(d) Ejection click
Correct answer: (b), see text page 320. A late diastolic sound caused by increased ventricular resistance to atrial contraction, a fourth heart sound commonly occurs in clients with hypertension.

8. Ben Harcourt, age 63, is admitted to the medical-surgical unit with congestive heart failure. His assessment findings include fatigue, shortness of breath, 10-lb weight gain over the past three days, blood pressure 170/98, pulse 120, respirations 24, S_3, and bibasilar crackles. To assess Mr. Harcourt further, the nurse places him at a 45-degree angle. In this position, what is the normal estimated central venous pressure?
(a) Less than 1 cm
(b) Less than 2 cm
(c) Less than 3 cm
(d) Less than 4 cm
Correct answer: (c), see text page 310. When estimating central venous pressure, the distance between the highest level of visible pulsation and the angle of Louis normally is less than 1¼″ (3 cm).

9. While auscultating Mr. Harcourt, the nurse detects a third heart sound. Which position facilitates auscultation of this heart sound?
(a) Supine position
(b) Prone position
(c) Sitting position
(d) Left-lateral recumbent position
Correct answer: (d), see text page 317. The left-lateral recumbent position is best for hearing low-pitched sounds related to atrioventricular problems, such as mitral valve murmurs and extra heart sounds.

10. To help differentiate the third heart sound from other heart sounds, the nurse listened closely to identify its timing. At what point in the cardiac cycle does S_3 occur?
(a) Early systole
(b) Late systole
(c) Early diastole
(d) Late diastole
Correct answer: (c), see text page 320. S_3 is a low-pitched heart sound that occurs early in diastole.

11. Which of the following statements can help the nurse differentiate split S_2 from S_3?
(a) Split S_2 is low-pitched; S_3 is high-pitched.
(b) S_3 occurs late in systole; split S_2, late in diastole.
(c) Split S_2 is heard best at the pulmonic area; S_3, at the apex.
(d) S_3 varies with respirations; split S_2 varies with position.
Correct answer: (c), see text page 318. Split S_2 is a high-pitched systolic sound heard best at the pulmonic area during inspiration. S_3 is a low-pitched diastolic sound heard best at the apex.

12. S_3 can be a sign of congestive heart failure. However, it can be a normal sound in which of the following clients?
(a) Healthy child
(b) Pregnant client
(c) Elderly client with arteriosclerosis
(d) Middle-aged adult client after exercise
Correct answer: (a), see text page 320. S_3 may be a normal filling sound in children and young adults.

13. Because Mr. Harcourt has tachycardia, the nurse should rely on which of the following facts to identify the timing of the cardiac cycle?
(a) S_1 is loudest at the base.
(b) S_1 occurs with the carotid pulse upstroke.
(c) S_1 occurs sometime during inspiration.
(d) S_1 is simultaneous with visible apical pulsations.
Correct answer: (b), see text page 318. S_1 can be identified by palpating the carotid pulse during auscultation. The pulse upstroke occurs almost simultaneously with S_1.

14. Dana Jenkins is 5 months pregnant. Auscultation normally may reveal which extra heart sound in Ms. Jenkins?
(a) Systolic murmur
(b) Third heart sound
(c) Fourth heart sound
(d) Diastolic murmur
Correct answer: (a), see text page 325. An innocent, or functional, systolic murmur may occur during pregnancy as a result of increased cardiac output.

15. Kathy Turner, age 36, has mitral valve prolapse with an ejection click. Which statement accurately characterizes ejection clicks?
(a) They are systolic sounds.
(b) They are low-pitched sounds.
(c) They are associated with palpable heaves.
(d) They are heard best in the supine position.
Correct answer: (a), see text page 325. Ejection clicks are high-pitched systolic sounds, heard best at the apical area with the client seated or standing.

16. In a client with mitral valve prolapse, murmurs may accompany ejection clicks. What produces the sound of murmurs?
(a) Valves closing
(b) Valves opening
(c) Turbulent blood flow
(d) Ventricular hypertrophy
Correct answer: (c), see text page 324. Murmurs, which are vibrating, blowing, or rumbling noises, result from turbulent blood flow in the heart.

17. Before admission for elective surgery, Patricia Roberts, age 44, undergoes a cardiovascular assessment. When palpating Ms. Roberts's peripheral pulses, the nurse should note which characteristic?
(a) Pitch
(b) Duration
(c) Amplitude
(d) Timing in the cardiac cycle
Correct answer: (c), see text page 310. During palpation, the nurse should identify the pulse rate, rhythm, symmetry, contour, strength, and amplitude.

18. Which peripheral pulse is located medial to the biceps tendon?
(a) Radial pulse
(b) Ulnar pulse
(c) Femoral pulse
(d) Brachial pulse
Correct answer: (d), see text page 313. The brachial pulse is located medial to the biceps tendon.

19. How would the pedal pulses of a healthy elderly client probably differ from those of Ms. Roberts?
(a) The pulses would be no different.
(b) The elderly client's pulses would be bounding.
(c) The elderly client's pulses would be weak.
(d) The younger client's pulses would have a palpable thrill.
Correct answer: (c), see text page 315. The pedal pulses in the elderly client commonly are weak.

20. The nurse also auscultates Ms. Roberts's carotid arteries to assess for bruits. Which technique is appropriate when auscultating these arteries?
(a) Use the bell of the stethoscope.
(b) Use the diaphragm of the stethoscope.
(c) Auscultate while the client inhales deeply.
(d) Palpate the radial pulse during auscultation.
Correct answer: (a), see text page 319. To auscultate the carotid arteries, the nurse should use the bell of the stethoscope while the client holds his or her breath.

21. Franklin Rogers, a 71-year-old Black male, is admitted to the critical care unit to rule out acute myocardial infarction (MI). His chief complaint is "recurrent, severe chest pain for the past hour relieved by nitroglycerin." His history includes hypertension, obesity, smoking, and hyperlipidemia. Physical assessment findings include: blood pressure 180/100, pulse 110, respirations 24, temperature 99° F, and S_4 on auscultation. Risk factors of cardiac disease may be unalterable, alterable, contributing, or other. Which of Mr. Rogers's history findings is a contributing factor?
(a) Race
(b) Hyperlipidemia
(c) Obesity
(d) Hypertension
Correct answer: (c), see text page 294. Obesity, inactivity, stress, and diet are contributing factors to cardiac disease.

22. Which finding would help differentiate anginal pain from that of an MI?
(a) The pain was provoked by stress.
(b) The pain affects the substernal region.
(c) The chest pain is severe.
(d) The pain is relieved by rest.
Correct answer: (d), see text page 296. Angina and MI may be provoked by stress and may cause severe pain in the substernal region. Anginal pain is relieved by rest; MI pain is not.

23. Which noninvasive diagnostic study would best locate ischemic changes in the myocardium?
(a) Lactic dehydrogenase test
(b) Total cholesterol level
(c) Chest X-ray
(d) Electrocardiography
Correct answer: (d), see text pages 328 and 330. Although all of these studies are helpful in assessing cardiac status, only electrocardiography can locate an MI and detect ischemia.

24. Several days after being admitted to the critical care unit with an MI, Rita Simons, age 66, develops a pericardial friction rub. Which fact about friction rubs can help the nurse differentiate them from other sounds?
(a) They are low-pitched sounds.
(b) They are heard best at the base.
(c) They occur with systole and diastole.
(d) They are accompanied by murmurs.
Correct answer: (c), see text page 328. A pericardial friction rub is a high-pitched sound that occurs during systole and diastole and is heard best at the lower left sternal border.

25. To enhance auscultation of the friction rub, the nurse should perform the assessment with Ms. Simons in which position?
(a) Supine position
(b) Seated, forward-leaning position
(c) Left-lateral recumbent position
(d) Prone position
Correct answer: (b), see text page 328. Auscultation with the client seated and leaning forward will enhance the sound of the friction rub by bringing the heart closer to the chest wall.

Test bank for Chapter 11, Cardiovascular System

1. Leonard Brown, age 70, is admitted to the critical care unit with uncontrolled hypertension. As part of the complete cardiovascular assessment, the nurse palpates Mr. Brown's point of maximum impulse (PMI) at the apex. What is the normal size of the left ventricular impulse?
(a) Less than 1 cm
(b) About 2 cm
(c) 3 to 4 cm
(d) More than 4 cm

2. The nurse continues the cardiovascular assessment by auscultating Mr. Brown's heart sounds. Which of the following actions produces the first heart sound (S_1)?
(a) Opening of the mitral and tricuspid valves
(b) Closing of the mitral and tricuspid valves
(c) Opening of the aortic and pulmonic valves
(d) Closing of the aortic and pulmonic valves

3. Which of the following actions produce the second heart sound (S_2)?
(a) Opening of the mitral and tricuspid valves
(b) Closing of the mitral and tricuspid valves
(c) Opening of the aortic and pulmonic valves
(d) Closing of the aortic and pulmonic valves

4. When auscultating Mr. Brown's heart sounds, the nurse should hear S_1 best at which auscultatory site?
(a) Pulmonic area
(b) Aortic area
(c) Erb's point
(d) Mitral area

5. The nurse should hear S_2 best at which auscultatory site?
(a) Mitral area
(b) Tricuspid area
(c) Erb's point
(d) Aortic area

6. When auscultating the tricuspid area, the nurse may hear which normal heart sound?
(a) Split first heart sound
(b) Split second heart sound
(c) Third heart sound
(d) Fourth heart sound

7. Because Mr. Brown has hypertension, the nurse can expect to hear which extra heart sound?
(a) Third heart sound
(b) Fourth heart sound
(c) Opening snap
(d) Ejection click

8. Ben Harcourt, age 63, is admitted to the medical-surgical unit with congestive heart failure. His assessment findings include fatigue, shortness of breath, 10-lb weight gain over the past three days, blood pressure 170/98, pulse 120, respirations 24, S_3, and bibasilar crackles. To assess Mr. Harcourt further, the nurse places him at a 45-degree angle. In this position, what is the normal estimated central venous pressure?
(a) Less than 1 cm
(b) Less than 2 cm
(c) Less than 3 cm
(d) Less than 4 cm

9. While auscultating Mr. Harcourt, the nurse detects a third heart sound. Which position facilitates auscultation of this heart sound?
(a) Supine position
(b) Prone position
(c) Sitting position
(d) Left-lateral recumbent position

10. To help differentiate the third heart sound from other heart sounds, the nurse listened closely to identify its timing. At what point in the cardiac cycle does S_3 occur?
(a) Early systole
(b) Late systole
(c) Early diastole
(d) Late diastole

11. Which of the following statements can help the nurse differentiate split S_2 from S_3?
(a) Split S_2 is low-pitched; S_3 is high-pitched.
(b) S_3 occurs late in systole; split S_2, late in diastole.
(c) Split S_2 is heard best at the pulmonic area; S_3, at the apex.
(d) S_3 varies with respirations; split S_2 varies with position.

12. S_3 can be a sign of congestive heart failure. However, it can be a normal sound in which of the following clients?
(a) Healthy child
(b) Pregnant client
(c) Elderly client with arteriosclerosis
(d) Middle-aged adult client after exercise

13. Because Mr. Harcourt has tachycardia, the nurse should rely on which of the following facts to identify the timing of the cardiac cycle?
(a) S_1 is loudest at the base.
(b) S_1 occurs with the carotid pulse upstroke.
(c) S_1 occurs sometime during inspiration.
(d) S_1 is simultaneous with visible apical pulsations.

14. Dana Jenkins is 5 months pregnant. Auscultation normally may reveal which extra heart sound in Ms. Jenkins?
(a) Systolic murmur
(b) Third heart sound
(c) Fourth heart sound
(d) Diastolic murmur

15. Kathy Turner, age 36, has mitral valve prolapse with an ejection click. Which statement accurately characterizes ejection clicks?
(a) They are systolic sounds.
(b) They are low-pitched sounds.
(c) They are associated with palpable heaves.
(d) They are heard best in the supine position.

16. In a client with mitral valve prolapse, murmurs may accompany ejection clicks. What produces the sound of murmurs?
(a) Valves closing
(b) Valves opening
(c) Turbulent blood flow
(d) Ventricular hypertrophy

17. Before admission for elective surgery, Patricia Roberts, age 44, undergoes a cardiovascular assessment. When palpating Ms. Roberts's peripheral pulses, the nurse should note which characteristic?
(a) Pitch
(b) Duration
(c) Amplitude
(d) Timing in the cardiac cycle

18. Which peripheral pulse is located medial to the biceps tendon?
(a) Radial pulse
(b) Ulnar pulse
(c) Femoral pulse
(d) Brachial pulse

19. How would the pedal pulses of a healthy elderly client probably differ from those of Ms. Roberts?
(a) The pulses would be no different.
(b) The elderly client's pulses would be bounding.
(c) The elderly client's pulses would be weak.
(d) The younger client's pulses would have a palpable thrill.

20. The nurse also auscultates Ms. Roberts's carotid arteries to assess for bruits. Which technique is appropriate when auscultating these arteries?
(a) Use the bell of the stethoscope.
(b) Use the diaphragm of the stethoscope.
(c) Auscultate while the client inhales deeply.
(d) Palpate the radial pulse during auscultation.

21. Franklin Rogers, a 71-year-old Black male, is admitted to the critical care unit to rule out acute myocardial infarction (MI). His chief complaint is "recurrent, severe chest pain for the past hour relieved by nitroglycerin." His history includes hypertension, obesity, smoking, and hyperlipidemia. Physical assessment findings include: blood pressure 180/100, pulse 110, respirations 24, temperature 99° F, and S_4 on auscultation. Risk factors of cardiac disease may be unalterable, alterable, contributing, or other. Which of Mr. Rogers's history findings is a contributing factor?
(a) Race
(b) Hyperlipidemia
(c) Obesity
(d) Hypertension

22. Which finding would help differentiate anginal pain from that of an MI?
(a) The pain was provoked by stress.
(b) The pain affects the substernal region.
(c) The chest pain is severe.
(d) The pain is relieved by rest.

23. Which noninvasive diagnostic study would best locate ischemic changes in the myocardium?
(a) Lactic dehydrogenase test
(b) Total cholesterol level
(c) Chest X-ray
(d) Electrocardiography

24. Several days after being admitted to the critical care unit with an MI, Rita Simons, age 66, develops a pericardial friction rub. Which fact about friction rubs can help the nurse differentiate them from other sounds?
(a) They are low-pitched sounds.
(b) They are heard best at the base.
(c) They occur with systole and diastole.
(d) They are accompanied by murmurs.

25. To enhance auscultation of the friction rub, the nurse should perform the assessment with Ms. Simons in which position?
(a) Supine position
(b) Seated, forward-leaning position
(c) Left-lateral recumbent position
(d) Prone position

12

Female and Male Breasts

Overview

Chapter 12 describes the anatomy and physiology of the female and male breasts and axillae, emphasizing important structures and functions and identifying normal developmental changes. It presents appropriate health history questions, describes the steps of a breast physical assessment, and discusses how to integrate assessment findings in the nursing process. Here are the chapter highlights:

• The human breasts are modified sebaceous glands located as a pair on the anterior chest. Each breast has a central nipple with surrounding areola.

• The female breast has 12 to 25 glandular lobes containing milk-producing alveoli. Hormones control breast tissue growth and lactation. Four major lymph node groups provide lymphatic drainage of the breasts.

• Maturational changes occurring at puberty affect the breasts. Sexual maturity ratings provide a general time frame for adolescent female breast development. Adolescent males may experience temporary breast changes.

• The health history should include questions that detect risk factors for breast cancer in females, including age, parity (number of pregnancies), and family history of breast cancer.

• The health history also should identify the client's drug use, because certain drugs can cause such breast changes as tenderness, pain, and fibrocystic disease.

• Physical assessment of the breasts includes inspection and palpation with the client seated and supine, and disrobed from the waist up. Deviations in size, symmetry, contour, sensitivity, and skin characteristics of the nipples, breasts, and axillae may indicate abnormalities. Position changes may elicit dimpling or retraction.

• Breast assessment provides an ideal opportunity to instruct the client in breast self-examination techniques.

• The nurse should document all assessment findings and use them in the nursing process to plan, implement, and evaluate the client's care.

• For more information about breast assessment, see pages 55PG through 59PG of the Photo Gallery in the text.

Suggested lecture topics

• Using audiovisual aids, review the anatomy and physiology of the breasts and axillae, including normal developmental changes. (For visual aids, see the transparency master, *Quadrants of the breast and associated lymph nodes,* as well as pages 55PG and 56PG in the text.)

• Discuss health history questions important to breast assessment, focusing on those that identify risk factors for breast cancer. Explain the reason for asking each question.

• Identify risk factors associated with breast cancer, and discuss ways in which a client can alter these factors.

• Using a breast examination simulator, demonstrate how to inspect and palpate the female breasts. (For visual aids, see pages 57PG and 58PG in the text.)

• Discuss normal breast assessment findings, including physiologic variations. Also discuss common abnormal findings, focusing on those that may suggest breast cancer. (For visual aids, see page 59PG in the text.)

Suggested critical thinking activities

• Have the students develop a breast self-examination teaching tool. Then pair the students and have them role-play a teaching session using the tool. Have each student evaluate the effectiveness of the partner's teaching tool and session.
• Using a simulator, have students practice breast inspection and palpation and describe all normal and abnormal findings.
• Using a case study, have the students identify a client's risk factors for breast cancer and plan ways to help the client reduce or eliminate these factors.
• Invite a speaker from the American Cancer Society to discuss breast cancer with the students.
• Have each student perform a breast self-examination and document the findings on the Skills Laboratory Assessment Guide. Then pair the students and have them critique each other's assessment findings.

Student study questions and answers

The following study questions are taken from text page 353 of Chapter 12, Female and Male Breasts. Their answers are based on information in that chapter.

1. Alice Rogers, age 68, comes to the clinic because her right breast has developed a sunken area above the areola. Which 10 pertinent health history questions would you ask Ms. Rogers when gathering subjective data?

Answer
1. How long have you had this problem?
2. Has the sunken appearance increased since you first noticed it?
3. Have you felt any pain or tenderness in the area?
4. Have you had any nipple discharge? If so, what were its characteristics?
5. Has anyone in your immediate family, such as your mother or sister, had breast cancer?
6. When was your last breast examination? What were the results?
7. When was your last mammogram (breast X-ray)?
8. Have you ever had breast surgery? If so, when and for what reason?
9. Are you currently taking any medications?
10. Have you ever given birth? If so, how many times? At what age did you first give birth?

2. Jimmy Allen, age 12, is brought to the clinic by his father. Mr. Allen and Jimmy are concerned because Jimmy has enlarged breasts. After performing an assessment, what would you probably tell them?

Skills laboratory guide: Health history

To collect information about the client's breasts, ask questions about health and illness patterns, health promotion and protection patterns, and role and relationship patterns. Sample questions from each category are listed below.

HEALTH AND ILLNESS PATTERNS

• How old are you?
• What changes, if any, have you noticed in your breasts? How would you describe these changes?
• Have you noticed any changes in your underarm area? If so, how would you describe these changes?
• Do you have breast pain or tenderness?
• Have you noticed any nipple discharge?
• Do you currently take any over-the-counter or prescription medications (including birth control pills or estrogen)? If so, which ones and how often do you take them?
• Have you ever had breast surgery?
• At what age did you begin to menstruate?
• Have you ever been pregnant? If you have children, at what age did you bear them? Did you breast-feed them?
• If you have gone through menopause, at what age did this occur?
• Do you have a history of cancer? Did your mother or any siblings ever have breast cancer?

HEALTH PROMOTION AND PROTECTION PATTERNS

• Do you perform breast self-examinations? If so, how often?
• Would you please demonstrate how you perform breast self-examination?
• When was your last mammogram (breast X-ray)?
• Have you recently changed your routine activities—for example, have you begun a new job or engaged in a new sport?

ROLE AND RELATIONSHIP PATTERNS

• How important are your breasts to a positive view of yourself?
• If you have breast tenderness or pain, how does it affect your sex life?

Answer
Young adolescent boys commonly have some temporary breast tissue growth (gynecomastia). Boys and girls alike produce the hormones estrogen and testosterone; until testosterone levels increase enough to override the effects of estrogen, a boy may experience enlargement in one or both breasts. Reassure Jimmy and his father that this condition usually is temporary and should resolve spontaneously as Jimmy matures.

3. Elisa Howell, age 18, goes to her college health clinic for a routine checkup. You note that she has large, pendulous breasts. Which four specific breast assessment steps should you perform to ensure a thorough breast assessment for Ms. Howell?

Skills laboratory guide: Physical assessment

This chart guides the student during assessment by identifying body areas, special considerations and techniques to be used, and normal findings.

BODY AREA	SPECIAL CONSIDERATIONS	NORMAL FINDINGS
Inspection		
Breasts	• Observe size, shape, symmetry, and color. Note any masses, lesions, unusual skin texture or venous pattern, edema, rashes, striae, retraction, dimpling, or flattening. • Inspect breasts with client seated with arms at the side, with hands on hips, and with arms over head. Ask a client with large breasts to lean forward. In women, one breast usually is smaller than the other. A neonate may exhibit transitory breast enlargement. An adolescent girl may have asymmetric breasts; an adolescent boy, gynecomastia. A pregnant client may have enlarged breasts with an increased venous pattern and striae.	• Appropriate breast size for client's age and sex • Symmetrical breasts with smooth, soft skin in a color consistent with body color • No masses, lesions, striae, asymmetrical venous distribution, edema, rashes, retraction, dimpling, or flattening
Nipples and areolae	• Note size, shape, color, symmetry, rashes, fissures, ulcerations, discharge, retraction, or inversion. An infant may have a milky, white discharge (witch's milk). A pregnant client's nipples and areolae may darken and discharge colostrum. • Note direction of nipples.	• Symmetric, round nipples and areolae that are equal in size and darker than breast tissue • No rashes, fissures, ulcers, discharge, retraction, or inversion • Symmetrical nipple direction—outward, slightly upward, and lateral
Axillae	• Note skin condition, rashes, lesions, unusual pigmentation, and hair growth.	• Intact axillary skin in a color consistent with overall skin pigmentation • No rashes or lesions • Appropriate hair growth for client's age and sex
Palpation		
Axillae	• Note tenderness, masses, or lymph node enlargement in the central, anterior, posterior, and lateral areas. • Palpate with the client's arm relaxed in the down position. If a node is palpable, note its size, shape, consistency, circumscription, mobility, tenderness, and location.	• No tenderness, masses, or lymph node enlargement
Breasts	• Ask the client to lie supine with a small pillow under the shoulder of the breast being examined and with the arm placed above the head. Palpate lightly with the middle three fingers in a systematic pattern. • Note consistency, masses, tenderness, induration, and inflammation. An adolescent client's breast should be firmer and more elastic than an elderly client's breast, which normally feels more granular. Breasts may be tender and nodular in a premenstrual client. • Chart findings by mentally dividing the breast into four quadrants or viewing it as a clock face.	• Breast consistency within normal limits for client's age and sex • No masses, tenderness, or induration • Firm inframammary ridge at lower edge of breast
Nipples and areolae	• Gently compress and milk the nipple between your thumb and index finger. Note discharge, tenderness, and masses. • Note the ducts through which any discharge appears and make a cytologic smear.	• No discharge, tenderness, or masses

Answer
• Inspect the breasts with Ms. Howell standing and leaning forward with her arms outstretched, so that her breasts swing forward freely.
• Palpate the breasts—in a circular fashion or across and down—with Ms. Howell sitting upright.
• Inspect and palpate the breasts with Ms. Howell in the supine position.
• Teach Ms. Howell how to examine her breasts, and instruct her to do so every month on the 5th to 7th day after her menstrual period begins.

4. Phyllis Anderson, a 35-year-old secretary, comes to the physician's office with the complaint of lumpy, tender breasts for the past 6 months. She says that the lumps are located in the upper outer areas of her breasts and the tenderness is worse before her menstrual period, which is due in 5 days. Because of job stress, Ms. Anderson drinks at least 5 cups of coffee daily. She has noticed no discharge from either nipple and no discharge occurs during palpation. Physical assessment reveals no masses, but several mobile, fairly well-defined, tender cystic nodules exist in both breasts in the upper outer quadrants. You find no other abnormalities. Ms. Anderson examines her breasts monthly and takes no medications.

How would you document the following information related to your nursing assessment of Ms. Anderson?
• subjective (history) assessment data
• objective (physical) assessment data
• assessment techniques and equipment
• two appropriate nursing diagnoses
• documentation of your findings

Answer

Subjective (history) assessment data
• Client complains of lumpy, tender breasts of 6 months' duration.
• Client reports that tenderness increases before onset of menses; her next menses is due in 5 days.
• Client reports no nipple discharge.
• Client drinks five or more cups of coffee daily.
• Client takes no medications.
• Client performs breast self-examination monthly.

Objective (physical) assessment data
• Female, age 35
• Multiple mobile, well-defined, tender cystic nodules palpated in upper outer quadrants of both breasts
• No nipple discharge elicited
• No other abnormalities noted

Assessment techniques and equipment
• Interview the client regarding current and past health history, family health history, and role and relationship patterns.
• Inspect and palpate the breasts, areolae, nipples, and axillae.
• No special equipment is needed.

Two appropriate nursing diagnoses
• Pain related to fibrocystic changes in both breasts
• Anxiety related to breast lumps

Documentation of findings
• S—Client complains of breast lumps and tenderness that have persisted for 6 months.
• O—Several mobile, well-defined, tender cystic nodules palpated in upper outer quadrants of both breasts
• A—Pain related to fibrocystic changes in both breasts

5. During a regular prenatal visit, Mrs. Hammersmith, age 25, mentions that her breasts have grown larger during pregnancy. She asks you what she can expect during the remainder of her pregnancy and when she breast-feeds the new baby. How do you respond?

Answer
Tell Mrs. Hammersmith that breast enlargement continues throughout pregnancy and that she should change her brassiere size to ensure adequate support. Also tell her that the nipples and areolae normally enlarge and darken, and that purplish streaks (striae gravidarum) may develop on the breasts as they enlarge. Explain that colostrum may leak from the nipples after the 6th week of pregnancy until the third day after delivery when milk production begins. Also explain that the breasts may become engorged and painful during the first few days after delivery, until milk production begins. Once the baby begins feeding regularly, milk production will continue and engorgement will subside.

Questions, answers, and rationales

1. Alice Conroy brings her daughter, Erin, age 12, to the physician's office. Both are concerned because Erin's breasts seem uneven. After performing an assessment, what would the nurse probably tell them about asymmetrical breast development?
(a) "It is normal during adolescence."
(b) "It results from an endocrine problem."
(c) "It results from a fibroadenoma."
(d) "It is a sign of an underlying mass."
Correct answer: (a), see text page 348. The breasts normally may develop asymmetrically during adolescence; they should become fairly equal with full development.

2. Ms. Conroy asks the nurse when Erin will begin menstruating. When does the onset of menses usually occur?
(a) Simultaneously with breast bud development
(b) Up to 1 year after breast bud development
(c) 1 to 2 years after breast bud development
(d) 2 to 3 years after breast bud development
Correct answer: (d), see text page 335. Usually, the time span from the beginning of breast buds (thelarche) to onset of menses is 2 to 3 years.

3. Susan Weiner, age 42, comes to the clinic because she has a small lump on her left breast. During the health history interview, the nurse asks when she began to menstruate. Menarche at which age would increase her risk of breast cancer?
(a) 11
(b) 13
(c) 15
(d) 17
Correct answer: (a), see text page 339. Menarche before age 12 increases breast cancer risk because the breast is exposed to estrogen for a longer-than-normal time.

4. The nurse also investigates Ms. Weiner's obstetric history. How is her risk of breast cancer affected by childbearing?
(a) The risk increases if she bears the first child before age 18.
(b) The risk decreases if she bears the first child between ages 18 and 30.
(c) The risk decreases if she bears the first child after age 30.
(d) The risk increases if she is childless.
Correct answer: (d), see text page 339. Having the first child before age 18 decreases the risk of breast cancer; childlessness or bearing a first child after age 30 increases it.

5. During the physical assessment, the nurse inspects Ms. Weiner's breasts. Which client position is most likely to reveal hidden breast dimpling?
(a) Sitting with her hands on her hips
(b) Lying supine with her arms at her sides
(c) Standing with her arms at her sides
(d) Leaning forward with her hands outstretched
Correct answer: (a), see text page 343. To inspect for hidden dimpling, the nurse should ask the seated client to place her hands against the hips.

6. Which inspection finding may be abnormal?
(a) Bilateral nipple inversion
(b) Nipples that point outward, slightly upward, and lateral
(c) Bilateral nipple eversion
(d) Unilateral nipple inversion
Correct answer: (d), see text pages 343 and 344. Nipples normally point outward, slightly upward, and lateral and may be everted or inverted. One inverted nipple (unless long present) should arouse suspicion.

7. How should the nurse position Ms. Weiner for palpation of the axillae and breasts?
(a) Supine with her arms at her sides
(b) Supine with her arms over her head
(c) Supine with a pillow under the shoulder of the side being examined and the arm on that side over the head
(d) Supine with a pillow under the opposite shoulder of the side being examined and the arm on that side over the head
Correct answer: (c), see text page 346. The client should lie supine with a small pad or pillow placed under the shoulder of the side being examined and with the arm on that same side over the head.

8. The nurse palpates Ms. Weiner's lymph nodes. Where should the nurse palpate to assess the lateral nodes?
(a) Anterior axillary fold
(b) Posterior axillary fold
(c) Infraclavicular area
(d) Inner aspect of upper arm
Correct answer: (d), see text pages 337 and 345. To palpate the lateral nodes, the nurse should press along the upper inner arm, trying to compress these nodes against the humerus.

9. During breast palpation, the nurse finds a small lump. Which characteristic of a lump suggests breast cancer?
(a) Tenderness
(b) Softness
(c) Irregularity
(d) Movability
Correct answer: (c), see text page 349. Breast cancer typically produces a nontender, firm, or hard lump that is irregularly shaped and fixed to skin or underlying tissue.

10. When assessing Ms. Weiner's nipples, which discharge suggests a serious disorder?
(a) Spontaneous discharge
(b) Manually expressed discharge
(c) Waxy discharge
(d) Any discharge
Correct answer: (a), see text pages 343, 344, and 347. Many women normally have a benign discharge on palpation, such as the waxy substance normally secreted by Montgomery's tubercles. However, spontaneous discharge in a nonlactating woman may indicate cancer.

11. Nipple discharge of which type of fluid is associated with breast cancer?
(a) Green
(b) White
(c) Bloody
(d) Yellow
Correct answer: (c), see text page 349. Breast cancer usually produces a bloody nipple discharge and a breast lump.

12. Which diagnostic study routinely is used to screen for breast cancer?
(a) Mammography
(b) Thermography
(c) Transillumination
(d) Computed tomography
Correct answer: (a), see text page 348. Because mammography detects lumps as small as 1 mm, it is useful for early detection. A baseline mammogram is recommended for all women age 35 to 40 followed by regular mammograms after age 40.

13. Terri Greenberg, age 41, comes to the clinic for her annual gynecologic examination. She has a history of fibrocystic breast disease. During the health history, the nurse asks her about breast self-examination (BSE). When should Ms. Greenberg perform BSE?
(a) On the 5th to 7th day of the cycle
(b) During the menstrual period
(c) Just before the menstrual period
(d) In the middle of the cycle
Correct answer: (a), see text page 341. The client should perform BSE on the 5th to 7th day after the first day of the menstrual period when breast tenderness and lumpiness are minimal.

14. The health history reveals that Ms. Greenberg has no family history of breast cancer or other risk factors. How frequently should she have a mammogram?
(a) Once as a baseline
(b) Once every 1 to 2 years
(c) Once every year
(d) Twice every year
Correct answer: (b), see text page 341. A client age 40 to 49 should have a mammogram every 1 to 2 years; a client over age 50, once a year.

15. After completing the health history, the nurse performs breast inspection. Because Ms. Greenberg's breasts are large and pendulous, the nurse should inspect them with the client in which position?
(a) Lying supine with her arms over her head
(b) Leaning forward with her hands on her hips
(c) Leaning forward with her arms outstretched
(d) Lying supine with her arms at her sides
Correct answer: (c), see text page 343. The nurse should inspect large or pendulous breasts with the client standing and leaning forward with her hands or arms outstretched. Both breasts should swing freely.

16. Because Ms. Greenberg has fibrocystic disease, the nurse should teach her to avoid which food?
(a) High-fat foods
(b) Caffeine-rich foods
(c) Dairy products
(d) Red meat
Correct answer: (b), see text page 349. Caffeine intake may exacerbate fibrocystic breast disease.

17. The physician aspirates Ms. Greenberg's breast cysts. Which type of fluid usually is aspirated from fibrocystic breasts?
(a) Gray-green
(b) Yellowish
(c) Bloody
(d) Clear
Correct answer: (a), see text page 349. In a client with fibrocystic disease, aspiration of cysts usually produces gray-green fluid.

18. JoAnne Craft, age 35, is 8 months pregnant. She comes to the clinic for a check-up. Which breast finding is normal in a pregnant client?
(a) Increased venous pattern
(b) Orange peel skin
(c) Dimpling
(d) Retraction
Correct answer: (a), see text page 348. Elevated estrogen levels during pregnancy cause a bilaterally prominent venous pattern on the breasts and upper trunk.

19. Three weeks after giving birth Ms. Craft develops mastitis. Which signs and symptoms does mastitis produce?
(a) Single, nontender mass
(b) Spontaneous, bloody nipple discharge
(c) Tender, hard, reddened breast
(d) Multiple painful masses
Correct answer: (c), see text page 349. Mastitis, which occurs in the third or fourth week postpartum, produces tenderness and pain; hard, reddened breasts; and enlarged axillary lymph nodes.

20. Helen Jordan, age 52, seeks care for an eczematous rash on her left nipple and areola. This type of rash is associated with which disorder?
(a) Fibrocystic disease
(b) Interductal papilloma
(c) Breast fibroadenoma
(d) Paget's disease
Correct answer: (d), see text page 344. Paget's disease may cause a red, scaly, eczema-like area over one nipple and areola.

21. John Hoffman, age 65, takes digoxin as prescribed for congestive heart failure. This cardiac glycoside may cause which adverse reaction?
(a) Galactorrhea
(b) Gynecomastia
(c) Mastalgia
(d) Breast atrophy
Correct answer: (b), see text page 340. Gynecomastia (male breast enlargement) may be an adverse reaction to a cardiac glycoside.

Test bank for Chapter 12, Female and Male Breasts

1. Alice Conroy brings her daughter, Erin, age 12, to the physician's office. Both are concerned because Erin's breasts seem uneven. After performing an assessment, what would the nurse probably tell them about asymmetrical breast development?
(a) "It is normal during adolescence."
(b) "It results from an endocrine problem."
(c) "It results from a fibroadenoma."
(d) "It is a sign of an underlying mass."

2. Ms. Conroy asks the nurse when Erin will begin menstruating. When does the onset of menses usually occur?
(a) Simultaneously with breast bud development
(b) Up to 1 year after breast bud development
(c) 1 to 2 years after breast bud development
(d) 2 to 3 years after breast bud development

3. Susan Weiner, age 42, comes to the clinic because she has a small lump on her left breast. During the health history interview, the nurse asks when she began to menstruate. Menarche at which age would increase her risk of breast cancer?
(a) 11
(b) 13
(c) 15
(d) 17

4. The nurse also investigates Ms. Weiner's obstetric history. How is her risk of breast cancer affected by childbearing?
(a) The risk increases if she bears the first child before age 18.
(b) The risk decreases if she bears the first child between ages 18 and 30.
(c) The risk decreases if she bears the first child after age 30.
(d) The risk increases if she is childless.

5. During the physical assessment, the nurse inspects Ms. Weiner's breasts. Which client position is most likely to reveal hidden breast dimpling?
(a) Sitting with her hands on her hips
(b) Lying supine with her arms at her sides
(c) Standing with her arms at her sides
(d) Leaning forward with her hands outstretched

6. Which inspection finding may be abnormal?
(a) Bilateral nipple inversion
(b) Nipples that point outward, slightly upward, and lateral
(c) Bilateral nipple eversion
(d) Unilateral nipple inversion

7. How should the nurse position Ms. Weiner for palpation of the axillae and breasts?
(a) Supine with her arms at her sides
(b) Supine with her arms over her head
(c) Supine with a pillow under the shoulder of the side being examined and the arm on that side over the head
(d) Supine with a pillow under the opposite shoulder of the side being examined and the arm on that side over the head

8. The nurse palpates Ms. Weiner's lymph nodes. Where should the nurse palpate to assess the lateral nodes?
(a) Anterior axillary fold
(b) Posterior axillary fold
(c) Infraclavicular area
(d) Inner aspect of upper arm

9. During breast palpation, the nurse finds a small lump. Which characteristic of a lump suggests breast cancer?
(a) Tenderness
(b) Softness
(c) Irregularity
(d) Movability

10. When assessing Ms. Weiner's nipples, which discharge suggests a serious disorder?
(a) Spontaneous discharge
(b) Manually expressed discharge
(c) Waxy discharge
(d) Any discharge

11. Nipple discharge of which type of fluid is associated with breast cancer?
(a) Green
(b) White
(c) Bloody
(d) Yellow

12. Which diagnostic study routinely is used to screen for breast cancer?
(a) Mammography
(b) Thermography
(c) Transillumination
(d) Computed tomography

13. Terri Greenberg, age 41, comes to the clinic for her annual gynecologic examination. She has a history of fibrocystic breast disease. During the health history, the nurse asks her about breast self-examination (BSE). When should Ms. Greenberg perform BSE?
(a) On the 5th to 7th day of the cycle
(b) During the menstrual period
(c) Just before the menstrual period
(d) In the middle of the cycle

14. The health history reveals that Ms. Greenberg has no family history of breast cancer or other risk factors. How frequently should she have a mammogram?
(a) Once as a baseline
(b) Once every 1 to 2 years
(c) Once every year
(d) Twice every year

15. After completing the health history, the nurse performs breast inspection. Because Ms. Greenberg's breasts are large and pendulous, the nurse should inspect them with the client in which position?
(a) Lying supine with her arms over her head
(b) Leaning forward with her hands on her hips
(c) Leaning forward with her arms outstretched
(d) Lying supine with her arms at her sides

16. Because Ms. Greenberg has fibrocystic disease, the nurse should teach her to avoid which food?
(a) High-fat foods
(b) Caffeine-rich foods
(c) Dairy products
(d) Red meat

17. The physician aspirates Ms. Greenberg's breast cysts. Which type of fluid usually is aspirated from fibrocystic breasts?
(a) Gray-green
(b) Yellowish
(c) Bloody
(d Clear

18. JoAnne Craft, age 35, is 8 months pregnant. She comes to the clinic for a check-up. Which breast finding is normal in a pregnant client?
(a) Increased venous pattern
(b) Orange peel skin
(c) Dimpling
(d) Retraction

19. Three weeks after giving birth Ms. Craft develops mastitis. Which signs and symptoms does mastitis produce?
(a) Single, nontender mass
(b) Spontaneous, bloody nipple discharge
(c) Tender, hard, reddened breast
(d) Multiple painful masses

20. Helen Jordan, age 52, seeks care for an eczematous rash on her left nipple and areola. This type of rash is associated with which disorder?
(a) Fibrocystic disease
(b) Interductal papilloma
(c) Breast fibroadenoma
(d) Paget's disease

21. John Hoffman, age 65, takes digoxin as prescribed for congestive heart failure. This cardiac glycoside may cause which adverse reaction?
(a) Galactorrhea
(b) Gynecomastia
(c) Mastalgia
(d) Breast atrophy

13

Gastrointestinal System

Overview

Almost everyone experiences a gastrointestinal (GI) problem at some time. Besides being common, GI problems can have wide-ranging metabolic implications, such as acid-base imbalance and nutritional deficits. To prepare the nurse to assess this important body system, Chapter 13 begins by reviewing its anatomy and physiology. Then it describes how to perform a thorough GI health history and physical assessment, identifying normal and abnormal findings as well as developmental considerations for pediatric, pregnant, and elderly clients. It concludes with documentation samples. Here are the chapter highlights:

- The GI system consists of the alimentary canal and accessory organs. The alimentary canal includes the mouth, pharynx, esophagus, stomach, small intestine, large intestine, and anus. Accessory organs that aid GI function include the liver, gallbladder and bile ducts, and pancreas. The GI tract functions to digest food and fluids into simple chemical forms and to eliminate waste products from the body.
- The GI health history should include questions about dietary intake, appetite, digestion, bowel elimination patterns, medication use, and history of GI disorders. The nurse should explore all GI complaints, even vague or seemingly mild ones, such as "heartburn" and "upset stomach." Such complaints may signal a serious underlying problem.
- When assessing the GI system, the nurse should auscultate the abdomen before performing palpation and percussion, which can change intestinal activity and interfere with bowel sound auscultation.

- Inspection helps assess abdominal contour, skin lesions, and the condition of the umbilicus. The nurse should note any visible arterial pulsations and peristaltic movements.
- The nurse should auscultate for bowel sounds with the diaphragm of the stethoscope and for vascular sounds with the bell of the stethoscope in all four quadrants of the abdomen.
- Percussion helps determine the size and location of abdominal organs and helps detect excessive accumulation of fluid and air in the abdomen.
- Palpation provides clues about the condition of the abdominal wall; the size, condition, and consistency of abdominal organs; the presence and nature of any abdominal masses; and the presence, degree, and location of any abdominal pain. Deep palpation helps detect organ location, masses, and areas of tenderness or increased muscular resistance.
- Advanced GI assessment skills include liver percussion, palpation, and hooking; rectal examination; and techniques that elicit abdominal pain, including eliciting rebound tenderness and testing for iliopsoas sign and obturator sign.
- To complete the GI assessment, the nurse should review any laboratory tests that may have been ordered, such as blood tests for bilirubin, cholesterol, and electrolyte levels; urine tests for bilirubin and urobilinogen levels; and fecal tests for occult blood, ova, and parasites.
- Finally, the nurse should document all assessment findings and use them to develop a nursing care plan.
- For more information about GI system assessment, see pages 60PG through 66PG of the Photo Gallery in the text.

Suggested lecture topics

- Review GI anatomy and physiology, highlighting usual variations in pediatric, pregnant, and elderly clients. (For visual aids, see the transparency master, *Structures of the gastrointestinal system,* as well as pages 60PG and 61PG in the text.)
- Discuss health history questions important to GI system assessment and the rationales for each.
- Using an anatomical simulator, demonstrate the appropriate techniques for assessing the abdomen and rectum. (For visual aids, see the transparency master, *Percussing the abdomen,* as well as pages 62PG through 65PG in the text.)
- Describe normal findings for abdominal and rectal assessments, highlighting usual variations in pediatric, pregnant, and elderly clients.
- Using audiovisual aids, discuss common abnormal findings for a GI system assessment. (For visual aids, see page 66PG in the text.)

Suggested critical thinking activities

- Pair the students and have them perform an abdominal assessment, including history and physical assessment, on each other.
- Have the students document their findings on the Skills Laboratory Assessment Guide.
- Have the entire class critique these assessment findings.
- Using an anatomical simulator, have the students demonstrate proper rectal examination technique and describe normal findings.
- Using a case study of a client with a GI disorder, have the students develop a nursing care plan.

Student study questions and answers

The following study questions are taken from text page 383 of Chapter 13, Gastrointestinal System. Their answers are based on information in that chapter.

1. What subjective and objective findings would you most often see in a client with diverticulitis? How do these contrast with the most likely findings in Crohn's disease?

Answer
- Subjective findings for a client with diverticulitis typically include occasional left lower quadrant pain, mild nausea, constipation with onset of pain, and a diet low in fiber. Objective findings may include abdominal tenderness on palpation and a low-grade fever.
- For a client with Crohn's disease, subjective findings commonly consist of cramping, right lower quadrant pain; nausea; and mild, urgent diarrhea. Other subjective find-

---

Skills laboratory guide: Health history

To collect information about the client's GI system, ask questions about health and illness patterns, health promotion and protection patterns, and role and relationship patterns. Sample questions from each category are listed below.

HEALTH AND ILLNESS PATTERNS

- Do you have any pain in your mouth, throat, abdomen, or rectum?
- If you have abdominal pain, when does it occur in relation to eating?
- What other symptoms accompany this pain?
- Do you have heartburn or indigestion?
- Have you had nausea and vomiting along with the pain? If so, did you notice any blood in the vomit? Did the vomited material have a fecal odor?
- Is the pain related to constipation and swelling in the abdomen?
- Have you had other problems, such as fever, at the same time?
- How often do you have bowel movements? Have you noticed any change in your normal pattern of bowel movements?
- What color are your stools?
- Have you recently had an unintentional weight loss, appetite loss, unexplained fatigue, or recurrent fever?
- Do you take any prescription or over-the-counter medications? If so, which drugs and at what dosages?
- Has anyone in your family ever had colorectal cancer or polyps?

HEALTH PROMOTION AND PROTECTION PATTERNS

- Do you smoke? If so, how much and for many years?
- Do you drink alcohol? If so, how much and how often?
- Do you drink coffee, tea, or cola, or use any other caffeine-containing products?
- How do you care for your teeth and gums?
- How do you spend a normal day? Do you participate in any regular exercise program?
- What do you do for a living? How do you feel about your job?

ROLE AND RELATIONSHIP PATTERNS

- Have you lived in or traveled to a foreign country? If so, when and where?
- In your family, who does the food shopping and who prepares the meals? Does the entire family eat together? Have these routines changed recently?
- Have you recently lost a loved one, experienced a breakup of a relationship, or undergone a similar stressful event?

---

ings may include a family history of Crohn's disease, emotional stress, flatulence, weight loss, weakness, malaise, and symptoms of uveitis. Objective findings are likely to include low-grade fever, abdominal tenderness on palpation, and a palpable mass in the right lower quadrant.

2. During the health history, a 32-year-old male client reports a history of bleeding hemorrhoids. You note that he has a hemoglobin of 12.2 g/dl and melena. Are these objective findings consistent with the client's history? What further assessment steps should you take?

Skills laboratory guide: Physical assessment

This chart guides the student during assessment by identifying body areas, special considerations and techniques to be used, and normal findings.

BODY AREA	SPECIAL CONSIDERATIONS	NORMAL FINDINGS
Inspection		
Abdomen	• Have client lie supine with a pillow under the head and arms at sides. Assess abdominal contour from foot of bed and client's side. • Note skin color, integrity, striae, lesions, scars, superficial veins, edema, and hair distribution. • Note bulges, symmetry, masses, distention, ascites, diastasis recti, and movement from peristalsis or arterial pulsations. • In a pregnant client, increased pigmentation at abdominal midline, striae, upward displacement of umbilicus abdominis, and diastasis recti are normal. In a young child, especially a Black child, diastasis recti normally occurs.	• Intact abdominal skin consistent with color of rest of body • No striae, lesions, scars, superficial veins, or edema • Appropriate hair distribution for client's age and sex • Flat, symmetrical abdomen with no bulges, masses, distention, or diastasis recti • Abdominal breathing in men and children • Slight visible pulsation in epigastric area; no visible peristalsis
Umbilicus	• Note position, contour (everted or inverted), inflammation, discoloration, and hernias. Detect hernias by having an adult client raise the head and shoulders while remaining supine; by observing a small child crying.	• Midline, concave umbilicus consistent with color of rest of abdomen • No inflammation, discoloration, or hernias
Auscultation		
Abdomen	• Use stethoscope diaphragm to detect bowel sounds. Listen in all four quadrants for 5 minutes before reporting absent bowel sounds. Note character, pitch, and frequency of bowel sounds. • Use stethoscope bell to detect bruits, venous hums, or friction rubs.	• Soft, medium-pitched bowel sounds in all four quadrants every 5 to 15 seconds • No borborygmi, hyperperistalsis, or hypoactive sounds • No bruits, venous hums, or friction rubs
Percussion		
Abdomen	• Do not percuss or palpate in clients with suspected abdominal aortic aneurysm or those who have received abdominal organ transplants. Perform these techniques cautiously in clients with suspected appendicitis. • Percuss over tender areas last. • Note tympany and dullness in all four quadrants. In a child, percussion notes are more tympanic. • Note tenderness, masses, or shifting dullness.	• Tympany in all four quadrants; dullness over liver and spleen. Normal percussion note may range from tympany to dullness, depending on intestinal and bladder contents. • No tenderness, masses, or shifting dullness
Palpation		
Abdomen	• Press fingertips gently about ½″ to ¾″ (1 to 2 cm) against the abdominal wall for light palpation. • Press fingertips about 1½″ (4 cm) against abdominal wall for deep palpation. • Use light, rapid bouncing or tapping of fingertips against abdominal wall for ballottement. • Note organ location, masses, and areas of tenderness or increased muscular resistance. • Note location, size, shape, consistency, border, tenderness, pulsations, and mobility of any mass. • In an elderly client, abdominal palpation is easier and the results more accurate. Because a child tends to be more ticklish and tense than an adult, distract the child during palpation.	• No masses or areas of tenderness or increased muscular resistance • No organ enlargement
Advanced assessment skills: Auscultation		
Liver	• Auscultate over inferior edge of liver; scratch below edge and work up until sound is clear.	• Inferior border of liver at costal margin • Positive scratch test

Skills laboratory guide: Physical assessment   *continued*

BODY AREA	SPECIAL CONSIDERATIONS	NORMAL FINDINGS
Advanced assessment skills: Percussion		
Liver	• Use fist percussion to detect tenderness over liver and gall-bladder. Use mediate percussion along the right midclavicular line (MCL) to estimate liver size.	• Nontender liver • Liver percussion (dullness) from a point at or just below the right costal margin to the 5th to 7th intercostal space at MCL
Advanced assessment skills: Palpation		
Liver	• Use bimanual or hooking technique; palpate during inspiration. • Note palpability, contour, tenderness, size, and consistency. In a child, the liver is palpable 1 to 2 finger breadths below ribs. In a client with emphysema or Riedel's lobe, the liver is lower and easier to palpate.	• Nonpalpable liver • If palpable, liver is smooth and firm with a rounded, regular edge
Advanced assessment skills: Rectal examination		
Rectum	• Have client bend over examination table or assume a knee-chest or left lateral Sims' position. • Inspect the anus for breaks in the skin, fissures, discharge, inflammation, lesions, scars, rectal prolapse, skin tags, and external hemorrhoids. Have client strain as though defecating to make visible internal hemorrhoids, polyps, rectal prolapse, or fissures. • Insert a gloved, lubricated finger 2½″ to 4″ (6 to 10 cm) to palpate internal rectum. Assess rectal wall for nodules, tenderness, irregularities, and fecal impaction. In a female client, note posterior side of uterus; in a male client, assess the prostate. In an infant or child, rectal palpation should be performed only when symptoms are present. A pregnant client may exhibit hemorrhoids; an elderly client, decreased sphincter tone. • Note fecal color and any blood or mucus after withdrawing your finger. Test feces for occult blood.	• Intact skin with no breaks, fissures, discharge, inflammation, lesions, scars, rectal prolapse, skin tags, hemorrhoids, or polyps • Smooth and soft rectal walls with no nodules, irregularities, or fecal impaction • Brown feces with no blood, mucus, or occult blood
Advanced assessment skills: Eliciting abdominal pain		
Rebound tenderness	• Position the client supine with knees flexed. Press deeply at McBurney's point, then release quickly. Note pain on release of pressure.	• No rebound tenderness
Iliopsoas sign	• Position the client supine with legs straight. Have the client raise one leg as you apply counter-pressure; test both legs. • Note increased abdominal pain.	• Negative iliopsoas sign
Obturator sign	• Position the client supine with right leg flexed 90 degrees at the hip and knee. • Hold client's leg just above the knee and at the ankle. Then gently rotate the leg laterally and medially. Note pain in the hypogastric region.	• Negative obturator sign

Answer

Hemorrhoidal bleeding may cause enough blood loss to result in mild anemia, but melena does not result from hemorrhoidal bleeding. Hemorrhoids, which are located in the anal area, may produce bright red bleeding. In contrast, melena produces tarry, black stools, which occur with upper GI tract bleeding. To assess the client's problem further, take these steps:

• Ask the client about feelings of lightheadedness or weakness, use of drugs or iron preparations, upper abdominal or back pain, and the relationship of pain to eating.
• Measure the client's vital signs.
• Perform a complete abdominal assessment.
• Perform a rectal examination.
• Test the client's stool for occult blood.
• Refer the client to the physician to rule out malignancy.

3. Mrs. Cavanaugh brings her 7-month-old daughter to the clinic, stating that the child has had 9 to 10 loose, liquid stools a day for 3 days and that she is taking her bottle poorly. What health history questions and physical assessment procedures will be most useful for this client?

Answer

Health history questions
• When did the diarrhea start? What does it look like? Is blood present? How many stools does the child have a day? How large are the stools? Does the child draw her knees up to her chest and cry?
• Is the child cranky? Has she had a fever? Has she been vomiting?
• How often does the child urinate? Has she been thirsty? How much and what types of fluids has she been drinking?
• What are her usual feeding patterns? What changes have occurred since the diarrhea started?

Physical assessment procedures
• Vital sign measurement. Vital signs can provide information about the child's fluid and electrolyte balance, which can be upset easily by excessive diarrhea.
• Inspection. Abdominal inspection may reveal distention, although the contour usually remains normal with short-term diarrhea. Rectal inspection may reveal local irritation in the perianal area. The nurse also should inspect for signs of dehydration, such as dry skin with poor turgor, dry mucous membranes, sunken fontanels; and signs of electrolyte loss, such as lethargy, weakness, and flaccidity.
• Auscultation. This technique may reveal hyperperistaltic bowel sounds.
• Percussion. Abdominal percussion may reveal tympany over all four quadrants.
• Palpation. This technique may detect areas of tenderness or localized pain. However, the nurse will have to watch for visible clues, such as abdominal guarding or facial grimacing, because the child cannot verbalize her feelings.
• Laboratory studies. Several studies may aid evaluation of the child's problem. Blood tests for electrolytes and pH can identify any electrolyte or acid-base imbalances that the diarrhea may have caused. The fecal occult blood test can detect GI bleeding that can result from persistent diarrhea. Visual inspection of the stool sample should detect any obvious signs of bleeding.

4. Which three types of clients are at greatest risk for constipation, and why?

Answer

Clients at greatest risk for constipation include pregnant clients, elderly clients, and those who take constipating medications.
• During pregnancy, the growing fetus displaces the colon, decreasing peristaltic activity. This commonly leads to GI problems, such as constipation and hemorrhoid formation.

• Aging decreases intestinal motility, leading to constipation in an elderly client. Decreased mobility and other problems associated with aging may interfere with the client's ability to use the bathroom effectively, possibly leading to constipation.
• Constipation may result from the use of many commonly prescribed medications, including certain antacids, antidepressants, antihypertensives, narcotic analgesics, phenothiazines, barium sulfate, ferrous sulfate, phenytoin sodium, and ranitidine hydrochloride.
• Other clients at risk for constipation include those with impaired mobility or who are on bed rest, clients who are poorly nourished or dehydrated, and pediatric clients.

5. Mrs. Stevens, a 71-year-old widow, comes to the outpatient clinic complaining of "constipation." She also complains of lack of appetite and occasional nausea, especially at bedtime. She states that since her husband died, she no longer cares to cook and no longer takes the long daily walks the couple used to share.

In the following categories, what information would you record regarding the nursing assessment of Mrs. Stevens?
• history (subjective) assessment data
• physical (objective) assessment data
• assessment techniques and equipment
• two appropriate nursing diagnoses
• documentation of findings.

Answer

History (subjective) assessment data
• Complains of constipation, lack of appetite, and occasional nausea (especially at bedtime)
• States that she no longer cooks or takes long daily walks since her husband died

Physical (objective) assessment data
• Female, age 71
• Abdomen convex and symmetrical with no distention
• Irritation in perianal area
• High-pitched, hypoactive bowel sounds
• Firm abdomen
• Dullness on percussion in lower quadrants
• No palpable fecal masses

Assessment techniques and equipment
• Interview client regarding past health history, current medications, dietary habits, activities of daily living, use of home remedies, and role and relationship patterns.
• Inspect the abdomen.
• Inspect the perianal area.
• Auscultate bowel sounds.
• Percuss the abdomen.
• Palpate the abdomen.

- Equipment should include gloves, tape, felt-tip marker, stethoscope, flashlight, measuring tape, and gown and drapes.

Two appropriate nursing diagnoses
- Constipation related to poor food and fluid intake
- Knowledge deficit related to prevention of constipation

Documentation of findings
- S—Client reports constipation, lack of appetite, and occasional nausea, especially at bedtime. Client describes a "lack of interest in cooking" and "depression" since husband died 2 years ago. Activity is decreased; client no longer takes long daily walks.
- O—T 99° F, P 84 and regular, R 20 and regular, BP 162/90. Abdomen convex with no distention, visible scars, lesions, or pulsations. Bowel sounds, high-pitched, hypoactive in all four quadrants (< every 20 seconds). Abdominal percussion dull in lower quadrants. Abdomen firm with no masses, rigidity, or palpable fecal masses.
- A—Constipation related to poor food and fluid intake

Questions, answers, and rationales

1. Frank Jacobs, age 41, seeks care because he has abdominal pain, fever, hematemesis, and melena. Which of these signs and symptoms is one of the most frequent GI problems?
(a) Pain
(b) Nausea
(c) Hematemesis
(d) Melena
Correct answer: (a), see text page 359. GI pain is one of the most common GI symptoms; it frequently is described as burning, squeezing, dull, or knot-like.

2. During the health history, the nurse reviews Mr. Jacobs's medication use. Which drug could cause GI bleeding?
(a) Methyldopa
(b) Digoxin
(c) Aspirin
(d) Codeine
Correct answer: (c), see text page 362. Adverse reactions to aspirin include GI disturbances, GI bleeding, and ulceration.

3. After obtaining health history data, the nurse should perform the physical assessment steps in which sequence?
(a) Inspection, palpation, percussion, and auscultation
(b) Inspection, percussion, palpation, and auscultation
(c) Auscultation, inspection, palpation, and percussion
(d) Inspection, auscultation, percussion, and palpation
Correct answer: (d), see text page 365. The GI system requires abdominal auscultation before percussion and palpation, which can alter intestinal activity and bowel sounds.

4. While inspecting Mr. Jacobs's abdomen, the nurse may see aortic pulsations in which area?
(a) Epigastric
(b) Right inguinal
(c) Hypogastric
(d) Left lumbar
Correct answer: (a), see text page 367. Aortic pulsations may be seen in the epigastric area.

5. To detect an umbilical or incisional hernia, the nurse should have Mr. Jacobs perform which maneuver?
(a) Flex the knees while remaining supine
(b) Raise the head and shoulders while remaining supine
(c) Raise the legs while remaining supine
(d) Assume Sims' position for 10 seconds
Correct answer: (b), see text page 367. True umbilical or incisional hernias may protrude when the client raises the head and shoulders while remaining supine.

6. The nurse auscultates Mr. Jacobs's bowel sounds. What is the normal frequency of bowel sounds?
(a) Every 5 to 15 seconds
(b) Every 15 to 30 seconds
(c) Every 30 to 60 seconds
(d) Every 5 to 7 minutes
Correct answer: (a), see text page 368. Normally, air and fluid moving through the bowel by peristalsis create soft, bubbling sounds and gurgles every 5 to 15 seconds.

7. Janet Dixon, age 48, is admitted to the hospital with right upper quadrant and right infrascapular pain caused by cholecystitis. This is an example of which type of pain?
(a) Referred pain
(b) Rebound pain
(c) Phantom pain
(d) Organ pain
Correct answer: (a), see text page 360. A gallbladder disorder is likely to cause referred pain (pain felt at a site different from that of the injured or diseased organ) in the right upper quadrant and right posterior infrascapular area.

8. Eddie Hobart, age 25, is rushed to the emergency department with blunt abdominal trauma caused by an automobile accident. The nurse performs a rapid physical assessment. Which finding suggests intra-abdominal bleeding?
(a) Borborygmi
(b) Everted umbilicus
(c) Visible peristaltic waves
(d) Bluish tint around the umbilicus
Correct answer: (d), see text page 367. A bluish tinge around the umbilicus may indicate intra-abdominal bleeding.

9. Donald Becker, age 63, is admitted to the hospital with hepatic cirrhosis. As part of the physical assessment, the nurse auscultates Mr. Becker's abdomen. Which sound suggests increased collateral circulation between the portal and systemic venous systems?
(a) Bruit
(b) Borborygmi
(c) Venous hum
(d) Friction rub
Correct answer: (c), see text page 368. A venous hum (continuous, medium-pitched tone created by blood flow in a large, engorged, vascular organ) suggests increased collateral circulation between the portal and systemic venous systems, as in hepatic cirrhosis.

10. When percussing Mr. Becker's liver, the nurse should expect to elicit which sound?
(a) Resonance
(b) Hyperresonance
(c) Dullness
(d) Tympany
Correct answer: (c), see text page 368. Percussion normally elicits dull sounds over the liver and spleen, a lower intestine filled with feces, and a bladder filled with urine.

11. During percussion along the right midclavicular line, the liver normally spans from the costal margin to which area?
(a) The 3rd to 5th intercostal space
(b) The 5th to 7th intercostal space
(c) The 7th to 9th intercostal space
(d) The 9th to 11th intercostal space
Correct answer: (b), see text page 375. Liver percussion along the right midclavicular line normally produces dullness from the costal margin to the 5th to 7th intercostal space.

12. The nurse may perform which other test to locate the inferior border of the liver?
(a) Fluid wave test
(b) Rebound test
(c) Obturator test
(d) Scratch test
Correct answer: (d), see text page 374. If locating the inferior border of the liver through percussion is difficult, the nurse may try the scratch test.

13. The nurse attempts to palpate Mr. Becker's liver. When is the liver in the best position for palpation?
(a) During deep inhalation
(b) During exhalation
(c) While the breath is held
(d) During quiet respiration
Correct answer: (a), see text page 375. The nurse should press gently in and up as the client inhales deeply. This maneuver may bring the liver edge down to a palpable position.

14. Bob and Stacy Harris bring their son Joey, age 8, to the emergency department for care. Joey has right lower quadrant pain, which suggests appendicitis. Where else may appendicitis pain occur?
(a) In the left lower quadrant
(b) In the right upper quadrant
(c) In the left upper quadrant
(d) Around the umbilicus
Correct answer: (d), see text page 377. A young child may experience the pain of appendicitis as diffuse or centered around the umbilicus, although it may localize later.

15. How could the nurse position Joey to elicit pain in the right lower quadrant?
(a) Supine with the knees flexed
(b) Side-lying with the knees pulled in to the chest
(c) Supine with the head raised against resistance
(d) Prone with the legs lifted slightly
Correct answer: (c), see text page 377. To elicit pain in the right lower quadrant, the supine child should try to raise the head while the nurse pushes back against the child's forehead.

16. The nurse may assess for which other signs to help detect appendicitis?
(a) Fluid wave
(b) Obturator sign
(c) Liver hooking
(d) Hepatojugular reflex
Correct answer: (b), see text page 376. A positive obturator sign (pain elicited in the hypogastric region) indicates obturator muscle irritation, which suggests appendicitis.

17. The nurse also attempts to elicit rebound tenderness. Which of the following indicates positive rebound tenderness?
(a) Pain during light palpation over the affected area
(b) Pain during deep palpation over the affected area
(c) Pain upon gradual withdrawal of fingers after light palpation
(d) Pain upon sudden withdrawal of fingers after deep palpation
Correct answer: (d), see text pages 370 and 376. Deep palpation may elicit rebound tenderness when the nurse suddenly withdraws the fingertips, a possible sign of peritoneal inflammation.

18. Mary Lane, age 72, is admitted to the hospital with a GI disorder. Which disorder would contraindicate abdominal palpation?
(a) Aortic aneurysm
(b) Bowel obstruction
(c) Cirrhosis
(d) Umbilical hernia
Correct answer: (a), see text pages 368 and 370. Abdominal palpation is contraindicated in a client with suspected aortic aneurysm because it may cause a rupture.

19. Which age-related change in Ms. Lane should make abdominal palpation easier and more accurate than in a younger client?
(a) Abdominal wall thickening
(b) Abdominal guarding
(c) Relaxed abdominal muscle tone
(d) Increased connective tissue
Correct answer: (c), see text page 374. Because the abdominal wall usually thins and abdominal muscle tone becomes more relaxed with aging, abdominal palpation may be easier and the results more accurate in an elderly client.

20. Ms. Lane also receives a rectal examination. Routine rectal examinations usually are performed only for clients in which age group?
(a) Under age 20
(b) Age 20 to 29
(c) Age 30 to 39
(d) Over age 40
Correct answer: (d), see text page 374. Usually, a routine rectal examination is performed only for a client over age 40. It also may be performed for any client with certain GI problems.

21. Melanie Stern, age 1 week, has projectile vomiting. Her physician suspects pyloric stenosis. The nurse should exclude which part of the GI assessment in this pediatric client?
(a) Abdominal palpation
(b) Rectal examination
(c) Vascular sound auscultation
(d) Liver palpation
Correct answer: (b), see text page 370. The nurse should not perform a rectal examination on a child, unless a specific sign or symptom, such as constipation, encopresis, or bleeding, is present.

22. Which physical finding suggests pyloric stenosis?
(a) Left-to-right peristaltic waves
(b) Abdominal distention
(c) Abdominal concavity
(d) Superficial abdominal veins
Correct answer: (a), see text page 370. Reverse (left-to-right) peristaltic waves may suggest pyloric stenosis, bowel malrotation, duodenal ulcer, or duodenal stenosis.

Test bank for Chapter 13, Gastrointestinal System

1. Frank Jacobs, age 41, seeks care because he has abdominal pain, fever, hematemesis, and melena. Which of these signs and symptoms is one of the most frequent GI problems?
(a) Pain
(b) Nausea
(c) Hematemesis
(d) Melena

2. During the health history, the nurse reviews Mr. Jacobs's medication use. Which drug could cause GI bleeding?
(a) Methyldopa
(b) Digoxin
(c) Aspirin
(d) Codeine

3. After obtaining health history data, the nurse should perform the physical assessment steps in which sequence?
(a) Inspection, palpation, percussion, and auscultation
(b) Inspection, percussion, palpation, and auscultation
(c) Auscultation, inspection, palpation, and percussion
(d) Inspection, auscultation, percussion, and palpation

4. While inspecting Mr. Jacobs's abdomen, the nurse may see aortic pulsations in which area?
(a) Epigastric
(b) Right inguinal
(c) Hypogastric
(d) Left lumbar

5. To detect an umbilical or incisional hernia, the nurse should have Mr. Jacobs perform which maneuver?
(a) Flex the knees while remaining supine
(b) Raise the head and shoulders while remaining supine
(c) Raise the legs while remaining supine
(d) Assume Sims' position for 10 seconds

6. The nurse auscultates Mr. Jacobs's bowel sounds. What is the normal frequency of bowel sounds?
(a) Every 5 to 15 seconds
(b) Every 15 to 30 seconds
(c) Every 30 to 60 seconds
(d) Every 5 to 7 minutes

7. Janet Dixon, age 48, is admitted to the hospital with right upper quadrant and right infrascapular pain caused by cholecystitis. This is an example of which type of pain?
(a) Referred pain
(b) Rebound pain
(c) Phantom pain
(d) Organ pain

8. Eddie Hobart, age 25, is rushed to the emergency department with blunt abdominal trauma caused by an automobile accident. The nurse performs a rapid physical assessment. Which finding suggests intra-abdominal bleeding?
(a) Borborygmi
(b) Everted umbilicus
(c) Visible peristaltic waves
(d) Bluish tint around the umbilicus

9. Donald Becker, age 63, is admitted to the hospital with hepatic cirrhosis. As part of the physical assessment, the nurse auscultates Mr. Becker's abdomen. Which sound suggests increased collateral circulation between the portal and systemic venous systems?
(a) Bruit
(b) Borborygmi
(c) Venous hum
(d) Friction rub

10. When percussing Mr. Becker's liver, the nurse should expect to elicit which sound?
(a) Resonance
(b) Hyperresonance
(c) Dullness
(d) Tympany

11. During percussion along the right midclavicular line, the liver normally spans from the costal margin to which area?
(a) The 3rd to 5th intercostal space
(b) The 5th to 7th intercostal space
(c) The 7th to 9th intercostal space
(d) The 9th to 11th intercostal space

12. The nurse may perform which other test to locate the inferior border of the liver?
(a) Fluid wave test
(b) Rebound test
(c) Obturator test
(d) Scratch test

13. The nurse attempts to palpate Mr. Becker's liver. When is the liver in the best position for palpation?
(a) During deep inhalation
(b) During exhalation
(c) While the breath is held
(d) During quiet respiration

14. Bob and Stacy Harris bring their son Joey, age 8, to the emergency department for care. Joey has right lower quadrant pain, which suggests appendicitis. Where else may appendicitis pain occur?
(a) In the left lower quadrant
(b) In the right upper quadrant
(c) In the left upper quadrant
(d) Around the umbilicus

15. How could the nurse position Joey to elicit pain in the right lower quadrant?
(a) Supine with the knees flexed
(b) Side-lying with the knees pulled in to the chest
(c) Supine with the head raised against resistance
(d) Prone with the legs lifted slightly

16. The nurse may assess for which other signs to help detect appendicitis?
(a) Fluid wave
(b) Obturator sign
(c) Liver hooking
(d) Hepatojugular reflex

17. The nurse also attempts to elicit rebound tenderness. Which of the following indicates positive rebound tenderness?
(a) Pain during light palpation over the affected area
(b) Pain during deep palpation over the affected area
(c) Pain upon gradual withdrawal of fingers after light palpation
(d) Pain upon sudden withdrawal of fingers after deep palpation

18. Mary Lane, age 72, is admitted to the hospital with a GI disorder. Which disorder would contraindicate abdominal palpation?
(a) Aortic aneurysm
(b) Bowel obstruction
(c) Cirrhosis
(d) Umbilical hernia

19. Which age-related change in Ms. Lane should make abdominal palpation easier and more accurate than in a younger client?
(a) Abdominal wall thickening
(b) Abdominal guarding
(c) Relaxed abdominal muscle tone
(d) Increased connective tissue

20. Ms. Lane also receives a rectal examination. Routine rectal examinations usually are performed only for clients in which age group?
(a) Under age 20
(b) Age 20 to 29
(c) Age 30 to 39
(d) Over age 40

21. Melanie Stern, age 1 week, has projectile vomiting. Her physician suspects pyloric stenosis. The nurse should exclude which part of the GI assessment in this pediatric client?
(a) Abdominal palpation
(b) Rectal examination
(c) Vascular sound auscultation
(d) Liver palpation

22. Which physical finding suggests pyloric stenosis?
(a) Left-to-right peristaltic waves
(b) Abdominal distention
(c) Abdominal concavity
(d) Superficial abdominal veins

14

Urinary System

Overview

Certain urinary complaints, such as hematuria and urinary frequency, immediately indicate the need for a urinary system assessment. Other findings, such as abdominal pain and edema, also may warrant such an assessment even though their connection to the urinary system may seem less obvious. In either case, Chapter 14 prepares the student to assess the urinary system. After providing a brief review of the anatomy and physiology of the urinary system, the chapter explains how to gather health history data, physical assessment findings, and laboratory results. Here are the chapter highlights:

• Urinary system structures include the kidneys, ureters, bladder, and urethra.

• The nephron—the basic functional unit of the kidney—regulates fluid and electrolyte balance via glomerular filtration, tubular reabsorption, and tubular secretion. It also rids the body of waste products by excreting urine.

• Important urine characteristics include pH (which normally ranges from 4.5 to 8.0); specific gravity (which normally ranges from 1.008 to 1.030); and urine volume (which normally ranges from 720 to 2,400 ml per 24 hours).

• When obtaining the health history, the nurse should establish a comfortable interview environment and use terms familiar to the client. Because urinary complaints may result from or cause problems in other body systems, the nurse should maintain a holistic approach by investigating complaints associated with related body structures.

• When obtaining the health history, the nurse also should explore the client's medication use. Such information may reveal whether the client is receiving treatment for a urinary dysfunction or suggest that an adverse drug reaction may have caused the dysfunction.

• Physical assessment should begin with measurement of weight and vital signs.

• During inspection, the nurse should examine the abdomen to detect any asymmetrical areas, hernias, veins, lesions, discolorations, bruises, scars, or signs of fluid retention, such as umbilical protrusion. The nurse also should inspect the client's urethral meatus for position, irritation, and discharge. Because signs of urinary dysfunction may appear in other body systems, the nurse also should inspect related body structures, such as the eyes, skin, hair, and nails.

• Physical assessment should include auscultation of renal arteries in the upper abdominal quadrants, with particular attention to any systolic bruits.

• Percussion over the costovertebral angle may reveal kidney pain or tenderness; percussion over the bladder helps determine bladder size and fullness.

• The nurse should try to palpate the client's kidneys and bladder, even though these organs usually cannot be palpated. When palpable, they normally feel smooth and firm with no lumps, masses, or tenderness.

• To complete the urinary system assessment, the nurse should review the results of any laboratory studies ordered to assess renal function.

• Finally, the nurse should document all assessment findings and use them in the nursing process to plan, implement, and evaluate the client's care.

• For more information about urinary system assessment, see pages 67PG through 70PG of the Photo Gallery in the text.

Suggested lecture topics

- Review the anatomical structures of the urinary system, using overhead transparencies or other audiovisual aids. (For a visual aid, see page 67PG in the text.)
- Discuss and diagram the role of the nephron in maintaining homeostasis.
- Using a chart, compare normal and abnormal laboratory findings related to renal function.
- Discuss health history questions important to urinary system assessment, explaining the rationales for asking them.
- Demonstrate how to inspect, auscultate, palpate, and percuss the urinary system. (For visual aids, see pages 68PG through 70PG in the text.)

Suggested critical thinking activities

- Pair the students by sex, and have them perform a urinary assessment, including history and physical assessment, on each other.
- Have the students document their assessment findings on the Skills Laboratory Assessment Guide.
- Have the class critique these assessment findings.
- Using a case study of a client with a urinary complaint, have the students develop a nursing care plan.

Student study questions and answers

The following study questions are taken from text page 412 of Chapter 14, Urinary System. Their answers are based on information in that chapter.

1. The nephron is the functional unit of the kidney. What are the structural components of the nephron and its three main activities?

Answer
The nephron consists of a glomerulus (inside Bowman's capsule), distal and proximal convoluted tubules, loop of Henle, and a collecting tubule. It performs three main functions: mechanical filtration of fluids, wastes, electrolytes, acids, and bases into the tubular system; reabsorption of selected molecules; and secretion of selected molecules.

2. Emily Augello, age 75, comes to the outpatient clinic complaining of pain and burning on urination, a fever of 100° F, and pain in the right kidney area. How would you document the following information related to your nursing assessment of Mrs. Augello?
- history (subjective) assessment data
- physical (objective) assessment data
- assessment techniques and special equipment used
- two appropriate nursing diagnoses
- documentation of your findings.

Skills laboratory guide: Health history

To collect information about the client's urinary system, ask questions about health and illness patterns, health promotion and protection patterns, and role and relationship patterns. Sample questions from each category are listed below.

HEALTH AND ILLNESS PATTERNS

- Do you ever have trouble starting or maintaining a urine stream?
- Do you ever experience urinary urgency—the feeling that you must urinate immediately? If so, do you ever experience this without urinating?
- Does your bladder feel full after you urinate?
- Do you ever feel a burning sensation when you urinate? If so, how often?
- Do you ever have pain when you urinate? If so, how often?
- What color is your urine? Does it appear dark yellow and opaque? Does it ever look red, brown, or black?

HEALTH PROMOTION AND PROTECTION PATTERNS

- Do you follow a special diet?
- Does the need to urinate awaken you at night? If so, how often? Does this happen only when you drink large amounts of liquid in the evening?
- How many times do you urinate daily? Have you noticed any change in frequency?
- Have you noticed any increase or decrease in the amount of urine you void each time?

ROLE AND RELATIONSHIP PATTERNS

- Can you carry out toileting independently?
- If you have urinary frequency or nocturia, does it affect any family members?
- Have you noticed any local tenderness when you cleanse yourself after voiding? Do you ever have pain during sexual intercourse?

Answer
History (subjective) assessment data
- Complaining of pain and burning on urination
- Complaining of pain in the right kidney area
Physical (objective) assessment data
- Female, age 75
- Fever of 100° F
Assessment techniques and equipment
- Interview client regarding past health history, current medications, and genital hygiene practices.
- Examine the urine.
- Inspect the urethral meatus.
- Palpate the kidneys and bladder.
- Percuss the kidneys and bladder.
- Auscultate the upper right and left quadrants.
Two appropriate nursing diagnoses
- Pain related to infection and inflammation
- Altered urinary elimination related to renal manifestations

Skills laboratory guide: Physical assessment

This chart guides the student during assessment by identifying body areas, special considerations and techniques to be used, and normal findings.

BODY AREA	SPECIAL CONSIDERATIONS	NORMAL FINDINGS
Inspection		
Head and neck	• Note orientation, level of consciousness, and neck vein distention. In infants and children, note position of ears; ears set at an unusual angle may indicate congenital kidney anomalies.	• Alert and oriented • No neck vein distention
Eyes	• Note thickened retinal vessels, blurred disk margins, and retinal hemorrhages.	• No retinal hemorrhage or infarction • No retinal nicking
Skin, hair, and nails	• Note skin color, ecchymosis, uremic frost, inflammation, turgor, mucous membrane dryness, pruritus, and edema.	• No ecchymosis, uremic frost, or inflammation • Normal skin turgor; moist lips, no cracks • No total body edema or pitting edema
Total body position	• Note body positioning, inability to lie flat, constant change of position.	• Able to lie flat in bed
Abdomen	• Note symmetry, skin lesions or discoloration, scars, distention, umbilical protrusion, striae. • Normally, an infant's abdomen is more rounded than an older child's or an adult's.	• Abdomen smooth, flat, and symmetrical • No hernias or prominent veins
Urethral meatus	• Note location, discharge, swelling, and ulceration.	• Male: centrally located at the end of the glans penis; no discharge • Female: located midline; no swelling or discharge
Auscultation		
Upper abdomen, in costovertebral areas	• Use bell of stethoscope lightly pressed against the upper right and upper left quadrants, beginning at the midline and moving laterally.	• No bruits
Percussion		
Kidneys	• For indirect percussion, place left palm over costovertebral angle and strike with right fist. • For direct percussion, strike the fist directly over the costovertebral angle.	• No flank pain • Client reports thudding sensation or pressure • No costovertebral tenderness
Bladder	• Perform mediate percussion 2″ (5 cm) above the symphysis pubis. Note dullness or tympany.	• Tympany in empty bladder, dullness in full bladder
Palpation		
Kidneys	• Use bimanual technique, with the left hand midway between the lower costal margin and the iliac crest and the right hand on the abdomen above the left hand. • Note shape, size, consistency, masses, and tenderness. • Kidneys normally are more easily palpable in elderly clients.	• Smooth, solid, elastic kidneys • No tenderness; equal in size • Left kidney higher than right • Right kidney easier to palpate than left
Bladder	• Have client void before palpating. Palpate 2″ above the symphysis pubis.	• In adults, the bladder is seldom palpable • Firm and smooth; no tenderness

Documentation of findings
- S—Client complains of pain and burning on urination along with pain in the right kidney area.
- O—T 100° F, P 90, R 22, B/P 130/80. Abdominal and suprapubic tenderness elicited on palpation. Urine appears cloudy and foul-smelling. Urethral meatus appears erythematous but with no discharge.
- A—Pain related to infection and inflammation

3. When Mrs. Augello leaves the outpatient clinic with a diagnosis of urinary tract infection, what instructions should you give her?

Answer
- Return for the scheduled follow-up visit.
- Continue taking the prescribed medication for the entire scheduled period.
- Wash the perineal area daily with an antibacterial soap to decrease the risk of infection.
- Avoid tub baths, especially bubble baths. Still water (as in tub baths) is a favorable bacterial medium; bubble baths cause urethral irritation.
- Clean the perineal area from front to back after bowel elimination to prevent bacterial transfer.
- Wear cotton underpants or underpants with a cotton crotch. Bacteria multiply best in a dark, moist environment; cotton underpants allow moisture to evaporate.
- Maintain good bladder habits, such as not holding urine. Urinate when the urge occurs—do not put it off. (Urinary stasis contributes to infection.)
- Report any discolored or cloudy urine.

4. A client complains of nausea and sudden onset of severe abdominal and left-sided pain. The client states, "This pain is awful. My father always said the worst pain he suffered was when he passed a kidney stone." In your nursing assessment of this client, which critical areas should you focus on?

Answer
- Past medical history—The previous medical records indicate that this client was hospitalized 1 year ago for renal calculi. At that time, the client passed one renal stone which was analyzed as calcium phosphate.
- Vital signs—Elevated BP, pulse, and respiration. Possible fever.
- Light abdominal palpation—Tenderness over left flank.
- Laboratory studies—Urinalysis: pH normal. Increased RBCs.

5. During your initial interview, a new client informs you that he has been taking furosemide (Lasix) for the past several months. Knowing this, what specific areas of the nursing assessment should you consider critical? What are the actions and possible adverse effects of furosemide?

Answer
- Medical history—Ask why furosemide therapy was started and what effects the client has noted.
- Vital signs, particularly the regularity of heart rate.
- General appearance, particularly noting edema or muscle weakness.
- Laboratory studies—Urinalysis: specific gravity, color, and clarity. Electrolytes: sodium, potassium, chloride. Osmolality.
- Furosemide is a potent loop diuretic that acts on the ascending loop of Henle, blocking sodium reabsorption and stimulating potassium and chloride excretion. Possible adverse effects include electrolyte imbalance, uricosuria, dehydration, and allergic interstitial nephritis.

Questions, answers, and rationales

1. Mary Barton, age 25, comes to the clinic for treatment of a recurrent urinary tract infection (UTI). Which sign or symptom suggests UTI?
(a) Burning on urination
(b) Urinary hesitancy
(c) Proteinuria
(d) Greenish-brown urine
Correct answer: (a), see text pages 392 and 404. Classic signs and symptoms of UTIs include urinary frequency and urgency, burning sensation and pain on urination, nocturia, and hematuria.

2. Joan Edwards, age 55, is being treated for obstructive jaundice. This disorder may cause her urine to turn which color?
(a) Blue-green
(b) Dark yellow
(c) Orange-red
(d) Pale straw
Correct answer: (c), see text page 392. Obstructive jaundice may cause the urine to become tea-colored (orange-red to orange-brown).

3. Matthew Blackburn, age 45, is admitted to the hospital with nephrolithiasis (renal calculi). Based on this admitting diagnosis, the nurse may expect him to report pain in which area?
(a) Upper quadrants
(b) Lower quadrants
(c) Shoulder
(d) Flank
Correct answer: (d), see text page 404. Nephrolithiasis typically causes severe radiating pain from the costovertebral angle to the flank, suprapubic region, and external genitalia.

4. To assess Mr. Blackburn for renal tenderness, the nurse performs blunt percussion over which area?
(a) Costovertebral angle
(b) Suprapubic area
(c) Either side of the umbilicus
(d) Symphysis pubis
Correct answer: (a), see text page 402. Blunt percussion over the costovertebral angle may elicit tenderness and pain, suggesting a renal disorder.

5. To palpate his kidneys, the nurse should use which technique?
(a) Lightly palpate the upper abdominal quadrants.
(b) Deeply palpate above the symphysis pubis.
(c) Bimanually palpate between the lower costal margin and the iliac crest to either side of the umbilicus.
(d) Lightly palpate at the costovertebral angle.
Correct answer: (c), see text page 403. For kidney palpation, the nurse uses bimanual palpation, placing the left hand under the lower back between the iliac crest and costal margin and the right hand on the abdomen directly above the left hand.

6. When are the kidneys most likely to be palpable?
(a) During normal respiration
(b) During deep inhalation
(c) During deep exhalation
(d) During shallow respiration
Correct answer: (b), see text page 403. Although the kidneys are difficult to palpate, they descend during deep inhalation, which facilitates palpation.

7. Sally Griffith, age 63, is receiving the aminoglycoside gentamicin as a part of treatment for pneumonia. This drug may cause which adverse urinary reaction?
(a) Renal calculi
(b) Nocturia
(c) Nephrotoxicity
(d) Glycosuria
Correct answer: (c), see text page 394. Aminoglycosides such as gentamicin may cause nephrotoxicity and acute tubular necrosis.

8. The physician is most likely to order which laboratory study to monitor Ms. Griffith's renal function?
(a) Albumin
(b) Creatinine
(c) Electrolytes
(d) Total protein
Correct answer: (b), see text page 406. Because renal impairment usually is the only cause of creatinine elevation, a creatinine test provides a sensitive measure of renal damage.

9. Kathleen O'Brien, age 35, is in her second trimester of pregnancy with her third child. During pregnancy, she is at greatest risk for developing which urinary disorder?
(a) UTI
(b) Renal calculi
(c) Glomerulonephritis
(d) Tubular necrosis
Correct answer: (a), see text page 396. UTI is the most common urinary problem during pregnancy.

10. What normal urinary changes may Ms. O'Brien experience during her pregnancy?
(a) Increased urine volume and frequency
(b) Mild-to-moderate proteinuria
(c) Mild-to-moderate glycosuria
(d) Increased urine specific gravity
Correct answer: (a), see text page 396. Pregnancy normally increases urine volume and frequency and decreases urine specific gravity.

11. Multiple births may cause which urinary problem?
(a) Stress incontinence
(b) Urine retention
(c) Urinary hesitancy
(d) Bladder distention
Correct answer: (a), see text pages 386 and 392. Stress incontinence suggests bladder dysfunction, which may occur in women who have had multiple births.

12. After giving birth to a healthy baby boy, Ms. O'Brien has difficulty voiding so the nurse assesses her for bladder distention. What percussion sound occurs over a distended bladder?
(a) Resonance
(b) Tympany
(c) Dullness
(d) Hyperresonance
Correct answer: (c), see text page 402. Bladder percussion normally produces a tympanic sound. Over a urine-filled bladder, it produces a dull sound.

13. The nurse also palpates Ms. O'Brien's bladder. Which finding is normal in an adult?
(a) The bladder is not palpable.
(b) The bladder is palpable 2″ to 5″ above the symphysis pubis.
(c) The bladder feels soft and smooth.
(d) The bladder feels hard and rough.
Correct answer: (a), see text page 403. An adult's bladder may not be palpable. If palpable, it normally feels firm and relatively smooth and lies 1″ to 2″ above the symphysis pubis.

14. The nurse palpates the bladder of Ms. O'Brien's son. Which finding is normal?
(a) The bladder is not palable.
(b) The bladder is palpable below the symphysis pubs.
(c) The bladder is palpable at the umbilicus.
(d) The bladder is palpable above the umbilicus.
Correct answer: (c), see text page 405. The bladder of a child under age 2 usually can be palpated and percussed to the umbilical level.

15. Alfred Kreiger, age 77, is scheduled for transurethral resection of the prostate to correct benign prostatic hypertrophy. Which urinary sign or symptom is associated with an enlarged prostate gland?
(a) Urinary hesitancy
(b) Polyuria
(c) Urethral discharge
(d) Flank pain
Correct answer: (a), see text page 391. Urinary hesitancy, or difficulty starting a urine stream, may result from a urethral stricture, such as from an enlarged prostate gland.

16. The nurse reviews Mr. Kreiger's medical history before surgery. Which medical problem may affect the urinary system?
(a) Hypothyroidism
(b) Chronic bronchitis
(c) Diabetes mellitus
(d) Coronary artery disease
Correct answer: (c), see text page 393. Diabetes mellitus can increase the risk of UTI and can lead to nephropathy.

17. When assessing Mr. Krieger, the nurse is likely to note which age-related finding?
(a) Easy-to-palpate kidneys
(b) Renal bruits
(c) Costovertebral angle tenderness
(d) Nonpalpable bladder
Correct answer: (a), see text page 405. In an elderly client, the kidneys are easier to palpate because of reduced abdominal muscle tone and mass.

18. The nurse is assessing George Somers, age 51, who has end-stage renal disease. In Mr. Somers, decreased erythropoietin production is likely to cause which skin color change?
(a) Cyanosis
(b) Erythema
(c) Bronze coloring
(d) Pallor
Correct answer: (d), see text page 399. End-stage renal failure reduces erythropoietin production, which decreases red blood cell production and causes pallor.

19. Because of his condition, Mr. Somers is confined to bed rest. During assessment, the nurse is most likely to find local, dependent edema in which area?
(a) Hands
(b) Ankles
(c) Sacrum
(d) Feet
Correct answer: (c), see text page 400. The nurse inspects for local edema on the lowest (dependent) body parts, such as the ankles, scrotum, and sacrum. In a client on bed rest, edema most likely occurs on the sacrum and scrotum.

20. The nurse also auscultates Mr. Somers's renal arteries. Auscultation of these arteries may reveal which sound?
(a) Venous hum
(b) Bruit
(c) Murmur
(d) Thrill
Correct answer: (b), see text page 401. Normally, auscultation of the renal arteries reveals no sounds. Abnormal findings include systolic bruits (whooshing sounds).

Test bank for Chapter 14, Urinary System

1. Mary Barton, age 25, comes to the clinic for treatment of a recurrent urinary tract infection (UTI). Which sign or symptom suggests UTI?
(a) Burning on urination
(b) Urinary hesitancy
(c) Proteinuria
(d) Greenish-brown urine

2. Joan Edwards, age 55, is being treated for obstructive jaundice. This disorder may cause her urine to turn which color?
(a) Blue-green
(b) Dark yellow
(c) Orange-red
(d) Pale straw

3. Matthew Blackburn, age 45, is admitted to the hospital with nephrolithiasis (renal calculi). Based on this admitting diagnosis, the nurse may expect him to report pain in which area?
(a) Upper quadrants
(b) Lower quadrants
(c) Shoulder
(d) Flank

4. To assess Mr. Blackburn for renal tenderness, the nurse performs blunt percussion over which area?
(a) Costovertebral angle
(b) Suprapubic area
(c) Either side of the umbilicus
(d) Symphysis pubis

5. To palpate his kidneys, the nurse should use which technique?
(a) Lightly palpate the upper abdominal quadrants.
(b) Deeply palpate above the symphysis pubis.
(c) Bimanually palpate between the lower costal margin and the iliac crest to either side of the umbilicus.
(d) Lightly palpate at the costovertebral angle.

6. When are the kidneys most likely to be palpable?
(a) During normal respiration
(b) During deep inhalation
(c) During deep exhalation
(d) During shallow respiration

7. Sally Griffith, age 63, is receiving the aminoglycoside gentamicin as a part of treatment for pneumonia. This drug may cause which adverse urinary reaction?
(a) Renal calculi
(b) Nocturia
(c) Nephrotoxicity
(d) Glycosuria

8. The physician is most likely to order which laboratory study to monitor Ms. Griffith's renal function?
(a) Albumin
(b) Creatinine
(c) Electrolytes
(d) Total protein

9. Kathleen O'Brien, age 35, is in her second trimester of pregnancy with her third child. During pregnancy, she is at greatest risk for developing which urinary disorder?
(a) UTI
(b) Renal calculi
(c) Glomerulonephritis
(d) Tubular necrosis

10. What normal urinary changes may Ms. O'Brien experience during her pregnancy?
(a) Increased urine volume and frequency
(b) Mild-to-moderate proteinuria
(c) Mild-to-moderate glycosuria
(d) Increased urine specific gravity

11. Multiple births may cause which urinary problem?
(a) Stress incontinence
(b) Urine retention
(c) Urinary hesitancy
(d) Bladder distention

12. After giving birth to a healthy baby boy, Ms. O'Brien has difficulty voiding so the nurse assesses her for bladder distention. What percussion sound occurs over a distended bladder?
(a) Resonance
(b) Tympany
(c) Dullness
(d) Hyperresonance

13. The nurse also palpates Ms. O'Brien's bladder. Which finding is normal in an adult?
(a) The bladder is not palpable.
(b) The bladder is palpable 2" to 5" above the symphysis pubis.
(c) The bladder feels soft and smooth.
(d) The bladder feels hard and rough.

14. The nurse palpates the bladder of Ms. O'Brien's son. Which finding is normal?
(a) The bladder is not palpable.
(b) The bladder is palpable below the symphysis pubis.
(c) The bladder is palpable at the umbilicus.
(d) The bladder is palpable above the umbilicus.

15. Alfred Kreiger, age 77, is scheduled for transurethral resection of the prostate to correct benign prostatic hypertrophy. Which urinary sign or symptom is associated with an enlarged prostate gland?
(a) Urinary hesitancy
(b) Polyuria
(c) Urethral discharge
(d) Flank pain

16. The nurse reviews Mr. Kreiger's medical history before surgery. Which medical problem may affect the urinary system?
(a) Hypothyroidism
(b) Chronic bronchitis
(c) Diabetes mellitus
(d) Coronary artery disease

17. When assessing Mr. Krieger, the nurse is likely to note which age-related finding?
(a) Easy-to-palpate kidneys
(b) Renal bruits
(c) Costovertebral angle tenderness
(d) Nonpalpable bladder

18. The nurse is assessing George Somers, age 51, who has end-stage renal disease. In Mr. Somers, decreased erythropoietin production is likely to cause which skin color change?
(a) Cyanosis
(b) Erythema
(c) Bronze coloring
(d) Pallor

19. Because of his condition, Mr. Somers is confined to bed rest. During assessment, the nurse is most likely to find local, dependent edema in which area?
(a) Hands
(b) Ankles
(c) Sacrum
(d) Feet

20. The nurse also auscultates Mr. Somers's renal arteries. Auscultation of these arteries may reveal which sound?
(a) Venous hum
(b) Bruit
(c) Murmur
(d) Thrill

15

Female Reproductive System

Overview

Female reproductive health concerns vary across the life span and range from menarchal problems and contraception to pregnancy and menopausal concerns. Chapter 15 prepares the nurse to assist clients with such concerns. It begins with a brief review of the female reproductive anatomy and physiology as well as developmental and maturational changes. Then it describes how to perform a complete assessment of the female reproductive system and how to integrate health history, physical assessment, and laboratory test data into nursing care. Here are the chapter highlights:

- The female reproductive system includes the external genitalia (labia minora, labia majora, and clitoris), adjacent structures (Bartholin's glands, Skene's glands, and the urethral meatus), and the internal genitalia (vagina, uterus, fallopian tubes, ovaries, and supporting structures).
- The female reproductive cycle functions via a complex network of hormonal substances produced by the hypothalamus, the pituitary, and the ovaries. The positive and negative feedback responses from these structures influence the menstrual cycle and ovulation. Decline of ovarian hormones eventually results in cessation of reproductive function at menopause.
- Depending on the reason for the assessment, health history questions should cover the areas of menstruation, procreation, contraception, sexually transmitted diseases (STDs), other reproductive system disorders, sexuality, and developmental concerns.
- Questions for females of specific age groups, such as the premenarchal girl and the elderly woman, should be focused to obtain accurate data in a sensitive manner.

- When obtaining the health history, the nurse should explore the client's use of medications, including oral contraceptives. Such information may reveal whether the client is receiving estrogen therapy for reproductive system dysfunction or whether an adverse drug reaction may have caused a dysfunction.
- A pelvic assessment requires careful psychological and physical preparation. Relaxation techniques may help the client during the gynecologic assessment. The nurse should prepare all assessment and diagnostic equipment before approaching the client.
- During the assessment, the nurse inspects the external genital structures and, using a vaginal speculum, the vagina and cervix. The nurse then palpates all external and internal structures, including the rectovaginal area.
- To complete the assessment, the nurse reviews the results of any laboratory tests (cultures or smears). The specimens most commonly obtained for laboratory study include cervical tissue for the Papanicolaou (Pap) test; exudate samples for culture and identification of *Neisseria gonorrhoeae, Chlamydia trachomatis,* and other sexually transmitted microorganisms; and wet mounts.
- Finally, the nurse documents all assessment findings and uses them in the nursing process to plan, implement, and evaluate the client's care.
- For more information about female reproductive system assessment, see pages 71PG through 72PG of the Photo Gallery in the text.

Suggested lecture topics

• Using audiovisual aids, review the anatomy and physiology of the female reproductive system, explaining normal variations that occur with age and pregnancy. (For a visual aid, see page 71PG in the text.)
• Discuss health history questions important to female reproductive system assessment, explaining the rationales for asking them.
• Using a pelvic examination simulator, demonstrate how to perform a complete physical assessment, including the use of the speculum and bimanual palpation.
• Discuss normal and common abnormal findings of a female reproductive system assessment, explaining the possible implications of abnormal findings. (For a visual aid, see page 72PG in the text.)

Suggested critical thinking activities

• Have the students prepare client-teaching aids that explain menstruation to preadolescent clients.
• Have the students prepare client-teaching aids that explain contraceptive methods to adolescent clients.
• Pair the students and have them perform a reproductive history on each other. Upon completion, have them critique each other's documentation of the history.
• Using a pelvic examination simulator, have the students perform a physical assessment of the female reproductive system.
• Using a case study of a woman with a reproductive system problem, have the students develop a nursing care plan.

Student study questions and answers

The following study questions are taken from text page 441 of Chapter 15, Female Reproductive System. Their answers are based on information in that chapter.

1. Maryellen Crowder, age 15, comes to the school clinic for information about contraception. Upon questioning her, you learn that she has little knowledge about the normal menstrual cycle and none about contraception. What basic facts about the menstrual cycle would you teach her?

Answer
The average menstrual cycle usually occurs over 28 days, although a normal cycle may range from 22 to 34 days. The cycle starts with the onset of menstruation on day 1. Menstruation usually lasts about 5 days. From day 6 to day 14, the uterine lining builds up in preparation to receive and nourish a fertilized egg. Around day 14, ovulation occurs when an egg is released from the ovary. Over the next week, the egg travels down the fallopian tube into the uterus. If the egg is not fertilized by a sperm, the uterine lining starts to shed, and the cycle begins again.

Skills laboratory guide: Health history

To collect information about the female client's reproductive system, ask questions about health and illness patterns, health promotion and protection patterns, and role and relationship patterns. Sample questions from each category are listed below.

HEALTH AND ILLNESS PATTERNS

• When was the first day of your last menstrual period? Was that period normal compared with your previous periods?
• How often do your periods occur? How long do they normally last?
• How would you describe your menstrual flow? How many pads or tampons do you use on each day of your period?
• Are you currently sexually active? If so, what contraceptive method do you use, if any?
• Do you have any unusual signs or symptoms of infection, such as discharge, itching, painful intercourse, sores or lesions, fever, chills, or swelling?
• Does your sexual partner have any signs or symptoms of infection, such as genital sores or penile discharge?
• Do you ever bleed between periods? If so, how much and for how long?
• Have you had any uncomfortable signs and symptoms before or during your periods?
• Have you ever had a sexually transmitted disease or other genital or reproductive system infection?
• Have you had surgery for a reproductive system problem?
• Have you ever been pregnant?
• Have you ever had problems conceiving?
• Has anyone in your family ever had reproductive problems?

HEALTH PROMOTION AND PROTECTION PATTERNS

• Do you eat a well-balanced diet?
• Do you have regular health checkups, including gynecologic examinations?
• When was your last Pap test?

ROLE AND RELATIONSHIP PATTERNS

• Have you noticed any changes in your sexual interest, frequency of intercourse, or sexual functioning?
• Are you experiencing any sexual problems?

---

2. Having her first gynecologic assessment today, Maryellen is frightened and anxious. What steps can you take to help her relax during the assessment?

Answer
• Instruct her to empty her bladder before the assessment begins.
• Ensure that the examination room is warm.
• Provide privacy and adequate draping.
• Using pictures and equipment, explain the assessment procedure so the client knows what to expect.
• Reassure her that, although the assessment may be uncomfortable, most women do not find it painful.

Skills laboratory guide: Physical assessment

This chart guides the student during assessment by identifying body areas, special considerations and techniques to be used, and normal findings.

BODY AREA	SPECIAL CONSIDERATIONS	NORMAL FINDINGS
Inspection		
External genitalia	• Have client empty bladder and assume lithotomy or Sims' position. Put on gloves. • Note pubic hair amount and distribution, color and condition of genitalia, clitoral size, and varicosities, lesions, organisms, edema, or discharge.	• Appropriate pubic hair distribution for client's age • Pink, moist external genitalia with no varicosities, lesions, organisms, edema, or abnormal discharge • Small amount of clear (preovulatory) or white (postovulatory) odorless discharge
Palpation		
Skene's glands and Bartholin's glands	• Palpate lightly, noting any discharge.	• No swelling, tenderness, or discharge
Vulva and perineum	• Note any masses or lesions. • Note integrity of the perineum.	• No masses, lesions, or anatomic deviations • Intact, smooth, thick tissue
Advanced assessment skills: Using the speculum		
Cervix	• Note cervical color, position, size, shape, and surface characteristics. Cervix may be pale in a menopausal client; bluish purple in a pregnant client. Note any lesions, nodules, masses, discharge, and bleeding. • Note shape and patency of cervical os. Cervical os is round in a nulliparous client; irregular in a multiparous client.	• Smooth, moist, shiny pink cervix, ¾" to 1¼" (2 to 3 cm) in diameter at the midline • No lesions, nodules, masses, discharge, or bleeding • Patent os
Vaginal walls	• Note color, condition, and presence of rugae. Note lesions, discharge, swelling, or masses.	• Pink, moist, rugose vaginal walls • No lesions, discharge, swelling, or masses
Advanced assessment skills: Bimanual palpation		
Vagina	• Palpate with palmar surfaces of fingers. Note any nodules, tenderness, or other abnormalities.	• Concentric rugae around vaginal wall • No nodules, tenderness, or other abnormalities
Cervix	• Note size, shape, position, consistency, regularity of contour, mobility, and sensitivity. In an older client, the cervix is smaller; in a pregnant client, it enlarges and softens.	• Firm, smooth, mobile, nontender cervix, ¾" to 1¼" in diameter and pointing posteriorly, anteriorly, or midplane • No masses or lesions
Uterus	• Place one hand on the abdomen between the umbilicus and symphysis pubis. Insert the first and second fingers of your other hand into the vagina, and tip the uterus upward. • Note position, size, shape, consistency, tenderness, mobility, and surface regularity.	• Appropriate uterine size for client's age and condition (pregnant or nonpregnant) • Firm, pear-shaped, symmetrical, and slightly mobile uterus that may be anteflexed, anteverted, retroflexed, retroverted, or midplane • No masses; tenderness only during menses
Ovaries and fallopian tubes	• If palpable, note size, shape, consistency, and tenderness. • The ovaries normally are not palpable in a prepubescent or postmenopausal client.	• Oval, smooth, mobile, firm, flattened ovaries about 1¼" x ¾" x ¼" (3 x 2 x 1 cm) in size and sensitive to palpation • Nonpalpable fallopian tubes
Rectovaginal area	• Change your gloves; then insert your index finger into the vagina, and your middle finger into the rectum. Note any hemorrhoids, painful areas, masses, or nodules. • Evaluate the posterior side of the uterus. • Note color of stool or presence of blood after withdrawing your gloved fingers.	• No hemorrhoids, painful areas, masses, or nodules • Firm, slightly mobile uterus

- During the assessment, explain what is occurring, what she can expect to feel, and what will occur next.
- Teach her how to relax by breathing slowly and deeply through the nose, exhaling through the mouth, and concentrating on breathing deeply.

3. How would you explain the actions of estrogen and progesterone during the menstrual cycle to a client?

Answer

The menstrual cycle is regulated by fluctuating levels of estrogen, progesterone, and other hormones. As the cycle begins, low estrogen and progesterone levels in the blood stimulate the hypothalamus (the hormone control center in the brain) to secrete gonadotropin-releasing hormone (GnRH). In turn, GnRH stimulates the pituitary gland (which is associated with the hypothalamus) to secrete follicle-stimulating hormone (FSH) and luteinizing hormone (LH).

During the second week of the cycle, FSH and LH stimulate the ovaries to increase estrogen secretion, which triggers the buildup of the endometrium, the blood-rich lining of the uterus that receives and nourishes a fertilized egg. Around day 14 of the cycle, estrogen levels decline, and the ovaries release an egg.

After the egg is released, estrogen and progesterone levels again increase. Increased progesterone levels stimulate the endometrium to thicken and become secretory in preparation to receive a fertilized egg. If fertilization does not occur, however, estrogen and progesterone levels begin to drop. When levels decrease sufficiently, the endometrium begins to shed, causing menstrual bleeding. Then, the decreased estrogen and progesterone levels stimulate the hypothalamus to secrete GnRH, causing the cycle to begin again.

4. What questions would you ask to obtain information about the female reproductive system of an adolescent and a menopausal client?

Answer

Adolescent client
- At what age did you first notice hair on your pubic area? When did you first notice your breasts growing?
- How do you feel you are developing physically compared with your friends?
- Have you noticed any moistness on your underpants?
- Have you experienced any new feelings or emotions? If so, would you like to talk about them?
- Have you noticed any blood on your underpants?
- When did you begin having menstrual periods?
- How old were you when you first had sex? Have you had pain with sex?

Menopausal client
- Do you experience hot flushes or flashes? If so, how bothersome are they?
- Do you experience vaginal dryness, pain, or itching during sexual intercourse?
- Are you experiencing menstrual irregularities?
- Do you practice contraception?
- Are you having any problems or changes you attribute to menopause? What are they? Could anything else be causing these problems or changes?
- How do you feel about menopause?
- Are you receiving hormone therapy for menopause?
- If you have completed menopause, do you have any vaginal bleeding?

5. Florence Devon, age 35 and married, complains of a white, thick vaginal discharge of 2 weeks' duration. Mrs. Devon reports that the discharge has no foul odor and that she has pain with intercourse and painful vaginal itching most of the time. She has tried a nonprescription cream but has had no relief. Physical assessment reveals erythematous (inflamed) and edematous (swollen) external genitalia, especially the labia. The vagina and cervix are also inflamed, swollen, and tender to the touch. A white, curdlike discharge appears on the internal surfaces. A 10% potassium hydroxide wet smear shows many hyphae and spores, indicative of *Candida albicans*.

How would you document the following information related to your nursing assessment of Mrs. Devon?
- history (subjective) assessment data
- physical (objective) assessment data
- assessment techniques and special equipment
- nursing diagnoses
- documentation.

Answer

History (subjective) assessment data
- Complains of white, thick, odorless vaginal discharge of 2 weeks' duration.
- Complains of pain during intercourse and painful vaginal itching.
- Reports no relief from over-the-counter (OTC) cortisone cream applied externally.

Physical (objective) assessment data
- Female, age 35
- Erythema, edema, and tenderness of external genitalia, vagina, and cervix
- White curdlike discharge on internal surfaces
- Wet smear positive for *Candida albicans* (hyphae and spores)

Assessment techniques and equipment
- Interview client regarding current and past health status, sexual practices, and current medication use.
- Inspect external genitalia.
- Using a vaginal speculum, inspect the vagina and cervix.

• Collect discharge specimen for wet smears (10% potassium hydroxide [KOH] and normal saline), using glass slides, coverslips, a cotton tipped applicator, and 10% KOH and normal saline solutions.

Nursing diagnoses

• Pain related to vaginal itching
• Sexual dysfunction related to painful intercourse

Documentation

• S—Client complains of white, thick, odorless vaginal discharge of 2 weeks' duration, along with pain during intercourse and painful vaginal itching that does not respond to OTC cortisone cream.
• O—Assessment reveals erythema, edema, and tenderness of external genitalia, vagina, and cervix, and a white curdlike discharge on internal genitalia. Wet smear positive for *Candida albicans* (hyphae and spores).
• A—Pain related to vaginal itching.

Questions, answers, and rationales

1. Pat Dwyer, age 25, comes to the clinic for her annual gynecologic examination. During the health history, the nurse learns that Ms. Dwyer uses oral contraceptives. Which factor increases the risk of cardiovascular disease in women using oral contraceptives?
(a) Smoking
(b) Barbiturate use
(c) Phenothiazine use
(d) High-protein diet
Correct answer: (a), see text page 420. Smoking increases the risk of cardiovascular disease and thrombi in women using oral contraceptives.

2. To assess Ms. Dwyer's reproductive system, the nurse should place her in which position?
(a) Supine
(b) Lithotomy
(c) Left lateral
(d) Dorsal recumbent
Correct answer: (b), see text page 427. For most clients, the lithotomy position is best for inspecting and palpating the genitalia.

3. The nurse performs a speculum examination. In a nulliparous client such as Ms. Dwyer, how should the cervical os appear?
(a) Round and open
(b) Round and closed
(c) Irregular and open
(d) Irregular and closed
Correct answer: (b), see text page 418. The cervical os appears round and closed in a nulliparous woman, and as an irregularly shaped slit in a parous woman.

4. Next, the nurse performs bimanual palpation. This technique is used to assess which structures?
(a) Skene's and Bartholin's ducts
(b) Ovaries and fallopian tubes
(c) Labia majora and minora
(d) Perineum and clitoris
Correct answer: (b), see text pages 416 and 433. Bimanual palpation is used to assess the internal genitalia, which include the uterus, ovaries, and fallopian tubes.

5. The nurse palpates Ms. Dwyer's vaginal wall. Which finding is normal?
(a) Smoothness
(b) Rugosity
(c) Nodularity
(d) Tenderness
Correct answer: (b), see text page 433. Rugae, a normal finding, feel like small ridges running concentrically around the vaginal wall.

6. The position of which structure or structures may help the nurse identify the uterine position?
(a) Fallopian tubes
(b) Ovaries
(c) Cervix
(d) Skene's glands
Correct answer: (c), see text page 434. A cervix pointing anteriorly indicates a retroverted uterus; a cervix pointing posteriorly, an anteverted uterus.

7. In a client such as Ms. Dwyer, how should the uterus normally feel during palpation?
(a) Pear-shaped and symmetrical
(b) Round and symmetrical
(c) Oval and asymmetrical
(d) Almond-shaped and asymmetrical
Correct answer: (a), see text page 435. In a nonpregnant client, the uterus normally is pear-shaped and symmetrical.

8. When palpating Ms. Dwyer's ovaries, the nurse should consider which finding normal?
(a) Sensitivity
(b) Round shape
(c) Softness
(d) Immobility
Correct answer: (a), see text page 435. If palpable, the ovaries are almond-shaped, firm, and mobile, and may be sensitive to palpation.

9. The nurse may perform which routine test to screen for cervical cancer?
(a) Enzyme immunoassay
(b) Complete blood count
(c) Papanicolaou (Pap) test
(d) Human chorionic gonadotropin test
Correct answer: (c), see text page 425. A Pap test can detect precancerous and cancerous cell changes in the cervix as well as certain infectious disorders.

10. Carol Berger, age 27, seeks care for a watery vaginal discharge and sores on her external genitalia. These signs suggest which disorder?
(a) Endometriosis
(b) Candidiasis
(c) Trichomonal infection
(d) Genital herpes
Correct answer: (d), see text page 429. Genital herpes causes watery discharge, lesions or sores and blisters on the external genitalia, and mild itching and pain.

11. Brenda White, age 31, schedules an appointment at the clinic because she believes she may be pregnant. In a pregnant client, the cervix is likely to be which color?
(a) Shiny pink
(b) Bright red
(c) Pale
(d) Bluish purple
Correct answer: (d), see text pages 428 and 431. During pregnancy, the cervix has a bluish purple cast (Chadwick's sign).

12. In a pregnant client, how does the cervix normally feel?
(a) Hard and enlarged
(b) Soft and enlarged
(c) Hard and recessed
(d) Soft and recessed
Correct answer: (b), see text page 433. A pregnant client's cervix usually is softened and enlarged.

13. Helen McCloskey, age 75, seeks care for irregular postmenopausal bleeding. Because of her age, she cannot assume the usual position for reproductive system assessment. The nurse should assist her into which alternate position?
(a) Supine
(b) Left lateral
(c) Fowler's
(d) Trendelenburg's
Correct answer: (b), see text page 427. An alternate position for the client who cannot assume the lithotomy position because of age, arthritis, or other reasons is Sims' (left lateral) position.

14. On inspection, Ms. McCloskey's external genitalia may display which normal age-related changes?
(a) Hypertrophy of labia majora
(b) Sparse, thin pubic hair
(c) Thick, coarse pubic hair
(d) Cystocele
Correct answer: (b), see text page 428. In the elderly client, the pubic hair becomes sparse, thin, brittle, gray, and straight.

15. When viewed through a speculum, Ms. McCloskey's cervix is likely to be which normal color?
(a) Pale
(b) Pink
(c) Red
(d) Blue
Correct answer: (a), see text page 431. In a postmenopausal client, the cervix normally may be pale.

16. Which structure normally is not palpable in a client of Ms. McCloskey's age?
(a) Rectum
(b) Uterus
(c) Ovaries
(d) Vagina
Correct answer: (c), see text page 435. The ovaries of a prepubertal girl or postmenopausal woman should not be palpable.

17. On cervical palpation, which finding is considered normal in a client of Ms. McCloskey's age?
(a) The cervix is smaller and recessed.
(b) The cervix is larger and harder.
(c) The cervix displays ectropion.
(d) The cervix displays eversion.
Correct answer: (a), see text page 433. The cervix of an older woman is smaller and usually is recessed.

18. Diagnostic tests confirm that Ms. McCloskey has ovarian cancer. Which assessment finding is associated with ovarian cancer?
(a) History of menstrual disturbances
(b) History of estrogen therapy
(c) History of diabetes
(d) Nulliparity
Correct answer: (d), see text page 429. Related assessment findings include early-stage menopause, postmenopause, and nulliparity.

19. Barbara Brooks, age 30, has been married for 5 years. She visits her physician because she has not become pregnant yet. In a client who engages in regular coitus without contraception, inability to conceive over which time period suggests a fertility problem?
(a) 3 to 6 months
(b) 6 to 9 months
(c) 9 to 12 months
(d) More than 12 months
Correct answer: (d), see text page 423. Lack of pregnancy after more than 1 year of regular coitus without contraception may indicate a fertility problem and the need for referral to a fertility specialist.

20. Linda Kellerman, age 22, comes to the clinic for treatment of a heavy, white, sweet-smelling vaginal discharge and pruritus. These signs and symptoms suggest which disorder?
(a) Candidiasis
(b) Ovarian cysts
(c) Genital herpes
(d) Endometriosis
Correct answer: (a), see text page 429. Candidiasis produces a heavy discharge with a yeasty, sweet odor (or no odor) as well as dysuria, pruritus, and dyspareunia.

Test bank for Chapter 15, Female Reproductive System

1. Pat Dwyer, age 25, comes to the clinic for her annual gynecologic examination. During the health history, the nurse learns that Ms. Dwyer uses oral contraceptives. Which factor increases the risk of cardiovascular disease in women using oral contraceptives?
(a) Smoking
(b) Barbiturate use
(c) Phenothiazine use
(d) High-protein diet

2. To assess Ms. Dwyer's reproductive system, the nurse should place her in which position?
(a) Supine
(b) Lithotomy
(c) Left lateral
(d) Dorsal recumbent

3. The nurse performs a speculum examination. In a nulliparous client such as Ms. Dwyer, how should the cervical os appear?
(a) Round and open
(b) Round and closed
(c) Irregular and open
(d) Irregular and closed

4. Next, the nurse performs bimanual palpation. This technique is used to assess which structures?
(a) Skene's and Bartholin's ducts
(b) Ovaries and fallopian tubes
(c) Labia majora and minora
(d) Perineum and clitoris

5. The nurse palpates Ms. Dwyer's vaginal wall. Which finding is normal?
(a) Smoothness
(b) Rugosity
(c) Nodularity
(d) Tenderness

6. The position of which structure or structures may help the nurse identify the uterine position?
(a) Fallopian tubes
(b) Ovaries
(c) Cervix
(d) Skene's glands

7. In a client such as Ms. Dwyer, how should the uterus normally feel during palpation?
(a) Pear-shaped and symmetrical
(b) Round and symmetrical
(c) Oval and asymmetrical
(d) Almond-shaped and asymmetrical

8. When palpating Ms. Dwyer's ovaries, the nurse should consider which finding normal?
(a) Sensitivity
(b) Round shape
(c) Softness
(d) Immobility

9. The nurse may perform which routine test to screen for cervical cancer?
(a) Enzyme immunoassay
(b) Complete blood count
(c) Papanicolaou (Pap) test
(d) Human chorionic gonadotropin test

10. Carol Berger, age 27, seeks care for a watery vaginal discharge and sores on her external genitalia. These signs suggest which disorder?
(a) Endometriosis
(b) Candidiasis
(c) Trichomonal infection
(d) Genital herpes

11. Brenda White, age 31, schedules an appointment at the clinic because she believes she may be pregnant. In a pregnant client, the cervix is likely to be which color?
(a) Shiny pink
(b) Bright red
(c) Pale
(d) Bluish purple

12. In a pregnant client, how does the cervix normally feel?
(a) Hard and enlarged
(b) Soft and enlarged
(c) Hard and recessed
(d) Soft and recessed

13. Helen McCloskey, age 75, seeks care for irregular postmenopausal bleeding. Because of her age, she cannot assume the usual position for reproductive system assessment. The nurse should assist her into which alternate position?
(a) Supine
(b) Left lateral
(c) Fowler's
(d) Trendelenburg's

14. On inspection, Ms. McCloskey's external genitalia may display which normal age-related changes?
(a) Hypertrophy of labia majora
(b) Sparse, thin pubic hair
(c) Thick, coarse pubic hair
(d) Cystocele

15. When viewed through a speculum, Ms. McCloskey's cervix is likely to be which normal color?
(a) Pale
(b) Pink
(c) Red
(d) Blue

16. Which structure normally is not palpable in a client of Ms. McCloskey's age?
(a) Rectum
(b) Uterus
(c) Ovaries
(d) Vagina

17. On cervical palpation, which finding is considered normal in a client of Ms. McCloskey's age?
(a) The cervix is smaller and recessed.
(b) The cervix is larger and harder.
(c) The cervix displays ectropion.
(d) The cervix displays eversion.

18. Diagnostic tests confirm that Ms. McCloskey has ovarian cancer. Which assessment finding is associated with ovarian cancer?
(a) History of menstrual disturbances
(b) History of estrogen therapy
(c) History of diabetes
(d) Nulliparity

19. Barbara Brooks, age 30, has been married for 5 years. She visits her physician because she has not become pregnant yet. In a client who engages in regular coitus without contraception, inability to conceive over which time period suggests a fertility problem?
(a) 3 to 6 months
(b) 6 to 9 months
(c) 9 to 12 months
(d) More than 12 months

20. Linda Kellerman, age 22, comes to the clinic for treatment of a heavy, white, sweet-smelling vaginal discharge and pruritus. These signs and symptoms suggest which disorder?
(a) Candidiasis
(b) Ovarian cysts
(c) Genital herpes
(d) Endometriosis

16

Male Reproductive System

Overview

Assessment of the male reproductive system is an essential part of a complete health assessment because many reproductive disorders pose serious physical and psychological consequences. To prepare the nurse for early detection of these disorders—and prevention of their consequences—Chapter 16 begins with a review of male reproductive system anatomy and physiology. Then it discusses the health history questions, physical assessment techniques, and laboratory tests that provide the necessary assessment data. Here are the chapter highlights:

• Male reproductive system structures include the penis, scrotum, prostate gland, and inguinal structures.

• The penis functions in urine elimination and sperm emission.

• The scrotum and its contents, including the testes, produce sperm and male sex hormones.

• Testosterone, the primary male sex hormone, affects sperm production, sexual function, and development of male secondary sexual characteristics, such as facial and body hair growth, increased muscle mass, and deepened voice.

• To ensure accurate and complete assessment findings, the nurse and the client must feel comfortable discussing sexual and reproductive function and assessing the genitalia and other structures.

• Assessing the male reproductive system begins with a comprehensive health history that focuses primarily on sexual and reproductive function. The health history also should assess the use of drugs that can affect the male reproductive system adversely, such as antidepressants and antihypertensives.

• Physical assessment of the male genitalia involves inspecting and palpating the penis and scrotum for structural abnormalities, inspecting and palpating the inguinal area for hernias, and palpating the prostate gland for enlargement, tenderness, and other abnormalities.

• To complete the assessment, the nurse should review the results of any laboratory tests ordered to evaluate reproductive system function, such as semen analysis or serum alpha-fetoprotein level.

• The nurse should document all assessment findings and use them in the nursing process to plan, implement, and evaluate the client's care.

• For more information about male reproductive system assessment, see pages 73PG through 75PG of the Photo Gallery in the text.

Suggested lecture topics

• Using audiovisual aids, review the anatomy and physiology of the male reproductive system, and explain normal developmental changes. (For a visual aid, see page 73PG in the text.)

• Discuss health history questions important to male reproductive system assessment, explaining the reasons for asking them.

• Using an anatomic simulator, demonstrate how to inspect, palpate, and transilluminate the male reproductive system. (For visual aids, see page 74PG in the text.)

• Describe normal and abnormal assessment findings for the male reproductive system as well as the implications of abnormal findings. (For visual aids, see page 75PG in the text.)

Skills laboratory guide: Health history

To collect information about the male client's reproductive system, ask questions about health and illness patterns, health promotion and protection patterns, and role and relationship patterns. Sample questions from each category are listed below.

HEALTH AND ILLNESS PATTERNS

- Have you noticed any changes in the color of the skin on your penis or scrotum?
- If you are uncircumcised, can you retract and replace the foreskin easily?
- Have you noticed the appearance of a sore, lump, or ulcer on your penis?
- Have you noticed any swelling in your scrotum?
- Are you experiencing any pain in your penis, testes, or scrotal sac?
- Have you felt a lump, painful sore, or tenderness in your groin?
- Do you have nocturia; urinary frequency, hesitancy, or dribbling; or pain in the area between your rectum and penis, or in your hips or lower back?
- Do you have any difficulty achieving and maintaining an erection during sexual activity?
- Do you have any difficulty with ejaculation?
- What prescription, over-the-counter, or street drugs do you take?
- Have you fathered any children?
- Have you ever had surgery on the genitourinary tract?
- Have you ever been diagnosed as having a sexually transmitted disease or any other genitourinary tract infection?
- Have you had diabetes mellitus, cardiovascular disease, neurologic disease, or malignancy in the genitourinary tract?
- Has anyone in your family had infertility problems?
- Has anyone in your family had a hernia?

HEALTH PROMOTION AND PROTECTION PATTERNS

- Do you examine your testes periodically?
- If you are sexually active, do you have more than one partner?
- Do you take any precautions to prevent contracting a sexually transmitted disease or acquired immunodeficiency syndrome (AIDS)?
- What is your job?
- Are you now or have you been exposed to radiation or toxic chemicals?
- Do you engage in sports or in any activity that requires heavy lifting or straining?
- Would you say you are under a lot of stress?

ROLE AND RELATIONSHIP PATTERNS

- What is your self-image? Do you consider yourself attractive to others?
- What is your cultural and religious background?
- Do you have a supportive relationship with another person?
- If you are experiencing sexual difficulty, is it affecting your emotional and social relationships?

Suggested critical thinking activities

- Have the students develop a client-teaching plan for testicular self-examination. Then pair the students and have them critique each other's teaching plan.
- Have male students perform a testicular self-examination and document their findings.
- Using an anatomic simulator or a live model, have the students perform a physical assessment of the male reproductive system and document their findings.
- Using a case study of a male client with a reproductive system problem, have the students develop a nursing care plan.

Student study questions and answers

The following study questions are taken from text page 461 of Chapter 16, Male Reproductive System. Their answers are based on information in that chapter.

1. How would you describe the regulation of male sex hormones?

Answer
In males, a negative feedback system controls the release of sex hormones. The hypothalamus secretes gonadotropin-releasing hormone (GnRH), which stimulates the anterior pituitary to release luteinizing hormone (LH) and follicle-stimulating hormone (FSH).

LH acts on the Leydig's cells in the testes, causing these cells to mature and secrete testosterone, the primary male sex hormone. FSH acts on the germinal epithelial cells of the seminiferous tubules to promote complete spermatogenesis. Male hormonal regulation is continuous. When testosterone concentrations rise, the body sends negative feedback messages to the hypothalamus to stabilize testosterone levels.

2. The nurse is assessing Mr. Yin, age 26, to rule out the presence of hernias. How would you proceed to inspect and palpate the inguinal area? What typical physical assessment findings for three types of hernias—inguinal, scrotal, and femoral—might you find?

Answer
To palpate a client's inguinal area for hernias, the nurse first should place the index finger and forefinger of each hand over each inguinal ring, and ask the client to bear down or cough to increase intra-abdominal pressure momentarily. Then, the nurse should insert the middle or index finger (for an adult) or the little finger (for a child) gently into the scrotal sac and follow the spermatic cord upward to the external inguinal ring at Hesselbach's triangle, an opening just above and lateral to the pubic tubercle. Holding the finger at this

Skills laboratory guide: Physical assessment

This chart guides the student during assessment by identifying body areas, special considerations and techniques to be used, and normal findings.

BODY AREA	SPECIAL CONSIDERATIONS	NORMAL FINDINGS
Inspection		
Penis	• Note skin color, integrity, and foreskin retractability. • Note lesions, inflammation, and discharge. • Note position of urethral meatus and drainage. Retract foreskin of an uncircumcised infant only enough to examine the urethral meatus. In a neonate, white cysts on the distal prepuce are normal.	• Penis color consistent with client's pigmentation • Intact skin with no lesions, inflammation, or discharge • Easy foreskin retraction if uncircumcised and client older than age 3 to 4 • Appropriate size for client's age
Scrotum	• Note presence and distribution of pubic hair. • Note scrotal appearance, size, and symmetry. During infancy, the scrotum is small, pink, wrinkled; after age 50, it is more pendulous. • Note lesions, ulcerations, indurations, or redness.	• Evenly distributed pubic hair • Coarser, darker skin than body skin • Appropriate scrotum size for client's age • Left testicle lower than right • No lesions, ulcerations, indurations, or redness
Inguinal area	• Observe for bulges as client bears down.	• No bulges (hernias)
Palpation		
Penis	• Note induration, tenderness, or lumps. • Palpate the length of the penis between your thumb and first two fingers.	• Appropriate penis size for client's age • Soft penis with no induration, tenderness, or lumps
Scrotum	• Note scrotal nodules, lesions, or ulcers. • Palpate the epididymis and vas deferens on the posterolateral surface. • Palpation may stimulate the cremasteric reflex, causing the testes to rise. • Note testicular size, shape, mobility, pressure-pain sensation, and masses. • Transilluminate any masses.	• Rough scrotal skin • No nodules, lesions, or ulcers • Firm epididymis lying vertically on testicular surface • Smooth, freely movable vas deferens • Small, oval, movable, smooth testes • Pressure-pain sensation only with testicular compression
Inguinal area	• Assess for an inguinal hernia by palpating into the scrotal sac to the inguinal ring; for a femoral hernia, palpating directly over the femoral artery. Have the client bear down or cough during palpation.	• No palpable masses or bulges (hernias)
Advanced assessment skills: Palpating the prostate gland		
Prostate	• Inspect the perineal, anal, and posterior scrotal areas. • Palpate the prostate on the anterior rectal wall using the pad of your gloved index finger. Note its size, shape, and consistency. • Grade an enlarged prostate as follows: Grade I, less than ½″ (1 cm) protrusion into the rectum; Grade II, ½″ to ¾″ (1 to 2 cm) protrusion; Grade III, ¾″ to 1½″ (2 to 3 cm) protrusion; Grade IV, greater than 1½″ (3 cm) protrusion.	• Intact, smooth skin with no masses • Walnut-sized, smooth, rubbery, and nontender prostate

spot, the nurse should ask the client to cough or bear down. An inguinal hernia, sometimes known as a scrotal hernia, will palpate as a mass or bulge.

To palpate for a femoral hernia, the nurse should place the right hand on the client's thigh with the index finger over the femoral artery. With the hand in this position, the nurse can locate the femoral canal under the ring finger in an adult and between the index and ring finger in a child. A hernia here will palpate as a soft bulge or mass.

3. How would you integrate a client's cultural and developmental background into the health history and physical assessment of the male reproductive system?

Answer

To integrate a client's cultural background into a male reproductive system assessment, the nurse should ask about the client's cultural and religious background and determine whether any cultural or religious factors influence his beliefs or practices regarding sexuality and reproduction. The client's answers to these questions can help the nurse identify potential problem areas and risk factors. For example, a cultural or religious prohibition of condom use may place the client at a higher risk for contracting acquired immunodeficiency syndrome (AIDS) or a sexually transmitted disease.

The nurse can integrate developmental considerations in the health history and physical assessment. During the health history, the nurse should phrase questions in terms appropriate to the client's level of understanding and development. Adolescent and adult males require a sensitive approach when asked questions about sexual development and function. During physical assessment, the nurse should keep in mind important developmental norms. The size and appearance of the penis and scrotum and the presence or absence of secondary sexual characteristics should match the client's developmental age.

4. Mr. Johnson, age 24, comes to the clinic complaining of a left testicular mass. How would you proceed with a complete assessment?

Answer

The nurse should begin with a symptom analysis of the client's chief complaint, using the PQRST method to obtain detailed information about the testicular mass. Then the nurse should ask about any related signs and symptoms, such as pain, lesions, or discharge. To complete the health history, the nurse should ask about the client's past health status, family health status, health promotion and protection patterns, and role and relationship patterns.

During the physical assessment, the nurse should inspect the scrotum, comparing the testes for symmetry and noting any obvious bulges, lumps, nodules, lesions, or ulcers. Next, the nurse should palpate and transilluminate the testicular mass. A serum alpha-fetoprotein test could provide further information.

Finally, the nurse should document the assessment findings, including the exact location, size, shape, consistency, and tenderness of the mass and the transillumination results.

5. Mr. Donovan, age 24, arrives in the emergency department complaining of a penile discharge and urethral redness. How would you document the following information related to your nursing assessment of Mr. Donovan?
• history (subjective) assessment data
• physical (objective) assessment data
• assessment techniques and any special equipment
• two appropriate nursing diagnosis
• documentation of your findings.

Answer

History (subjective) assessment data
• Complaining of penile discharge and urethral tenderness

Physical (objective) assessment data
• Male, age 24
• Milky white penile discharge and inflamed urethral meatus
Assessment techniques and equipment
• Interview the client about current and past health history and sexual practices.
• Inspect the penis and urethral meatus.
• Obtain a urethral discharge specimen for culture and sensitivity testing.
• Equipment should include gloves and appropriate specimen equipment.
Two appropriate nursing diagnoses
• Pain related to urethral inflammation
• Potential impaired skin integrity related to penile discharge
Documentation of findings
• S—Client complains of penile discharge and urethral tenderness.
• O—Male, age 24. Urethral meatus reddened. Milky white penile discharge present.
• A—Pain related to urethral inflammation

Questions, answers, and rationales

1. Raymond Trainer, age 32, seeks care for a testicular lump he discovered during self-examination. At what age is a client at highest risk for testicular cancer?
(a) Under age 15
(b) Age 15 to 30
(c) Age 30 to 45
(d) Over age 45
Correct answer: (b), see text page 450. Testicular cancer is the most common type of cancer in males between ages 15 and 30.

2. When inspecting Mr. Trainer's scrotum, the nurse should consider which finding normal?
(a) The testes hang evenly and freely.
(b) The left testicle is larger than the right.
(c) The right testicle hangs lower than the left.
(d) The left testicle hangs lower than the right.
Correct answer: (d), see text page 453. The left testicle usually hangs slightly lower than the right; both should hang freely in the scrotum.

3. When the nurse palpates the testes, how should they feel?
(a) Rough and hard
(b) Rubbery and smooth
(c) Nodular and soft
(d) Granular and firm
Correct answer: (b), see text page 451. The normal testis is egg-shaped, rubbery-firm, movable within the scrotum; it should feel smooth, with no lumps.

4. Which laboratory study is likely to be ordered to detect testicular cancer?
(a) Serum alpha-fetoprotein
(b) Serum alkaline phosphatase
(c) Serum acid phosphatase
(d) Serum uric acid
Correct answer: (b), see text page 459. By measuring the glycoprotein produced by tumors, the serum alpha-fetoprotein test helps detect—and monitor treatment for—testicular cancer.

5. Donna and Joseph Brownlee have been married for 5 years and have not been able to conceive. They undergo a complete fertility assessment. The prostate gland produces which substance that affects fertility?
(a) Hormones that stimulate sperm development
(b) Acidic fluid that neutralizes vaginal secretions
(c) Alkaline fluid that enhances sperm mobility
(d) Mucoid fluid that nourishes and protects sperm
Correct answer: (c), see text page 445. Prostatic fluid adds volume to the semen and enhances sperm mobility and possibly fertility by neutralizing urethral and vaginal acidity.

6. Which hormone is required for spermatogenesis?
(a) Testosterone
(b) Luteinizing hormone
(c) Follicle-stimulating hormone
(d) Gonadotropin-releasing hormone
Correct answer: (a), see text page 445. Testosterone, which is responsible for the development and maintenance of male sex organs and secondary sex characteristics, is required for spermatogenesis.

7. Howard Woods, age 55, is admitted to the hospital for treatment of benign prostatic hypertrophy. This disorder commonly produces which sign or symptom?
(a) Urination pattern changes
(b) Large scrotal mass
(c) Blood-tinged semen
(d) Low back pain
Correct answer: (a), see text page 457. Benign prostatic hypertrophy may cause changes in urination pattern, such as hesitancy, incontinence with dribbling, reduced caliber and force of urine stream, and urine retention.

8. The nurse assesses Mr. Woods to obtain baseline data. Where should the nurse palpate the prostate gland?
(a) Behind the scrotum
(b) In the inguinal canal
(c) In the femoral canal
(d) On the rectal wall
Correct answer: (d), see text page 458. Using the pad of the index finger, the nurse should palpate the prostate gland on the anterior rectal wall, just past the anorectal ring.

9. In a client with benign prostatic hypertrophy such as Mr. Woods, how should the nurse expect the prostate to feel?
(a) Soft and boggy
(b) Hard and fixed
(c) Soft and tender
(d) Hard and nodular
Correct answer: (a), see text page 459. In benign prostatic hypertrophy, the prostate is enlarged, protrudes into the rectum, and feels soft, boggy (nonfirm, mushy), and non-tender.

10. In a client with a normal prostate gland, how should the nurse expect it to feel?
(a) Hard and nodular
(b) Rubbery and smooth
(c) Soft and smooth
(d) Hard and tender
Correct answer: (b), see text page 458. The prostate gland should feel smooth and rubbery and usually is about the size of a walnut.

11. In a client with prostatic cancer, how should the nurse expect the prostate gland to feel?
(a) Soft and tender
(b) Hard and fixed
(c) Rubbery and smooth
(d) Soft and nodular
Correct answer: (b), see text page 459. In prostatic cancer, palpation typically reveals a hard, fixed, firm prostate or a fixed lesion on the prostate.

12. Mr. Woods undergoes several laboratory tests. An above-normal level of serum acid phosphatase suggests which disorder?
(a) Benign prostatic hypertrophy
(b) Prostatic cancer
(c) Prostatitis
(d) Priapism
Correct answer: (b), see text page 459. Because this test measures the phosphatase enzymes produced by prostatic tumors, an above-normal level may indicate prostatic cancer.

13. Stephen Caldwell, age 56, has an inguinal hernia. To accentuate the hernia during assessment, the nurse may ask him to perform which maneuver?
(a) Bend to the side
(b) Flex the knees
(c) Bear down
(d) Stretch
Correct answer: (c), see text page 456. Bearing down or coughing increases the intra-abdominal pressure momentarily, causing the hernia to become more palpable as a mass or bulge.

14. During an annual check-up, Barry Gordon, age 62, complains of decreased libido. Which drugs may affect the libido adversely?
(a) Antihypertensives
(b) Thyroid hormones
(c) Antipyretics
(d) Corticosteroids
Correct answer: (a), see text page 449. Antihypertensives, such as clonidine, methyldopa, nadolol, and resperpine, may decrease libido or cause impotence.

15. When inspecting Mr. Gordon's genitalia, the nurse may note which normal age-related change?
(a) Pendulous scrotum
(b) Testicular atrophy
(c) Testicular hypertrophy
(d) Taut scrotal skin
Correct answer: (a) see text page 458. Around age 50, the male client may display grey or white pubic hair and a more pendulous scrotum.

16. Glenda Bower, age 21, has just given birth to a healthy male infant, whom she names Bobby. During Bobby's initial assessment, the nurse should consider which finding abnormal?
(a) Pink, smooth penis
(b) Small white cysts on prepuce
(c) Undescended testes
(d) Pink, wrinkled scrotum
Correct answer: (c), see text page 458. Cryptorchidism (undescended testes) is a congenital malformation that should be reported.

17. The prepuce (foreskin) of an uncircumcised male should be completely retractable by what age?
(a) At birth
(b) Age 1 or 2
(c) Age 3 or 4
(d) Age 5 or 6
Correct answer: (c), see text page 458. By age 3 or 4, the child's prepuce should be completely retractable.

18. During transillumination of Bobby's scrotum, the nurse detects a large, translucent mass. This finding suggests which disorder?
(a) Epispadias
(b) Hypospadias
(c) Hydrocele
(d) Paraphimosis
Correct answer: (c), see text page 457. Hydrocele can produce a large scrotal mass that appears translucent on transillumination and may be painful and tender.

19. After Harold Cummings, age 26, is admitted to the hospital with priapism, the nurse assesses his medical history. Which disorder commonly is associated with this presenting sign?
(a) Diabetes
(b) Hypertension
(c) Vascular disease
(d) Sickle cell anemia
Correct answer: (d), see text page 457. A history of sickle cell anemia or spinal cord lesion commonly accompanies priapism (painful, constant erection without sexual desire).

20. Donald Porter, age 20, comes to the health clinic for treatment of dysuria and a white discharge from the penis. Which disorder is most likely to cause these signs and symptoms?
(a) Genital herpes
(b) Orchitis
(c) Gonorrhea
(d) Syphilis
Correct answer: (c), see text page 457. Gonorrhea can cause dysuria, urinary frequency, and white or yellow discharge from a swollen urethral meatus.

Test bank for Chapter 16, Male Reproductive System

1. Raymond Trainer, age 32, seeks care for a testicular lump he discovered during self-examination. At what age is a client at highest risk for testicular cancer?
(a) Under age 15
(b) Age 15 to 30
(c) Age 30 to 45
(d) Over age 45

2. When inspecting Mr. Trainer's scrotum, the nurse should consider which finding normal?
(a) The testes hang evenly and freely.
(b) The left testicle is larger than the right.
(c) The right testicle hangs lower than the left.
(d) The left testicle hangs lower than the right.

3. When the nurse palpates the testes, how should they feel?
(a) Rough and hard
(b) Rubbery and smooth
(c) Nodular and soft
(d) Granular and firm

4. Which laboratory study is likely to be ordered to detect testicular cancer?
(a) Serum alpha-fetoprotein
(b) Serum alkaline phosphatase
(c) Serum acid phosphatase
(d) Serum uric acid

5. Donna and Joseph Brownlee have been married for 5 years and have not been able to conceive. They undergo a complete fertility assessment. The prostate gland produces which substance that affects fertility?
(a) Hormones that stimulate sperm development
(b) Acidic fluid that neutralizes vaginal secretions
(c) Alkaline fluid that enhances sperm mobility
(d) Mucoid fluid that nourishes and protects sperm

6. Which hormone is required for spermatogenesis?
(a) Testosterone
(b) Luteinizing hormone
(c) Follicle-stimulating hormone
(d) Gonadotropin-releasing hormone

7. Howard Woods, age 55, is admitted to the hospital for treatment of benign prostatic hypertrophy. This disorder commonly produces which sign or symptom?
(a) Urination pattern changes
(b) Large scrotal mass
(c) Blood-tinged semen
(d) Low back pain

8. The nurse assesses Mr. Woods to obtain baseline data. Where should the nurse palpate the prostate gland?
(a) Behind the scrotum
(b) In the inguinal canal
(c) In the femoral canal
(d) On the rectal wall

9. In a client with benign prostatic hypertrophy such as Mr. Woods, how should the nurse expect the prostate to feel?
(a) Soft and boggy
(b) Hard and fixed
(c) Soft and tender
(d) Hard and nodular

10. In a client with a normal prostate gland, how should the nurse expect it to feel?
(a) Hard and nodular
(b) Rubbery and smooth
(c) Soft and smooth
(d) Hard and tender

11. In a client with prostatic cancer, how should the nurse expect the prostate gland to feel?
(a) Soft and tender
(b) Hard and fixed
(c) Rubbery and smooth
(d) Soft and nodular

12. Mr. Woods undergoes several laboratory tests. An above-normal level of serum acid phosphatase suggests which disorder?
(a) Benign prostatic hypertrophy
(b) Prostatic cancer
(c) Prostatitis
(d) Priapism

13. Stephen Caldwell, age 56, has an inguinal hernia. To accentuate the hernia during assessment, the nurse may ask him to perform which maneuver?
(a) Bend to the side
(b) Flex the knees
(c) Bear down
(d) Stretch

14. During an annual check-up, Barry Gordon, age 62, complains of decreased libido. Which drugs may affect the libido adversely?
(a) Antihypertensives
(b) Thyroid hormones
(c) Antipyretics
(d) Corticosteroids

15. When inspecting Mr. Gordon's genitalia, the nurse may note which normal age-related change?
(a) Pendulous scrotum
(b) Testicular atrophy
(c) Testicular hypertrophy
(d) Taut scrotal skin

16. Glenda Bower, age 21, has just given birth to a healthy male infant, whom she names Bobby. During Bobby's initial assessment, the nurse should consider which finding abnormal?
(a) Pink, smooth penis
(b) Small white cysts on prepuce
(c) Undescended testes
(d) Pink, wrinkled scrotum

17. The prepuce (foreskin) of an uncircumcised male should be completely retractable by what age?
(a) At birth
(b) Age 1 or 2
(c) Age 3 or 4
(d) Age 5 or 6

18. During transillumination of Bobby's scrotum, the nurse detects a large, translucent mass. This finding suggests which disorder?
(a) Epispadias
(b) Hypospadias
(c) Hydrocele
(d) Paraphimosis

19. After Harold Cummings, age 26, is admitted to the hospital with priapism, the nurse assesses his medical history. Which disorder commonly is associated with this presenting sign?
(a) Diabetes
(b) Hypertension
(c) Vascular disease
(d) Sickle cell anemia

20. Donald Porter, age 20, comes to the health clinic for treatment of dysuria and a white discharge from the penis. Which disorder is most likely to cause these signs and symptoms?
(a) Genital herpes
(b) Orchitis
(c) Gonorrhea
(d) Syphilis

17

Nervous System

Overview

The nurse may encounter signs and symptoms of nervous system disorders in clients of any age. Because nervous system disorders can cause or result from problems in other body systems, Chapter 17 prepares the nurse to perform a thorough nervous system assesssment. After reviewing the anatomy and physiology of the nervous system, the chapter describes how to perform a neurologic health history and a complete and partial (screening) physical assessment, comparing normal and abnormal findings and developmental considerations. Finally, it explains how to integrate history and physical data with that from laboratory studies. Here are the chapter highlights:

- The nervous system consists of the central nervous system (CNS)—which includes the brain and spinal cord—and the peripheral nervous system (PNS)—which includes the cranial and spinal nerves and the autonomic nervous system.
- Reflex responses are the normal reactions of the nervous system to stimuli. These responses occur automatically, without any brain involvement, to protect the body.
- When obtaining a neurologic health history, the nurse should ask questions about the client's general well-being and body function because nervous system disorders can cause or result from problems in other body systems. When appropriate, the nurse should verify critical or questionable information with the client's family members or previous medical records.
- A complete neurologic assessment provides information about five broad areas of neurologic function: cerebral function, cranial nerves, motor system and cerebellar functions, sensory system, and reflexes. A neurologic screening

includes evaluation of level of consciousness (LOC), selected cranial nerve assessment, motor screening, and sensory screening.
- The nurse should begin with an assessment of cerebral functioning, including LOC, communication, and, briefly, mental status. LOC evaluation includes assessment of level of arousal and orientation. Communication assessment includes evaluation of verbal responsiveness. Advanced assessment of cerebral function includes formal language skills and complete mental status evaluations.
- Cranial nerve assessment provides information about the functioning of the CNS, particularly the brain stem. The neurologic screening evaluates 4 of the 12 cranial nerves (CN II, III, IV, and VI), because they are the most vulnerable to the effects of increasing intracranial pressure (ICP).
- Motor system and cerebellar function assessment evaluates the integrity of the cerebral cortex, the pyramidal and extrapyramidal pathways, the corticospinal tracts, the lower motor neurons, muscle condition, the cerebellum, and the basal ganglia. The neurologic screening of the motor system assesses muscle strength, arm and leg movement, and gait. A complete neurologic assessment evaluates motor functions (muscle size, tone, strength, and movement), cerebellar functions (balance and coordination), and gait.
- Sensory system assessment evaluates the sensory receptors, the afferent nerves, the sensory tracts, and the sensory, interpretive, and integrative areas of the cerebral cortex. Neurologic screening of the sensory system evaluates light touch sensation in the extremities. Complete assessment of sensory function evaluates superficial pain, temperature sensation, response to vibration, proprioception, stereognosis, number identification, two-point discrimination, point localization, and extinction.

Skills laboratory guide: Health history

To collect information about the client's nervous system, ask questions about health and illness patterns, health promotion and protection patterns, and role and relationship patterns. Sample questions from each category are listed below.

HEALTH AND ILLNESS PATTERNS

- Do you have headaches? If so, how would you describe them?
- Have you noticed a change in your ability to remember things?
- Have you noticed a change in your mental alertness or ability to concentrate?
- Have you ever fainted or blacked out? Do you have difficulty remembering blocks of time?
- Do you experience blurred vision, double vision, or any other visual disturbances, such as blind spots?
- How would you rate your muscle strength? Have you recently noticed any change in strength?
- Have you noticed a change in your ability to feel textures or any numbness, tingling, or other unusual sensations?
- Have you ever had a head injury? If so, when? How would you describe what happened? Do you have any lasting effects?
- Have you ever been treated by a neurologist or neurosurgeon? If so, why?
- Have any of your immediate family members (mother, father, or siblings) had high blood pressure or a stroke?

HEALTH PROMOTION AND PROTECTION PATTERNS

- What do you do with your leisure time? Do you enjoy reading or listening to music?
- Do you have difficulty following conversations or television programs?
- How would you describe an emotionally stressful situation? How would you handle such a situation?
- Do you need to rest during the day?
- Do you use alcohol or other mood-altering drugs?

ROLE AND RELATIONSHIP PATTERNS

- How has your disability affected you?
- Can you do the things for yourself that you would like to do?
- Can you fulfill your usual family responsibilities?
- How has your illness or disability affected members of your family emotionally and financially?
- Have you noticed any change in your sexuality?

- Assessment of deep tendon and superficial reflexes evaluates the sensory receptor organ and evaluates how well a sensory message is relayed through the system. Reflex evaluation is only done as part of the complete neurologic assessment.
- The nurse should integrate laboratory test results with history and physical assessment findings, documenting them and using them to develop a nursing care plan for the client.
- For more information about nervous system assessement, see pages 76PG through 85PG of the Photo Gallery in the text.

Suggested lecture topics

- Review the anatomy and physiology of the nervous system, including developmental considerations. (For a visual aid, see the transparency master *Structures of the central nervous system* and page 76PG in the text.)
- Discuss health history questions important to a nervous system assessment, explaining the rationales for asking them.
- Demonstrate how to use the equipment needed for nervous system assessment.
- Using a student volunteer, demonstrate nervous system assessment techniques and discuss normal findings. (For visual aids, see pages 77PG through 85PG of the Photo Gallery in the text.)
- Using audiovisual aids, discuss common abnormal findings related to nervous system assessment.

Suggested critical thinking activities

- Pair the students and have them perform a nervous system assessment, including a health history and physical assessment, on each other.
- Have the students document their findings on the Skills Laboratory Assessment Guide.
- Have the entire class critique these findings.
- Using audiovisual aids, have the students identify which findings vary with developmental status.
- Using a case study of a client with a neurologic problem, have the students develop a nursing care plan.

Student study questions and answers

The following study questions are taken from text pages 508 and 509 of Chapter 17, Nervous System. Their answers are based on information in that chapter.

1. Thomas Wilson, age 28, has just been brought to the emergency department after a motorcycle accident. Despite wearing a helmet, Mr. Wilson sustained a head injury and was unconscious for approximately 20 minutes at the scene of the accident. He is now awake, but restless and disoriented.

Mr. Wilson needs a rapid assessment of the nervous system; however, his condition does not allow a complete examination of all cranial nerves. Considering the nature of his injuries, which cranial nerves are essential to assess? (For each cranial nerve, identify its name, describe which function[s] require evaluation, and explain why the assessment is essential.)

(Text continues on page 150.)

Skills laboratory guide: Physical assessment

This chart guides the student during assessment by identifying neurologic function, special considerations and techniques to be used, and normal findings.

NEUROLOGIC FUNCTION	SPECIAL CONSIDERATIONS	NORMAL FINDINGS
Cerebral function		
Level of consciousness (LOC)	• Note level of arousal (including response to stimuli) and orientation to person, place, and time. A psychiatric disturbance can cause bizarre confusion patterns. In an elderly client, disorientation may result from decreased visual and auditory acuity. • Assess level of arousal by starting with a minimal (auditory) stimulus and increasing its intensity, as needed, to tactile and finally painful stimuli. In a child, assess LOC by observing behavior.	• Alert and oriented to person, place, and time • Appropriate behavior
Communication	• Note quality, quantity, and appropriateness of verbal responses. • Note language client speaks. • Note dysphasia, aphasia, dysarthria, dysphonia, and use of neologisms.	• Appropriate verbal responses • No dysphasia, aphasia, dysarthria, dysphonia, or use of neologisms
Mental status	• Ask ten screening questions, each addressing one area of the complete mental status examination.	• Appropriate answers to screening questions
Advanced assessment skills: Cerebral function		
Complete mental status	• Evaluate general appearance, behavior, mood, affect, cognitive functions, attention, memory, intellectual skills (general knowledge, vocabulary, and calculation skills), abstract reasoning, judgment, and thought processes and content.	• Appropriate general appearance, behavior, mood, and affect • Intact cognitive functions • Normal attention span • Intact immediate, remote, and recent memory • Intact intellectual skills, abstract reasoning, judgment, and thought processes and content that are appropriate for client's age
Cranial nerves		
Olfactory nerve (CN I)	• Check sense of smell in both nostrils.	• Intact sense of smell in both nostrils
Optic (CN II) and oculomotor (CN III) nerves	• Check visual acuity, visual fields, and retinal structures.	• Pupils equal, round, and reactive to light and accommodation, direct and consensual
Oculomotor (CN III), trochlear (CN IV), and abducens (CN VI) nerves	• Test extraocular eye movement.	• Smooth, yoked eye movement in all six directions
Trigeminal (CN V) nerve	• Assess sensory portion by testing response to light touch and sharp stimuli in three facial areas. • Assess motor portion by testing client's clenched jaws. • Assess the corneal reflex.	• Intact light touch and sharp stimuli sensations bilaterally • Symmetrically clenched jaws that remain closed against resistance • Both eyelids close when cotton is stroked across one cornea
Facial (CN VII) nerve	• Test motor functions of face. • Test taste sensations on anterior two-thirds of tongue.	• Symmetric facial movements • Symmetric taste sensations to salt and sugar
Acoustic (CN VIII) nerve	• Test gross hearing acuity. • Observe eye movements and balance.	• Ability to hear whispered voice or watch tick • No nystagmus or disturbed balance

continued

Skills laboratory guide: Physical assessment *continued*

NEUROLOGIC FUNCTION	SPECIAL CONSIDERATIONS	NORMAL FINDINGS
Cranial nerves *continued*		
Glossopharyngeal (CN IX) and vagus (CN X) nerves	• Evaluate voice quality, position of soft palate, and gag reflex. • Test taste sensations on posterior third of tongue.	• Strong, clear voice • Rising soft palate and uvula when client says "ah"; intact gag reflex • Symmetric taste sensations to sour and bitter
Spinal accessory (CN XI) nerve	• Test neck and shoulder strength.	• Neck and shoulders easily overcome resistance • Bilaterally equal ROM
Hypoglossal (CN XII) nerve	• Note tongue position and mobility. Note ability to articulate the sounds d, l, n, and t.	• Midline, freely movable tongue • Clear speech
Advanced assessment skills: Cranial nerves		
Oculocephalic (doll's eyes) reflex (CN III and CN VI)	• Perform procedure only on an unconscious client, never on a client with suspected cervical spine injury. • Note how eyes move in response to head movement.	• Eye movement in opposite direction from head movement
Oculovestibular reflex (ice water or cold calorics) (CN VIII)	• Make sure client's eardrum is intact. • Note client's eye movements.	• Nystagmus; eye movement away from stimulated ear
Motor function	• Note muscle size, strength, and symmetry. • Note gait, voluntary and involuntary movements, weakness, atrophy, and paralysis. • In an infant, fine tremors and involuntary movements normally occur up to age 2 months; flexor tone persists to age 3 months. • A child normally develops hand preference after age 2, and has a wide-based gait until age 6. An elderly client normally experiences decreased muscle mass and strength, limited range of motion, reduced mobility, fine motor tremors, and slowed gait.	• Appropriate, symmetrical muscle size and strength in upper and lower extremities • Coordinated, rhythmic gait; purposeful movements; no involuntary movements, weakness, atrophy, or paresis
Advanced assessment skills: Cerebellar function		
Balance	• Have client perform the Romberg test, heel and toe walking, and tandem-gait (heel-to-toe) walking. A toddler cannot walk on heels or toes for more than 5 to 6 seconds; a child cannot tandem walk until age 7.	• Slight swaying with eyes closed (Romberg test) • Coordinated, balanced heel and toe walking and tandem walking
Coordination	• Test client's ability to perform rapid alternating movements, point-to-point localization, and leg coordination.	• Intact rapid alternating movements bilaterally • Intact ability to touch items indicated with eyes open and closed • Intact ability to slide heel down shin bilaterally
Sensory system		
Light touch	• Test with client's eyes closed. • Evaluate light touch sensation in all extremities. • Compare arms and legs for symmetry of sensation. • Note any numbness or tingling.	• Present, symmetrical light touch sensations in all extremities • No numbness or tingling
Advanced assessment skills: Sensory system		
Superficial pain	• Test with client's eyes closed. • Lightly touch—but do not puncture—client's skin with a sharp object. Note response. • Compare distal and proximal portions of all extremities.	• Intact pain response in all areas
Temperature sensation	• Note client's ability to sense hot and cold. • Perform only if client displays abnormal pain sensation.	• Correct identification of hot and cold

Skills laboratory guide: Physical assessment *continued*

NEUROLOGIC FUNCTION	SPECIAL CONSIDERATIONS	NORMAL FINDINGS
Advanced assessment skills: Sensory system *continued*		
Response to vibration	• Place vibrating tuning fork on bony prominences, proceeding from distal to proximal areas. Note client's ability to sense vibrations. If client has intact distal vibration sensation, further testing is unnecessary.	• Intact vibration sensation in all areas
Sense of position (proprioception)	• Note client's ability to sense position changes of toes and fingers. If client exhibits impaired sense of position, repeat procedure on next joint of extremity.	• Intact sense of position
Sense of touch (stereognosis)	• Note client's ability to identify objects by touch.	• Intact sense of touch
Number identification	• Note client's ability to recognize, by touch, a large number traced on the palm.	• Correct identification of number
Two-point discrimination	• Touch one or two sharp objects to the client's skin. Note whether the client can feel one or two points and smallest distance between the two points at which the client still can discriminate the presence of two points. Acuity varies in different body areas.	• Two-point discrimination less than 5 mm on fingertips
Point localization	• With the client's eyes closed, briefly touch a point on the skin. Note the client's ability to identify the point touched.	• Correct identification of point touched
Extinction	• Note client's ability to identify two corresponding areas that you touch simultaneously.	• Intact ability to sense touch in both areas
Advanced assessment skills: Deep tendon reflexes		
Biceps reflex	• Tap the reflex hammer over your finger placed on the biceps tendon. Note elbow movement. • The biceps reflex should be present at birth. • Grade all deep tendon reflexes as follows: 0, absent; +, diminished; ++, normal; +++, increased; ++++, hyperactive or clonic. Record the reflex grade on a stick figure. • Facilitate deep tendon reflex testing by having the client perform isometric muscle contractions.	• Brisk elbow flexion; ++ bilaterally
Triceps reflex	• Tap the reflex hammer directly on the triceps tendon at its insertion point. Note elbow and triceps muscle movement. The triceps reflex should appear by age 6 months.	• Brisk elbow extension and triceps muscle contraction; ++ bilaterally
Brachioradialis (supinator) reflex	• Tap the reflex hammer on the styloid process of the radius 1" to 2" (2.5 to 5 cm) above the wrist. Note elbow, forearm, finger, and hand movement.	• Elbow flexion, forearm supination, and finger and hand flexion; ++ bilaterally
Quadriceps (knee-jerk or patellar) reflex	• Tap the patellar tendon with the reflex hammer. Note knee and quadriceps movement. • The quadriceps reflex should be present at birth; it may be decreased in an elderly client.	• Knee extension and quadriceps contraction; ++ bilaterally
Achilles (ankle-jerk) reflex	• Tap the Achilles tendon with the reflex hammer. Note foot movement. The Achilles reflex should appear by age 4 months; it may be diminished or absent in an elderly client.	• Plantar flexion followed by muscle relaxation; ++ bilaterally
Advanced assessment skills: Superficial reflexes		
Pharyngeal (gag) reflex	• Touch posterior wall of the pharynx with a tongue depressor. Note client's response.	• Gagging

continued

Skills laboratory guide: Physical assessment *continued*

NEUROLOGIC FUNCTION	SPECIAL CONSIDERATIONS	NORMAL FINDINGS
Advanced assessment skills: Superficial reflexes *continued*		
Abdominal reflex	• Stroke each side of the client's upper and lower abdomen. • Note umbilicus and abdominal muscle movement. The abdominal reflex should appear by age 6 months; it may be decreased or absent in an elderly client. • Grade the following superficial reflexes as follows: 0, absent; +, normal. Record the reflex grade on a stick figure.	• Umbilicus deviation toward stimulated side and abdominal muscle contraction; + abdominal reflex
Cremasteric reflex	• Assess this reflex in males only. • Scratch each inner thigh with a tongue depressor. Note testicular movement.	• Testicular elevation; + cremasteric reflex
Anal reflex	• Scratch side of anus with a blunt instrument. Note anal puckering.	• Anal puckering; + anal reflex
Bulbocavernous reflex	• Assess this reflex in males only. • Gently pinch the foreskin or glans. Note bulbocavernous muscle movement.	• Bulbocavernous muscle contraction; + bulbocavernous reflex
Pathologic reflexes		
Grasp reflex	• Stimulate the client's palm with your fingers. Note hand grasping.	• No grasp reflex
Sucking reflex	• Stimulate the client's lips with a mouth swab. Note sucking movement.	• No sucking reflex
Snout reflex	• Gently percuss the oral area with your fingers. Note lip puckering.	• No snout reflex
Babinski reflex	• Stroke the lateral aspect of the client's sole. Note toe dorsiflexion and fanning.	• No Babinski reflex
Vital sign measurements		
Vital signs	• Note temperature, pulse, respirations, and blood pressure.	• All vital signs within normal ranges for client's age

Answer
• Cranial nerves II, III, IV, and VI are the key cranial nerves to assess because they are the most vulnerable to the effects of increasing ICP, which may occur if this client develops intracranial bleeding or edema from cerebral contusions. Because a client who is restless, disoriented, or unconscious is at risk for aspiration, the nurse should check the gag reflex, which is controlled by cranial nerves IX and X.
• Optic nerve (CN II). Assess the optic disc and response to light. A raised or bulging optic disc (papilledema) or tortuous or distended retinal venules signal increased ICP.
• Oculomotor nerve (CN III). Assess pupil size, shape, and response to light. Changes in these factors may indicate increased ICP and impending cerebral herniation. Also, establishing the client's baseline pupil status allows accurate interpretation of future observations.
• Oculomotor nerve (CN III), trochlear nerve (CN IV), and abducens nerve (CN VI). Assess extraocular eye move-

ments. Impaired extraocular eye movements may indicate brain stem compression related to increased ICP and impending brain herniation.

2. Joseph Jones, age 83, is a farmer from rural North Carolina. Over the past two months, Mr. Jones's family has become concerned over subtle changes in his behavior. They brought him to the clinic, where he is now being evaluated.

According to the health history, Mr. Jones has had no formal education beyond the second grade. Although he needs a complete mental status examination (MSE), you realize that the usual MSE will need to be adapted to the client's socioeconomic and educational background to elicit meaningful information.

How would you modify each of the following aspects of the complete MSE for Mr. Jones's assessment? What questions or procedures would you use to test each of the cognitive functions listed below?
• vocabulary

- general knowledge
- abstract reasoning
- calculations
- attention span.

Answer
- Vocabulary. Ask Mr. Jones to define words with which he would be familiar as a farmer in a rural area. Progress from common words to less familiar ones—for example: seed, road, field, tractor, thunder, plough, drought, harvest, surplus, commodity.
- General knowledge. Avoid questions that require formal learning, such as capitals of foreign countries, remote historical facts, or abstract scientific principles. Instead, choose questions that relate to Mr. Jones's life experience. For example:
—At what temperature does the pond freeze?
—What is the warmest season of the year?
—What is daylight saving time?
—What is the capital of North Carolina?
—What is the name of the ocean at the North Carolina coast?
- Abstract reasoning. Avoid using proverbs. Instead, ask the client to identify similarities. For example:
—How are dogs and cats alike?
—How are tobacco and cigarettes alike?
—How are seeds and sand alike?
—You also might ask Mr. Jones to interpret some local names with abstract meanings; for example, Why are the Smoky Mountains called "smoky"?
- Calculations. Have Mr. Jones perform calculations he might use on a typical day. For example, ask, "If your groceries cost $9.75 and you give the clerk $10, how much change should you get?"
- Attention span. Because Mr. Jones's formal mathematical education is limited, avoid using mathematical tests of attention span. Instead, use lists that are familiar to him. For example, you might say, "Starting with December, name the months of the year backwards," or "Beginning with a, tell me the letters of the alphabet skipping every other letter. Here's the start: a-c-e. Now you tell me the rest."

3. You are performing a complete assessment of Mary Kelly, age 93. You know that nervous system anatomy and physiology change with age, which, in turn, affects neurologic function.

When assessing the following neurologic functions, what normal changes would you expect to see in this client?
- proprioception (position) sense
- vibration sense
- auditory acuity
- superficial abdominal reflexes
- pupil size
- muscle size
- muscle strength

- recent memory
- coordination
- sense of taste.

Answer
- Proprioception. Diminished or absent in the feet and ankles.
- Vibration sensation. Diminished or absent in the feet and ankles.
- Auditory acuity. Decreased.
- Superficial abdominal reflexes. Decreased or absent.
- Pupil size. Decreased.
- Muscle size. Decreased bilaterally and symmetrically.
- Muscle strength. Decreased.
- Recent memory. Relatively intact.
- Coordination. Movements even and rhythmic. (An elderly client will perform rapid alternating movements more slowly and less easily than a young client.)
- Sense of taste. Diminished. (Loss of taste buds is a normal consequence of aging.)

4. Mrs. Wilkins brings her daughter Beth, age 14, to the hospital for evaluation of difficulty walking. Beth's gait is unsteady, she cannot walk without assistance, and her mother reports that she has already fallen twice at home. At this time, the etiology of Beth's problem is unknown.

Which five specific aspects of a complete nervous system assessment are especially important to emphasize when evaluating Beth?

Answer
- Muscle size. Weakness usually accompanies the decreased muscle mass that is associated with neuromuscular degenerative disorders, myopathies, neuropathies, or disuse.
- Extremity strength and movement. Weakness or difficulty moving a leg may alter the gait. Altered strength and movement can result from disorders of the CNS upper motor neurons (stroke, tumor, cerebral or spinal cord trauma) or from disorders of the PNS lower motor neurons (neuropathies, Guillain-Barré syndrome, amyotrophic lateral sclerosis). Movement disorders caused by extrapyramidal tract dysfunction (such as Parkinson's disease) typically affect leg movement, posture, and muscle tone, ultimately impairing gait.
- Acoustic nerve (CN VIII). Disorders of the vestibular branch impair balance, which can cause an unsteady gait.
- Reflexes. Reflex impairment can alter gait. Hyperactive lower extremity reflexes can cause a spastic gait; decreased lower extremity reflexes produce footdrop.
- Proprioception. Loss of proprioception impairs detection of a body part in relation to other body parts, which can impair gait.

5. Elizabeth Jamison, age 37, is the mother of two small children and the vice president of a branch office of a well-known bank. She has been experiencing recurrent severe headaches lasting 18 to 36 hours, usually accompanied by nausea and dizziness. Most distressing to her is that the headaches make work and care of her children impossible. How would you document the following information related to your assessment of Mrs. Jamison?
• history (subjective) assessment data
• physical (objective) assessment data
• assessment techniques and any special equipment
• two appropriate nursing diagnoses
• documentation of your findings.

Answer
History (subjective) assessment data
• Client complains of recurrent, severe headaches, accompanied by nausea and dizziness.
• Client reports headaches one or more times a week. Each one lasts 18 to 36 hours.
• Client reports headaches make work and child care impossible.
Physical (objective) assessment data
• Female, age 37
• Alert and oriented to person, place, and time; concentration, memory, calculation skills, abstract reasoning, and judgment intact; no language expression or comprehension deficit; appears tense; speech rapid
• Cranial nerves II through XII intact
• Extremities are strong and move on command; no abnormal movements; gait stable; negative Romberg; performs rapid alternating movements easily; right-handed
• Light touch, superficial pain, vibration, and position sensations intact; stereognosis intact (correctly identifies coin as heads or tails); temperature not tested
• Deep tendon and superficial reflexes present
Assessment techniques and equipment
• Interview the client regarding past and family health history, coping strategies and stress, role and relationship patterns, and occupational health patterns.
• Observe client to assess cerebral functioning.
• Assess cranial nerves.
• Assess muscle strength, arm and leg movement, balance and coordination, and gait.
• Evaluate light touch, pain, vibration sensation, and stereognosis.
• Test reflexes using reflex hammer.
• Equipment should include a penlight, cotton, a sharp object, pungent-smelling substances, test tubes, salt, sugar, a sour substance, a bitter substance, tongue depressors, a coin, a paper clip, a reflex hammer, a tuning fork, and an ophthalmoscope.
Two appropriate nursing diagnoses
• Pain related to recurrent, severe headaches
• Altered role performance related to disabling effects of migraine headache

Documentation of findings
• S—Client complains of recurrent, severe headaches lasting 18 to 36 hours accompanied by dizziness and nausea. Client reports that headaches interfere with work and child care.
• O—Alert and oriented to person, place, and time; cranial nerves II through XII intact; no visual field deficit apparent; motor and sensory system intact; reflex activity normal
• A—Pain related to recurrent, severe headaches

Questions, answers, and rationales

1. Jane Bryant, age 29, seeks care for recurrent headaches. During the health history, the nurse obtains a complete description of the headaches. Which ones may be an early warning sign of a brain tumor?
(a) Cluster headaches
(b) Migraine headaches
(c) Early morning headaches
(d) Late evening headaches
Correct answer: (c), see text page 471. Early morning headaches that are present upon awakening and disappear after arising may be an early warning sign of a brain tumor.

2. Which history question helps assess cerebral function?
(a) "How would you describe your eyesight?"
(b) "Have you noticed a change in your ability to remember?"
(c) "Have you noticed a change in your muscle strength?"
(d) "Have you noticed a change in your coordination?"
Correct answer: (b), see text page 471. All of these questions assess neurologic function, but asking about memory specifically assesses cerebral function.

3. Ms. Bryant undergoes a complete neurologic examination, including cranial nerve assessment. When evaluating the trigeminal nerve (CN V), the nurse assesses which reflex?
(a) Corneal reflex
(b) Corneal light reflex
(c) Gag reflex
(d) Cough reflex
Corrrect answer: (a), see text page 488. The nurse assesses the sensory portion of the trigeminal nerve by testing sensation on the face and head and assessing the corneal reflex.

4. To assess the motor portion of the facial nerve (CN VII), the nurse should ask the client to perform which action?
(a) Swallow
(b) Clench the jaws
(c) Raise and lower the eyebrows
(d) Raise the shoulders against resistance
Correct answer: (c), see text page 489. The nurse assesses the motor portion of the facial nerve by asking the client to wrinkle the forehead, raise and lower the eyebrows, smile to show teeth, and puff out the cheeks.

5. When assessing the vagus nerve (CN X), the nurse evaluates which other cranial nerve?
(a) Facial (CN VII)
(b) Acoustic (CN VIII)
(c) Glossopharyngeal (CN IX)
(d) Hypoglossal (CN XII)
Correct asnwer: (c), see text page 489. The glossopharyngeal (CN IX) and vagus (CN X) nerves are assessed together because they have overlapping functions.

6. Which cranial nerve controls the pupillary response?
(a) CN II
(b) CN III
(c) CN IV
(d) CN V
Correct answer: (b), see text page 488. The oculomotor nerve (CN III) controls pupil size, pupil shape, and pupillary response to light.

7. Leonard Carpenter, age 48, has a degenerative cerebellar disorder. Which health history question helps assess cerebellar function?
(a) "Do you have problems with balance?"
(b) "Have you noticed any change in your muscle strength?"
(c) "Do you have difficulty speaking or expressing yourself?"
(d) "Do you have any difficulty swallowing?"
Correct answer: (a), see text page 472. Poor balance implies a cerebellar disorder or impairment of the vestibular portion of cranial nerve VIII.

8. Which assessment finding usually is associated with cerebellar dysfunction?
(a) Ataxia
(b) Anosmia
(c) Aphasia
(d) Paresthesia
Correct answer: (a), see text page 472. An impaired gait (ataxia) is the primary sign of cerebellar dysfunction.

9. Which assessment finding would be abnormal in Mr. Carpenter, but normal in a child under age 6?
(a) Shuffling gait
(b) Wide-based gait
(c) Scissors gait
(d) Ataxic gait
Correct answer: (b), see text page 492. A child normally has a wide-based gait until age 6. A wide-based gait after that age could indicate a neuromuscular or cerebellar disorder.

10. To evaluate Mr. Carpenter's balance, the nurse should assess his ability to perform which activity?
(a) Tandem-gait walking
(b) Point-to-point localization
(c) Rapid alternating movements
(d) Leg coordination
Correct answer: (a), see text page 493. To assess balance, the nurse should have the client perform tandem-gait (heel-to-toe) walking, the Romberg test, and heel and toe walking.

11. To perform the Romberg test, the nurse should give Mr. Carpenter which instructions?
(a) "With your feet together and arms at your sides, try to hold your balance with your eyes open. Now do it with them closed."
(b) "First, walk on your heels across the room. Now walk on your toes to come back."
(c) "Use the thumb of one hand to touch each finger on that hand. Now do the same thing on the other hand."
(d) "Lie flat on your back. Now slide your heel down the shin of the opposite leg, moving slowly from the knee to the ankle."
Correct answer: (a), see text page 493. In the Romberg test, the nurse has the client stand with feet together, arms at sides, and without support. Then the nurse observes the client's ability to maintain balance with both eyes open and with them closed.

12. George Johnson, age 57, is admitted to intensive care unit with a head injury caused by an automobile accident. To assess Mr. Johnson's level of consciousness, the nurse should use which stimulus *first*?
(a) Olfactory
(b) Auditory
(c) Tactile
(d) Painful
Correct answer: (b) see text page 478. When assessing level of consciousness, the nurse always starts with a minimal (auditory) stimulus, increasing its intensity, as needed.

13. What is the best technique to test a response to painful stimuli?
(a) Stick the client with a pin.
(b) Pinch the Achilles tendon.
(c) Apply supraorbital pressure.
(d) Rub the sternum.
Correct answer: (b), see text page 478. Techniques to test response to painful stimuli include application of firm pressure over a nailbed or a firm pinch of the Achilles tendon.

14. The nurse uses the Glasgow Coma Scale in Mr. Johnson's neurologic assessment. What does this tool assess?
(a) Muscle strength
(b) Cerebellar function
(c) Range of motion
(d) Level of consciousness
Correct answer: (d), see text page 480. The Glasgow Coma Scale is used to assess level of consciousness. It rates the client's eye, motor, and verbal responses.

15. To assess for increasing ICP, the nurse should assess which key cranial nerves?
(a) CN II, III, IV, and VI
(b) CN I, V, VII, and IX
(c) CN V, VIII, XI, and XII
(d) CN IX, X, XI, and XII
Correct answer: (a), see text page 486. Because of their anatomic locations, the optic (CN II), oculomotor (CN III), trochlear (CN IV), and abducens (CN VI) nerves are most vulnerable to the effects of increasing ICP.

16. The nurse also assesses Mr. Johnson's orientation to time. A bizarre response, such as "The year 2020," may suggest which disorder?
(a) Increased intracranial pressure
(b) Psychiatric disorder
(c) Alzheimer's disease
(d) Early senility
Correct answer: (b), see text page 480. Bizarre answers, such as 1756 or 2020, may indicate a possible psychiatric disturbance or simple uncooperativeness.

17. Why does the nurse assess Mr. Johnson's deep tendon reflexes (DTRs) and other reflexes?
(a) To assess muscle strength
(b) To assess spinal cord intactness
(c) To assess the tendons
(d) To assess dermatome sensitivity
Correct answer: (b), see text page 498. Reflex assessment helps evaluate the intactness of specific cervical, thoracic, lumbar, and sacral spinal segments.

18. What is the normal response to biceps reflex assessment?
(a) Elbow flexion
(b) Elbow extension
(c) Forearm supination
(d) Hand pronation
Correct answer: (a), see text page 498. Assessment of the biceps reflex should elicit brisk elbow flexion that is visible and palpable.

19. What is the normal response to Achilles reflex assessment?
(a) Plantar flexion
(b) Dorsiflexion
(c) Foot eversion
(d) Toe fanning
Correct answer: (a), see text page 499. Assessment of the Achilles reflex should elicit plantar flexion followed by muscle relaxation.

20. The nurse has difficulty eliciting some DTRs in Mr. Johnson. To facilitate reflex testing of the arms, the nurse should give him which instruction?
(a) "Flex your arms."
(b) "Clasp your hands together."
(c) "Make a fist."
(d) "Clench your teeth."
Correct answer: (d), see text page 502. To improve arm reflex response, the nurse should have the client clench his teeth or squeeze one thigh with the hand not being evaluated.

21. Robert Howard, age 57, takes isoniazid as prescribed for tuberculosis. This drug is associated with which adverse neurologic effect?
(a) Nervousness
(b) Lightheadedness
(c) Speech disturbances
(d) Peripheral neuropathy
Correct answer: (d), see text page 473. Isoniazid and nitrofurantoin may cause peripheral neuropathy as an adverse reaction.

22. Alma Blackburn, age 75, is admitted to the medical unit with speech disturbance and weakness on her right side. The nurse assesses this elderly client thoroughly. Which normal age-related changes may affect Ms. Blackburn's orientation?
(a) Decreased visual and auditory acuity
(d) Decreased attention span
(c) Decreased ability to remember
(d) Decreased intellectual ability
Correct answer: (a), see text page 481. Decreased visual and auditory acuity related to aging can prevent the elderly client from properly recognizing or interpreting stimuli in the hospital environment.

23. The nurse performs a mental status screening of Ms. Blackburn. Which question may the nurse use to assess recent memory?
(a) "When is your birthday?"
(b) "Where were you born?"
(c) "What did you have for breakfast?"
(d) "What was your mother's maiden name?"
Correct answer: (c), see text page 481. This question is best for assessing recent memory; the others are better for testing remote memory.

24. To assess Ms. Blackburn's response to vibration, where should the nurse place a vibrating tuning fork?
(a) On a bony prominence
(b) On a tendon
(c) On a muscle
(d) On a dermatome
Correct answer: (a), see text page 496. If the client does not respond to a vibrating tuning fork on an interphalangeal joint, the nurse tests the next most proximal bony prominence.

25. The nurse should consider which finding normal in a client of Ms. Blackburn's age?
(a) Increased pain perception in the arms
(b) Increased temperature perception in the legs
(c) Decreased proprioception in the legs
(d) Decreased vibration sensation in the arms
Correct answer: (c), see text page 495. In an elderly client vibration sensation and proprioception may diminish or disappear in the distal lower extremities.

Test bank for Chapter 17, Nervous System

1. Jane Bryant, age 29, seeks care for recurrent headaches. During the health history, the nurse obtains a complete description of the headaches. Which ones may be an early warning sign of a brain tumor?
(a) Cluster headaches
(b) Migraine headaches
(c) Early morning headaches
(d) Late evening headaches

2. Which history question helps assess cerebral function?
(a) "How would you describe your eyesight?"
(b) "Have you noticed a change in your ability to remember?"
(c) "Have you noticed a change in your muscle strength?"
(d) "Have you noticed a change in your coordination?"

3. Ms. Bryant undergoes a complete neurologic examination, including cranial nerve assessment. When evaluating the trigeminal nerve (CN V), the nurse assesses which reflex?
(a) Corneal reflex
(b) Corneal light reflex
(c) Gag reflex
(d) Cough reflex

4. To assess the motor portion of the facial nerve (CN VII), the nurse should ask the client to perform which action?
(a) Swallow
(b) Clench the jaws
(c) Raise and lower the eyebrows
(d) Raise the shoulders against resistance

5. When assessing the vagus nerve (CN X), the nurse evaluates which other cranial nerve?
(a) Facial (CN VII)
(b) Acoustic (CN VIII)
(c) Glossopharyngeal (CN IX)
(d) Hypoglossal (CN XII)

6. Which cranial nerve controls the pupillary response?
(a) CN II
(b) CN III
(c) CN IV
(d) CN V

7. Leonard Carpenter, age 48, has a degenerative cerebellar disorder. Which health history question helps assess cerebellar function?
(a) "Do you have problems with balance?"
(b) "Have you noticed any change in your muscle strength?"
(c) "Do you have difficulty speaking or expressing yourself?"
(d) "Do you have any difficulty swallowing?"

8. Which assessment finding usually is associated with cerebellar dysfunction?
(a) Ataxia
(b) Anosmia
(c) Aphasia
(d) Paresthesia

9. Which assessment finding would be abnormal in Mr. Carpenter, but normal in a child under age 6?
(a) Shuffling gait
(b) Wide-based gait
(c) Scissors gait
(d) Ataxic gait

10. To evaluate Mr. Carpenter's balance, the nurse should assess his ability to perform which activity?
(a) Tandem-gait walking
(b) Point-to-point localization
(c) Rapid alternating movements
(d) Leg coordination

11. To perform the Romberg test, the nurse should give Mr. Carpenter which instructions?
(a) "With your feet together and arms at your sides, try to hold your balance with your eyes open. Now do it with them closed."
(b) "First, walk on your heels across the room. Now walk on your toes to come back."
(c) "Use the thumb of one hand to touch each finger on that hand. Now do the same thing on the other hand."
(d) "Lie flat on your back. Now slide your heel down the shin of the opposite leg, moving slowly from the knee to the ankle."

12. George Johnson, age 57, is admitted to intensive care unit with a head injury caused by an automobile accident. To assess Mr. Johnson's level of consciousness, the nurse should use which stimulus *first*?
(a) Olfactory
(b) Auditory
(c) Tactile
(d) Painful

13. What is the best technique to test a response to painful stimuli?
(a) Stick the client with a pin.
(b) Pinch the Achilles tendon.
(c) Apply supraorbital pressure.
(d) Rub the sternum.

14. The nurse uses the Glasgow Coma Scale in Mr. Johnson's neurologic assessment. What does this tool assess?
(a) Muscle strength
(b) Cerebellar function
(c) Range of motion
(d) Level of consciousness

15. To assess for increasing ICP, the nurse should assess which key cranial nerves?
(a) CN II, III, IV, and VI
(b) CN I, V, VII, and IX
(c) CN V, VIII, XI, and XII
(d) CN IX, X, XI, and XII

16. The nurse also assesses Mr. Johnson's orientation to time. A bizarre response, such as "The year 2020," may suggest which disorder?
(a) Increased intracranial pressure
(b) Psychiatric disorder
(c) Alzheimer's disease
(d) Early senility

17. Why does the nurse assess Mr. Johnson's deep tendon reflexes (DTRs) and other reflexes?
(a) To assess muscle strength
(b) To assess spinal cord intactness
(c) To assess the tendons
(d) To assess dermatome sensitivity

18. What is the normal response to biceps reflex assessment?
(a) Elbow flexion
(b) Elbow extension
(c) Forearm supination
(d) Hand pronation

19. What is the normal response to Achilles reflex assessment?
(a) Plantar flexion
(b) Dorsiflexion
(c) Foot eversion
(d) Toe fanning

20. The nurse has difficulty eliciting some DTRs in Mr. Johnson. To facilitate reflex testing of the arms, the nurse should give him which instruction?
(a) "Flex your arms."
(b) "Clasp your hands together."
(c) "Make a fist."
(d) "Clench your teeth."

21. Robert Howard, age 57, takes isoniazid as prescribed for tuberculosis. This drug is associated with which adverse neurologic effect?
(a) Nervousness
(b) Lightheadedness
(c) Speech disturbances
(d) Peripheral neuropathy

22. Alma Blackburn, age 75, is admitted to the medical unit with speech disturbance and weakness on her right side. The nurse assesses this elderly client thoroughly. Which normal age-related changes may affect Ms. Blackburn's orientation?
(a) Decreased visual and auditory acuity
(d) Decreased attention span
(c) Decreased ability to remember
(d) Decreased intellectual ability

23. The nurse performs a mental status screening of Ms. Blackburn. Which question may the nurse use to assess recent memory?
(a) "When is your birthday?"
(b) "Where were you born?"
(c) "What did you have for breakfast?"
(d) "What was your mother's maiden name?"

24. To assess Ms. Blackburn's response to vibration, where should the nurse place a vibrating tuning fork?
(a) On a bony prominence
(b) On a tendon
(c) On a muscle
(d) On a dermatome

25. The nurse should consider which finding normal in a client of Ms. Blackburn's age?
(a) Increased pain perception in the arms
(b) Increased temperature perception in the legs
(c) Decreased proprioception in the legs
(d) Decreased vibration sensation in the arms

18

Musculoskeletal System

Overview

Although musculoskeletal assessment usually is a small portion of the overall physical assessment, a complete assessment of this body system is necessary when the general assessment or history suggests a musculoskeletal problem. Chapter 18 prepares the nurse for either type of musculoskeletal assessment. After providing a brief overview of musculoskeletal anatomy and physiology, the chapter explains how to perform a complete health history and physical assessment, highlighting normal and abnormal findings and developmental considerations. It concludes by describing how to document assessment findings and integrate them into the nursing process. Here are the chapter highlights:

- The musculoskeletal system consists of skeletal muscles, ligaments, tendons, bones, cartilage, joints, and bursae.
- Because the health history is crucial to care plan formulation, the nurse must collect complete information for a client with a musculoskeletal complaint.
- Throughout the assessment, the nurse remains alert for findings not identified during the health history and asks additional questions as necessary.
- The nurse should conduct the musculoskeletal system physical assessment in a way that conserves client strength and ensures client comfort. It begins with general observations of the symmetry of shape, size, position, and movement of body parts. Finer evaluations of posture, gait, and coordination follow.
- Physical assessment continues with evaluation of muscle strength, mass, and tone.
- The nurse also assesses joint and bone characteristics, and then evaluates joint range of motion (ROM).

- Specific musculoskeletal problems, such as scapular winging or meniscal tears in the knee, require advanced assessment skills.
- To complete the musculoskeletal system assessment, the nurse evaluates relevant laboratory test results.
- Finally, the nurse documents all assessment findings and uses them in the nursing process to plan, implement, and evaluate the client's care.
- For more information about musculoskeletal system assessment, see pages 86PG through 92PG of the Photo Gallery in the text.

Suggested lecture topics

- Using audiovisual aids, review the anatomy and physiology of the musculoskeletal system. (For visual aids, see pages 86PG to 87PG in the text.)
- Discuss health history questions important to musculoskeletal system assessment, explaining the reasons for asking them.
- Demonstrate how to inspect and palpate the musculoskeletal system, comparing normal and abnormal findings. (For visual aids, see pages 88PG to 90PG in the text.)
- Invite an orthopedic specialist to explain screening for early detection of musculoskeletal disorders.
- Invite a pediatric nurse practitioner to discuss normal and abnormal musculoskeletal assessment findings in infants, children, and adolescents. (For visual aids, see page 91PG in the text.)

Suggested critical thinking activities

• Pair the students and have them perform a musculoskeletal assessment, including health history and physical assessment, on each other.
• Have the students document their findings on the Skills Laboratory Assessment Guide.
• Have the entire class critique these findings.
• Using a case study of a client with a musculoskeletal problem, have the students develop a nursing care plan.

Student study questions and answers

The following study questions are taken from text pages 544 and 546 of Chapter 18, Musculoskeletal System. Their answers are based on information in that chapter.

1. After you have assessed 82-year-old Joseph Dolan, a Black retired accountant, your documented findings include:
• dorsal kyphosis of the thoracic spine
• short, shuffling walk
• right shoulder crepitus and pain with movement
• a weak (rating 3) effort resisting nurse's effort to push down on arms abducted to 90 degrees
• a hard, bony ridge on the left clavicle, 2″ (5 cm) lateral to the sternoclavicular joint.

For each physical finding, state whether the deviation from normal is related to developmental, sexual, or racial factors.

What are the anatomic and physiologic bases for each finding?

Answer
• Dorsal kyphosis is a developmental change that typically occurs with aging. As vertebrae lose height and the intervertebral discs narrow, the spinal curvature develops exaggerated convexity.
• Another developmental change, a gait with short steps and uneven rhythm also commonly occurs in elderly clients. Contributing factors include loss of muscle strength and coordination, poor vision, a fear of falling, and painful arthritic changes in the hip, knee, or ankle joints.
• Shoulder crepitus and pain on movement are common abnormal findings in elderly clients. Pain and crepitus typically result from roughened articular cartilages irritating nerve endings in the joint.
• Mr. Dolan's weak resistance to the nurse's effort indicates decreased deltoid muscle strength. Common in elderly clients, this abnormal finding may be caused by muscle atrophy from physical inactivity or inadequate nutritional intake to maintain muscle mass and strength.
• Asymmetrical size or contour of the clavicles, such as a bony ridge on the left clavicle, is an abnormal finding at any age. Such a finding may indicate a fracture.

Skills laboratory guide: Health history

To collect information about the client's musculoskeletal system, ask questions about health and illness patterns, health promotion and protection patterns, and role and relationship patterns. Sample questions from each category are listed below.

HEALTH AND ILLNESS PATTERNS

• Can you point to the area where you feel pain?
• How would you describe the pain; for instance, aching, burning, stabbing, or throbbing?
• When you have this pain, do you also have pain in any other location?
• When did this pain begin? What were you doing at the time?
• What activities seem to decrease or increase the pain?
• Do you have any other unusual sensations, such as tingling, with the pain?
• Will you describe your weakness? When did you first notice muscle weakness? Did it begin in the same muscles where you notice it now?
• When did you first notice swelling? Did you injure this area?
• When did the stiffness begin? Has stiffness increased or been constant?
• Is pain associated with the stiffness? Do you ever hear a grating sound?
• What methods have you tried to reduce the stiffness?
• Are you taking any prescription or over-the-counter drugs or using home remedies to treat the problem? If so, which ones, at what strengths, and for how long?
• Have you ever had any injury to a bone, muscle, ligament, cartilage, joint, or tendon?
• Have you ever had surgery or other treatment involving bone, muscle, ligament, cartilage, joint, or tendon?

HEALTH PROMOTION AND PROTECTION PATTERNS

• How much alcohol do you drink daily? How much coffee, tea, or other caffeine-containing beverages?
• Does your current problem ever prevent you from falling asleep, or does it awaken you during the night?
• Do you follow an exercise schedule? If so, describe it. How has your current problem affected your usual exercise routine?
• Have any of your usual activities, such as dressing, grooming, climbing stairs, or rising from a chair, become difficult or impossible for you?
• Are you now using, or do you think you would be helped by, an assistive device, such as a cane, walker, or brace?
• Do you supplement your diet with vitamins, calcium, protein, or other products?
• Do weather changes seem to affect the problem—for example, does pain increase in cold or damp weather?

ROLE AND RELATIONSHIP PATTERNS

• Has this problem adversely affected your hobbies, leisure pursuits, or social life?
• Do you feel stress because of your current problem?
• What effect, if any, does this problem have on your sexual relationship?

Skills laboratory guide: Physical assessment

This chart guides the student during assessment by identifying body areas, special considerations and techniques to be used, and normal findings.

BODY AREA	SPECIAL CONSIDERATIONS	NORMAL FINDINGS
Inspection		
Posture	• Note overall body symmetry and posture. • Note spinal curvature with client standing straight and bending forward from the waist. A toddler normally has an exaggerated lumbar concavity; an elderly client, an exaggerated thoracic convexity. An adolescent may exhibit lateral curvature. • Note knee position and symmetry. Genu valgum is common in the first year of walking. Genu varum is normal in children from ages 2 to 3½.	• Erect posture and symmetrical body • Midline spine without lateral deviation • Appropriate cervical, thoracic, lumbar, and sacral curvatures for client's age • Symmetrical knees that face forward and are less than 1″ (2.5 cm) apart
Gait	• Note phases of gait, cadence, stride length, base of support, posture, arm swing, and toeing in or out. A toddler or an elderly, obese, or pregnant client may have a wide support base; an elderly client, an uneven rhythm and short steps.	• Smooth, rhythmic gait with appropriate movement through all phases • Approximately 12″ stride length with a 2″ to 4″ base of support; erect posture with midline trunk, arms swung in opposition, and no toeing in or out
Coordination	• Note movement coordination and any involuntary movements, ataxia, spasticity, or tremors.	• Coordinated, smooth movements with no involuntary movements, ataxia, spasticity, or tremors
Inspection and palpation		
Muscle tone	• Palpate muscles at rest and during passive range of motion (ROM). Note muscle tone, consistency, tenderness, atony, hypotonicity, or hypertonicity.	• Soft, pliable muscles when relaxed; firm, nontender muscles when contracted • No atony, hypotonicity, or hypertonicity
Muscle mass	• Measure circumference of upper midarm, thigh, and calf at rest at same location on each side. Note atrophy or hypertrophy. Dominant side may be up to ½″ (1 cm) larger.	• Bilaterally equal circumferences with no atrophy or hypertrophy
Muscle strength	• Note the client's ability to perform active ROM against resistance for cervical spine and neck, shoulders, upper arms and elbows, wrists and hands, hips and pelvis, legs, knees, ankles and feet, and toes. Grade muscle strength on this scale: 0, no contraction; 1, slight contraction; 2, passive ROM without gravity; 3 to 4, active ROM with light-to-moderate resistance; and 5, active ROM with full resistance.	• In all muscle groups, 5 for active ROM with full resistance. • In all paired muscle groups, 5 for bilaterally equal resistance
Arms and legs	• Measure arm length and leg length. Bilateral differences in length should not exceed ⅜″ (1 cm).	• Bilaterally equal arm length • Bilaterally equal leg length
All joints and bones	• Note skin condition, ROM, pain, tenderness, deformity, crepitation, swelling, ankylosis, contractures, stability, erythema, warmth, and nodules.	• Intact skin over all joints and bones • Stable joints with full, active ROM bilaterally • No pain, tenderness, deformity, crepitus, swelling, ankylosis, contractures, erythema, warmth, or nodules
Cervical spine and neck joints	• Inspect cervical spine posteriorly, laterally, and anteriorly with client sitting or standing.	• Midline cervical spine and head • 45° flexion, 55° extension, 40° lateral bending, 70° rotation
Clavicles	• Note bone condition.	• Firm, smooth, continuous bone
Scapulae	• Note scapular location and symmetry.	• Placement over thoracic ribs 2 through 7 • Equal distance from medial scapular edges to midspinal line; no scapular winging
Ribs	• Note bone condition.	• Firm, smooth, continuous bone
Shoulders	• Note freedom of movement during ROM. Compare left side to right.	• 180° forward flexion, 50° to 60° backward extension, 180° abduction, 45° to 50° adduction, 90° internal and external rotation

Skills laboratory guide: Physical assessment *continued*

BODY AREA	SPECIAL CONSIDERATIONS	NORMAL FINDINGS
Inspection and palpation *continued*		
Upper arm and elbow	• Assess elbow joint contour and ROM.	• Smooth contour • 150° flexion, 90° supination and pronation
Wrists	• Check for Tinel's sign (an indicator of carpal tunnel syndrome) by tapping over the median nerve. • Assess joint ROM.	• No Tinel's sign • 70° hyperextension, 90° flexion, 20° radial deviation, 30° to 50° ulnar deviation
Fingers and thumbs	• Note Heberden's nodes and deformities, such as webbing or extra digits. • Assess joint ROM.	• No Heberden's nodes or deformities • 30° hyperextension, 90° flexion, 20° abduction between fingers, fingers touching in adduction
Thoracic and lumbar spine	• Note thoracic, lumbar, and sacral curvatures. • Assess joint ROM.	• Appropriate thoracic, lumbar, and sacral curvatures • 30° hyperextension, 75° to 90° flexion, 35° lateral bending, 30° rotation
Hips and pelvis	• Assess joint ROM. In an infant, the hips may rotate externally 60° to 175°. In an elderly client, the hips may be partially adducted and flexed and may have reduced ROM.	• 120° flexion, 45° to 50° abduction, 20° to 30° adduction, 30° hyperextension, 40° internal rotation, and 45° external rotation
Knees	• Note knee movements and assess joint ROM.	• Smooth knee movements • 120° to 130° flexion
Ankles and feet	• Note calluses or deformities. • Assess joint ROM. Forefoot adduction is common in neonates.	• No calluses or deformities • 20° hyperextension, 45° to 50° plantar flexion, 5° eversion and inversion, 10° abduction, 20° adduction
Toes	• Note calluses, bunions, and deformities. • Assess joint ROM.	• No calluses, bunions, or deformities • 40° hyperextension and flexion
Advanced assessment skills		
Joint ROM	• Use a goniometer to measure joint movement.	• See above for normal ROM in all joints
Spine	• Perform the straight leg test to detect herniated lumbar disk: raise the supine client's straightened leg with foot dorsiflexed. Note low back pain.	• Negative straight leg test bilaterally
Hip	• Perform the Thomas test, noting extended leg movement as client draws opposite knee to chest. • Perform the Trendelenburg test, noting levels of iliac crests as client balances on each foot.	• Negative Thomas test bilaterally • Negative Trendelenburg test bilaterally
Knee	• To detect fluid in the knee joint, test for bulge sign by pressing the area above the client's patella. • To assess ligament integrity, perform the drawer test. With client supine, flex and stabilize the knee. Gently attempt anterior and posterior movement. Then place one hand on the lower leg and the other over the fibula head and apply medial pressure. • To assess for torn meniscus (cartilage), perform the McMurray test. With client supine and the flexed knee stabilized, hold the heel and internally—then externally—rotate to full extension.	• Negative bulge sign bilaterally • Negative drawer test bilaterally • Negative McMurray test bilaterally

2. Jenny Nice, a 16-year-old Caucasian high school student, has an appointment at the outpatient clinic. Her reason for the visit is left arm pain.

List 10 questions you should ask Jenny to obtain a thorough history. How would you word these questions so that Jenny can understand them?

Answer

The nurse should word all health history questions in terms that are appropriate to the client's level of understanding and should avoid unfamiliar medical or technical terms. The

nurse should use the PQRST method to clarify the client's current musculoskeletal complaint and any others. Appropriate questions for Jenny would include:
• Can you show me exactly where your arm hurts?
• What does the pain feel like? For instance, does it burn or ache?
• Do you have any idea what is causing the pain?
• Do you have pain anywhere else; for instance, in your neck or back?
• Do you have any other unusual feelings in your arm or hand, such as weakness, numbness, or tingling?
• On a scale of 1 to 10, with 10 being the most and 1 the least, how would you rate your pain right now? What rating would you give your pain when it hurts the most?
• Does anything seem to make your arm hurt less or more?
• When did you first notice this pain? What were you doing at the time?
• Are you taking any medicine for this pain? If so, what are you taking and how long have you been taking it? Does this medicine help decrease the pain?
• Have you noticed other symptoms now or when your pain is at its worst? For instance, have you had a fever or noticed any rash since the pain began?

3. Michael Birdsong, a 35-year-old Native American psychiatrist, has just had a long leg cast removed after 4 months. The cast was applied after torn right knee ligaments were repaired. His stated concerns are: "I can't bend my knee as far as I used to, and I can't straighten it completely. My leg is stiff, sore, and weak. It feels like it won't support my weight." You need to obtain a baseline assessment before Dr. Birdsong begins physical therapy.

How would you document the following information related to your nursing assessment of Dr. Birdsong?
• history (subjective) assessment data
• physical (objective) assessment data
• assessment techniques and equipment
• two appropriate nursing disgnoses
• documentation of your findings.

Answer
History (subjective) assessment data
• Client complains that he cannot bend his knee or straighten it completely.
• Client reports that his right leg is "stiff, sore, and weak" and that it "feels like it can't support my weight."
Physical (objective) assessment data
• Male, age 35
• Long leg cast has just been removed
Assessment techniques and equipment
• Interview the client regarding current health status, past health status, sleep and wakefulness patterns, exercise and activity patterns, socioeconomic patterns, and social support.
• Observe knee position and overall posture.

• Assess gait and coordination.
• Inspect knee for swelling and discoloration.
• Palpate thigh and calf muscles bilaterally to assess muscle tone.
• Using a tape measure, measure circumference of the thigh and calf bilaterally to assess muscle mass.
• Test muscle strength of knee extensors bilaterally.
• Using a goniometer, measure knee extension and flexion.
Two appropriate nursing diagnoses
• Impaired physical mobility related to right knee pain, stiffness, and decreased range of motion
• Anxiety related to feeling that right leg will not support weight
Documentation of findings
• S—Client reports "I can't bend my knee as far as I used to, and I can't straighten it completely. My leg is stiff, sore, and weak. It feels like it won't support my weight."
• O—Decreased ROM in right knee; decreased muscle tone, mass, and strength in right leg
• A—Impaired physical mobility related to right knee pain, stiffness, and decreased range of motion

4. You have three clients who are to have selected body areas and characteristics assessed. The clients are Sandy Jones, age 2; George Hurd, age 30; and Agnes Friend, age 92. What findings would you expect for each in gait, posture, and arm and hand strength?

Answer
Gait
• Sandy's movements will rely on a wide support base, with her feet spaced more than 4″ (10 cm) apart. She may be knock-kneed.
• George's movements should be smooth and coordinated throughout the swing and stance phases of gait. His posture should be erect with approximately 2″ (5 cm) to 4″ (10 cm) between his feet as he walks.
• At age 92, Agnes's gait may have an uneven rhythm, a wide support base, and short steps.
Posture
• Lumbar concavity (lordosis) is common in children of Sandy's age. Knee deviations, such as genu valgum (knock-knees), may be present if Sandy has been walking for less than 1 year.
• George should exhibit a normal adult spinal curvature with a convex thoracic curvature and a concave lumbar curvature. The spine should be midline. The iliac crests, shoulders, and scapulae should be at the same level horizontally. When George bends over, his spine should be straight with no unilateral thoracic or flank prominence (hump).
• Agnes's spine should be straight in the upright and flexed (bent over) positions. Her iliac crests, shoulders, and scapulae should be at the same horizontal level. She may have

a normal adult curvature or a dorsal kyphosis (an exaggerated thoracic convexity), which is common in elderly clients.

Arm and hand strength
- Sandy should have a firm grasp bilaterally, as demonstrated by grasping the nurse's finger and by holding objects.
- For George, all muscles should have a strength rating of 5.
- Agnes's muscle strength may be less than 5 because of the decreased muscle mass and tone associated with decreased use and normal age-related atrophy.

5. For these clients, what differences would you plan in your overall examination and assessment techniques?

Answer
For all three clients, make sure the examination room is warm and private. Obtain a health history directly from George and Agnes (if her memory is intact). Direct Sandy's health history questions to her parent or guardian.

When assessing Sandy, use toys to prevent restlessness and to evaluate movement and strength. Plan to perform parts of the examination with Sandy on her parent's lap. Palpate tender areas last to gain her cooperation.

For George, perform a standard head-to-toe assessment, simultaneously evaluating the muscle and joint function of each body area. Divide the assessment into observation of posture, gait, and coordination and inspection and palpation of muscles, joints, and bones.

Expect to modify Agnes's physical assessment to conserve her energy. Conduct tests with Agnes seated or reclining whenever possible. Keep in mind that Agnes may move slowly and need rest periods between tests. Plan to ask more history questions, as needed, based on physical findings.

Questions, answers, and rationales

1. Tom Mooney, age 42, seeks care for low back pain. To assess spinal curvature, the nurse should inspect the spine with Mr. Mooney in which two positions?
(a) Sitting up and standing straight
(b) Lying supine and in a lateral recumbent position
(c) Standing straight and lying supine
(d) Standing straight and bending forward from the waist
Correct answer: (d), see text page 522. The nurse should inspect the spine with the client standing straight and bending forward from the waist with the arms relaxed and dangling.

2. The nurse assesses the range of motion (ROM) of Mr. Mooney's spine. Besides flexion, hyperextension, and lateral bending, spinal ROM includes which other movement?
(a) Rotation
(b) Circumduction
(c) Inversion
(d) Protraction
Correct answer: (a), see text page 531. Spinal ROM normally includes flexion (75° to 90°), hyperextension (30°), left and right lateral bending (35°) and left and right rotation (30°).

3. How can the nurse assess Mr. Mooney for a herniated disc?
(a) Assess iliac crest levels with the client on one foot.
(b) Compress the area just above the client's patella.
(c) Dorsiflex the foot while raising a straightened leg.
(d) Perform McMurray's test on each leg.
Correct answer: (c), see text page 538. The nurse raises the client's leg in a straightened position and dorsiflexes the foot. Pain during this maneuver indicates a herniated disc.

4. Joey Olivera, age 2, is brought to the clinic for a routine physical examination. When assessing his spine, the nurse may observe which normal developmental change?
(a) Kyphosis
(b) Lordosis
(c) Scoliosis
(d) Kyphoscoliosis
Correct answer: (b), see text pages 523 and 541. A toddler normally will have lumbar concavity (lordosis) when learning how to walk.

5. Which variation in gait is normal for a child of Joey's age?
(a) Shuffling gait
(b) Increased stride length
(c) Wide support base
(d) Toeing-in
Correct answer: (c), see text page 523. A toddler's gait normally involves a wide support base—that is, with feet wide apart.

6. Helen Moss, age 72, has osteoporosis. Which factor might have predisposed her to this musculoskeletal disorder?
(a) Large stature
(b) Inadequate calcium intake
(c) Late menopause
(d) Vigorous exercise
Correct answer: (b), see text page 540. Predisposing factors for osteoporosis include inadequate intake of calcium and Vitamin D, decreased estrogen levels, and small stature.

7. When assessing Ms. Moss, the nurse obtains a drug history. Use of which drug increases the risk of osteoporosis?
(a) Colchicine
(b) Diazepam
(c) Prednisone
(d) Furosemide
Correct answer: (c), see text page 519. Prednisone may cause adverse reactions, such as muscle weakness, muscle wasting, and osteoporosis.

8. When inspecting Ms. Moss's spinal curvature, the nurse is likely to note which age-related change?
(a) Scoliosis
(b) Lordosis
(c) Dorsal kyphosis
(d) Kyphoscoliosis
Correct answer: (c), see text page 523. A dorsal kyphosis (exaggerated convexity of the thoracic curvature) typically accompanies aging.

9. In an elderly client, such as Ms. Moss, which joint commonly displays reduced ROM?
(a) Hip
(b) Ankle
(c) Knee
(d) Finger
Correct answer: (a), see text page 541. A partially adducted and flexed hip joint commonly is noted in elderly clients, as is reduced ROM during rotation and hyperextension.

10. The nurse should use which instrument to measure joint ROM for Ms. Moss?
(a) Goniometer
(b) Skinfold calipers
(c) Tape measure
(d) Ruler
Correct answer: (a), see text page 541. To quantify joint ROM, the nurse uses a goniometer.

11. When assessing Ms. Moss, nurse measures her limbs. Where should the nurse measure arm length?
(a) From the humerus to the tip of the middle finger
(b) From the humerus to the wrist
(c) From the acromion process to the tip of the middle finger
(d) From the acromion process to the wrist
Correct answer: (c), see text page 525. Each arm should be measured from the acromion process to the tip of the middle finger.

12. Where should the nurse measure leg length?
(a) From the posterior superior iliac spine to the medial tibialis
(b) From the posterior superior iliac spine to the medial malleolus
(c) From the anterior superior iliac spine to the medial tibialis
(d) From the anterior superior iliac spine to the medial malleolus
Correct answer: (d), see text page 525. Each leg should be measured from the anterior superior iliac spine to the medial malleolus with the tape crossing at the medial side of the knee.

13. The nurse detects a difference in Ms. Moss's leg lengths. Which difference is normal?
(a) No difference
(b) 0.8 cm
(c) 1.2 cm
(d) 2.0 cm
Correct answer: (b), see text page 525. More than 3/8″ (1 cm) disparity in length between each limb is abnormal.

14. Margaret Mayer, age 42, has carpal tunnel syndrome. Which findings are associated with this disorder?
(a) Numbness and tingling of thumb, index, and middle fingers
(b) Hypertrophy of the thenar eminences
(c) Sharp pain over palm of hand
(d) Paralysis of hand
Correct answer: (a), see text page 540. Carpal tunnel syndrome may produce pain that worsens after manual activity or at night and numbness, burning, or tingling of the thumb, index, and middle fingers.

15. During Ms. Mayer's assessment, how does the nurse elicit Tinel's sign?
(a) Briskly tap over the palmar surface of the hand
(b) Briskly tap the wrist over the median nerve
(c) Briskly tap the proximal interphalangeal joint
(d) Briskly tap the thumb and then each finger
Correct answer: (b), see text page 537. A positive Tinel's sign (tingling sensations in the thumb, index, and middle finger), which is elicited by briskly tapping the client's wrist over the median nerve, may indicate carpal tunnel syndrome.

16. Joan Block, age 65, has degenerative joint disease of the right knee. To assess for effusion (fluid collection) in the knee joint, the nurse should use which test sign?
(a) Bulge test
(b) Thomas test
(c) Apley's test
(d) Trendelenburg test
Correct answer: (a), see text page 539. The nurse assesses for effusion by compressing the area just above the client's patella. If an effusion exists, a bulge will appear to the sides or below the patella, or in both places.

17. The nurse performs the drawer test on Ms. Block. What does this test assess?
(a) Range of motion
(b) Muscle strength
(c) Degree of edema
(d) Joint stability
Correct answer: (d), see text page 539. The drawer test assesses anterior, posterior, medial, and lateral knee stability.

18. After injuring his knee during a basketball game, Michael Brown, age 16, is brought to the emergency department. Assessment reveals that he has a positive McMurray's test. What does the finding indicate?
(a) Torn cartilage
(b) Effusion in the joint
(c) Bruised patella
(d) Joint instability
Correct answer: (a), see text page 539. A positive McMurray's test may indicate torn meniscus (curved fibrous cartilage in the knee).

19. Alice Green, age 35, has rheumatoid arthritis. Assessment reveals grade-4 muscle strength in her hands. What does this finding indicate?
(a) Partial paralysis
(b) Paresis
(c) Mild weakness
(d) Normal strength
Correct answer: (c), see text page 526. The nurse grades muscle strength on a scale of 0 (paralysis) to 5 (normal). Grade 4 indicates mild weakness.

20. Samuel Clark, age 71, has gouty arthritis. Gout is most likely to cause abnormal findings in which laboratory test?
(a) Urine uric acid
(b) Bence John protein
(c) Serum creatine phosphokinase
(d) Serum glutamic-pyruvic transaminase
Correct answer: (a), see text page 545. This test reflects the excretion of uric acid, which typically falls below normal in clients with gout.

Test bank for Chapter 18, Musculoskeletal System

1. Tom Mooney, age 42, seeks care for low back pain. To assess spinal curvature, the nurse should inspect the spine with Mr. Mooney in which two positions?
(a) Sitting up and standing straight
(b) Lying supine and in a lateral recumbent position
(c) Standing straight and lying supine
(d) Standing straight and bending forward from the waist

2. The nurse assesses the range of motion (ROM) of Mr. Mooney's spine. Besides flexion, hyperextension, and lateral bending, spinal ROM includes which other movement?
(a) Rotation
(b) Circumduction
(c) Inversion
(d) Protraction

3. How can the nurse assess Mr. Mooney for a herniated disc?
(a) Assess iliac crest levels with the client on one foot.
(b) Compress the area just above the client's patella.
(c) Dorsiflex the foot while raising a straightened leg.
(d) Perform McMurray's test on each leg.

4. Joey Olivera, age 2, is brought to the clinic for a routine physical examination. When assessing his spine, the nurse may observe which normal developmental change?
(a) Kyphosis
(b) Lordosis
(c) Scoliosis
(d) Kyphoscoliosis

5. Which variation in gait is normal for a child of Joey's age?
(a) Shuffling gait
(b) Increased stride length
(c) Wide support base
(d) Toeing-in

6. Helen Moss, age 72, has osteoporosis. Which factor might have predisposed her to this musculoskeletal disorder?
(a) Large stature
(b) Inadequate calcium intake
(c) Late menopause
(d) Vigorous exercise

7. When assessing Ms. Moss, the nurse obtains a drug history. Use of which drug increases the risk of osteoporosis?
(a) Colchicine
(b) Diazepam
(c) Prednisone
(d) Furosemide

8. When inspecting Ms. Moss's spinal curvature, the nurse is likely to note which age-related change?
(a) Scoliosis
(b) Lordosis
(c) Dorsal kyphosis
(d) Kyphoscoliosis

9. In an elderly client, such as Ms. Moss, which joint commonly displays reduced ROM?
(a) Hip
(b) Ankle
(c) Knee
(d) Finger

10. The nurse should use which instrument to measure joint ROM for Ms. Moss?
(a) Goniometer
(b) Skinfold calpers
(c) Tape measure
(d) Ruler

11. When assessing Ms. Moss, nurse measures her limbs. Where should the nurse measure arm length?
(a) From the humerus to the tip of the middle finger
(b) From the humerus to the wrist
(c) From the acromion process to the tip of the middle finger
(d) From the acromion process to the wrist

12. Where should the nurse measure leg length?
(a) From the posterior superior iliac spine to the medial tibialis
(b) From the posterior superior iliac spine to the medial malleolus
(c) From the anterior superior iliac spine to the medial tibialis
(d) From the anterior superior iliac spine to the medial malleolus

13. The nurse detects a difference in Ms. Moss's leg lengths. Which difference is normal?
(a) No difference
(b) 0.8 cm
(c) 1.2 cm
(d) 2.0 cm

14. Margaret Mayer, age 42, has carpal tunnel syndrome. Which findings are associated with this disorder?
(a) Numbness and tingling of thumb, index, and middle fingers
(b) Hypertrophy of the thenar eminences
(c) Sharp pain over palm of hand
(d) Paralysis of hand

15. During Ms. Mayer's assessment, how does the nurse elicit Tinel's sign?
(a) Briskly tap over the palmar surface of the hand
(b) Briskly tap the wrist over the median nerve
(c) Briskly tap the proximal interphalangeal joint
(d) Briskly tap the thumb and then each finger

16. Joan Block, age 65, has degenerative joint disease of the right knee. To assess for effusion (fluid collection) in the knee joint, the nurse should use which test sign?
(a) Bulge test
(b) Thomas test
(c) Apley's test
(d) Trendelenburg test

17. The nurse performs the drawer test on Ms. Block. What does this test assess?
(a) Range of motion
(b) Muscle strength
(c) Degree of edema
(d) Joint stability

18. After injuring his knee during a basketball game, Michael Brown, age 16, is brought to the emergency department. Assessment reveals that he has a positive McMurray's test. What does the finding indicate?
(a) Torn cartilage
(b) Effusion in the joint
(c) Bruised patella
(d) Joint instability

19. Alice Green, age 35, has rheumatoid arthritis. Assessment reveals grade-4 muscle strength in her hands. What does this finding indicate?
(a) Partial paralysis
(b) Paresis
(c) Mild weakness
(d) Normal strength

20. Samuel Clark, age 71, has gouty arthritis. Gout is most likely to cause abnormal findings in which laboratory test?
(a) Urine uric acid
(b) Bence John protein
(c) Serum creatine phosphokinase
(d) Serum glutamic-pyruvic transaminase

19

Immune System and Blood

Overview

Chapter 19 describes a complete assessment of the immune system and blood. Unlike other body systems, the immune system and blood are not composed of simple organ groups. The immune system consists of billions of circulating cells and specialized structures, such as lymph nodes, that are located throughout the body. The blood includes fluid and formed elements that circulate throughout the body. Because disorders of the immune system and blood can produce multisystemic and sometimes vaque signs and symptoms, the nurse must be prepared to assess these areas thoroughly. Here are the chapter highlights:

- The immune system, a complex network of specialized cells and organ tissues, recognizes and defends against attacks by foreign microorganisms. It preserves the body's internal environment by scavenging dead or damaged cells and by recognizing its own elements (self) as distinct from a foreign substance (nonself). Its three main defensive mechanisms are protective surface phenomena, general host defenses, and specific immune responses.
- Immune system organs include the bone marrow, lymph nodes, spleen, and accessory organs (tonsils, adenoids, appendix, thymus, and Peyer's patches).
- Protective surface phenomena include pH changes and defensive secretions at accessible entry sites.
- General host defenses are nonspecific, responding in the same way to all invaders. They stimulate phagocytosis and inflammatory responses.
- Specific immune responses exhibit memory for and response to specific microorganisms via humoral and cell-mediated immunity. Humoral immunity requires B cells; cell-mediated immunity requires T cells.

- Blood, a tissue composed of formed elements (blood cells) suspended in a fluid medium (plasma), transports gases, nutrients, wastes, and other substances to and from the body's cells and tissues.
- During hematopoiesis, the following cells develop from the multipotential stem cells in the bone marrow: erythrocytes (red blood cells, or RBCs), thrombocytes (platelets), and five kinds of leukocytes (white blood cells, or WBCs).
- RBCs contain hemoglobin, which allows them to transport oxygen and carbon dioxide. Antigens on RBC membranes determine blood group or type. The major blood groups are A, B, AB, and O. Blood of any type also may include the Rh antigen.
- Platelets contribute to hemostasis by controlling bleeding and maintaining intravascular integrity. Four major plasma components and several plasma and tissue factors participate in coagulation.
- WBCs play an important part in the body's defense against invasive microorganisms. Identified by their nuclear and cytoplasmic characteristics, WBCs are categorized as granulocytes (neutrophils, eosinophils, and basophils) and agranulocytes (monocytes and lymphocytes).
- Migratory and mainly phagocytic, granulocytes engulf, ingest, and digest foreign materials, or assist with this function. They constitute the body's first line of cellular defense.
- Monocytes are phagocytic and may be migratory or fixed. Outside the bloodstream in tissues that filter large amounts of body fluids, monocytes are called macrophages. They defend against invading organisms. Lymphocytes differentiate into B cells and T cells.
- Immune and blood disorders typically cause abnormal bleeding, lymphadenopathy, fatigue, weakness, fever, and

joint pain. The nurse should assess for these effects during the health history. Because immune and blood disorders can cause multisystem effects, the nurse also should evaluate effects on other body structures and systems.

- The health history should explore the client's medication history because over-the-counter (OTC) and prescription drugs can induce hematopoietic problems, blood dyscrasias, and impaired immune responses.
- Physical assessment of the immune system and blood should incorporate assessment of related body structures and systems, such as the skin and oral mucosa and the respiratory and nervous systems.
- The physical assessment also should include inspection and palpation of the superficial lymph nodes. Red streaks, palpable nodes, and lymphedema may indicate a lymphatic disorder; enlarged nodes suggest current or recent inflammation. Tender nodes usually indicate infection; hard or fixed nodes, malignant tissue. General lymphadenopathy can result from inflammation or a neoplastic disorder.
- To complete the assessment, the nurse reviews all laboratory test results—for example, blood and bone marrow studies and immunocompetence studies.
- Finally, the nurse documents all assessment findings and uses them in the nursing process to plan, implement, and evaluate client care.
- For more information about immune system and blood assessment, see pages 93PG through 100PG of the Photo Gallery in the text.

Suggested lecture topics

- Using audiovisual aids, review the anatomy and physiology of the immune system and blood, highlighting developmental variations. (For visual aids, see the transparency master *Structures of the immune system* and pages 93PG through 95PG in the text.)
- Discuss health history questions important to immune system and blood assessment, explaining the rationales for asking them.
- Using a live model, demonstrate how to assess the immune system and blood through inspection, palpation, and percussion. (For visual aids, see pages 96PG through 99PG in the text.)
- Compare normal and abnormal assessment findings for the immune system and blood. (For visual aids, see pages 96PG through 100PG in the text.)

Suggested critical thinking activities

- Ask the students to explain the function and diagram the drainage of a selected lymph node group.
- Pair the students and have them perform an immune system and blood assessment—including a health history and physical assessment—on each other.

Skill Laboratory guide: Health history

To collect information about the client's immune system and blood, ask questions about health and illness patterns, health promotion and protection patterns, and role and relationship patterns. Sample questions from each category are listed below.

HEALTH AND ILLNESS PATTERNS

- Have you noticed any unusual bleeding, for example, frequent nosebleeds or bruises?
- Have you noticed any bleeding from your gums?
- Have you noticed any rash or skin discolorations? If so, on which part of your body?
- Have you noticed any swelling in your neck, armpits, or groin?
- Do you ever feel tired? If so, are you tired all the time or only after exertion?
- Have you noticed any sores that heal slowly?
- Are you bothered by a persistent or recurrent cough or cold? Do you cough up sputum? Do you feel chest pain when you cough, breathe deeply, or laugh?
- Has your appetite changed recently? Do you experience nausea, flatulence, or diarrhea?
- Have you vomited recently? If so, how would you describe the vomitus?
- Have you noticed any blood in your bowel movements or have you had any black, tarry bowel movements?
- Have you noticed any change in how your urine looks or in your urination pattern?
- Have you recently suffered from emotional instability, headaches, irritability, or depression?
- Do you recall being seriously ill as a child or having a long illness requiring frequent visits to a physician?
- Have you ever had surgery? Have you had an organ transplant?
- Have you ever had a blood transfusion?
- How would you describe the health of your blood relatives?

HEALTH PROMOTION AND PROTECTION PATTERNS

- What is your typical daily diet? What types and amounts of food do you eat at each meal?
- Do you drink alcoholic beverages?
- How would you rate your stress level?
- Have you ever used intravenous (I.V.) drugs? If so, which ones and under what conditions?
- Have you ever been in military service? If so, when and where did you serve?
- What type of work do you do? In what kind of environment do you work?

ROLE AND RELATIONSHIP PATTERNS

- How supportive are your family members and friends?
- Are you sexually active? If so, are you involved in a monogamous relationship?
- Have you noticed any change in your usual pattern of sexual functioning? If so, can you describe this change?
- What is your sexual preference? Do you or have you engaged in anal intercourse?

Skills laboratory guide: Physical assessment

This chart guides the student during assessment by identifying body areas, special considerations and techniques to be used, and normal findings.

BODY AREA	SPECIAL CONSIDERATIONS	NORMAL FINDINGS
Inspection, palpation, percussion, auscultation		
General appearance	• Note general physical appearance, facial features, height, weight, posture, movements, gait, and vital signs.	• Well-groomed client in no acute distress • Appropriate appearance for client's stated age; appropriate facial expression • Erect posture with rhythmic gait, smooth movements, and no involuntary movements • Height, weight, and vital signs within normal limits for client's age and sex
Skin, hair, and nails	• Observe skin color and integrity, noting pallor, cyanosis, erythema, petechiae, and lesions. In a light-skinned client, check for petechiae in pressure areas, such as the elbows, waistline, and upper arms. In a dark-skinned client, check the oral mucosa and conjunctiva. • Note hair texture and distribution. • Note nail color, shape, and texture.	• Appropriate skin, hair, and nail color for client's race • No pallor, cyanosis, erythema, or petechiae • Intact skin with no lesions • Appropriate hair distribution with no alopecia • Pink, smooth, slightly convex nails with no clubbing
Head and neck	• Note color and condition of nasal mucosa, turbinates, oral mucosa, gums, and tongue.	• Pink nasal mucosa and turbinates with no lesions • Pink, moist, smooth, oral mucosa with no lesions • Pink, moist, slightly irregular gums with no spongy or edematous areas • Pink, slightly rough tongue
Eyes and ears	• Check fields of gaze and accommodation. • Note color of conjunctiva and sclera, and eyelid condition. • Check for aneurysms, hemorrhages, and vessel tortuosity during ophthalmoscopic examination. • Test gross hearing acuity. • Note tympanic membrane color and condition during otoscopic examination.	• Intact extraocular movements; positive accommodation • Pink conjunctiva; white sclera; no ptosis or eyelid inflammation • No aneurysms, hemorrhages, or tortuous vessels • Normal hearing bilaterally • Pearly gray, intact tympanic membrane with no bulging or retraction
Respiratory system	• Note respiratory rate and rhythm. • Percuss for resonance, noting dullness or hyperresonance. • Auscultate breath sounds.	• Respiratory rate and rhythm within normal limits for client's age • Resonance over lung tissue; no dullness or hyperresonance • Vesicular breath sounds throughout periphery of lung fields; no adventitious sounds
Cardiovascular system	• Note pulse rate and rhythm. • Palpate the point of maximal impulse (PMI). • Auscultate for extra heart sounds, murmurs, and rubs. • Note color of extremities and peripheral pulses.	• Appropriate pulse rate and rhythm for client's age; no tachycardia or dysrhythmias • PMI at 5th intercostal space (ICS), left midclavicular line (MCL); no displacement • No extra heart sounds, murmurs, or rubs • Warm extremities, colored to match the rest of the body • Symmetrical, regular peripheral pulses bilaterally
Gastrointestinal system	• Auscultate bowel sounds, noting any hyperactivity. • Percuss and palpate the liver, noting any enlargement. • Note color of anus. Defer internal rectal examination if platelet count is less than 50,000/mm^3.	• Normal bowel sounds in all 4 quadrants with no hyperactivity • Dullness over liver 2⅜" to 4¾" (6 to 12 cm) in right MCL • Nonpalpable, nontender liver; no hepatomegaly • Pink anus without inflammation or breaks
Urinary system	• Note urine color, clarity, and odor. • Note color, discharge from, or inflammation of urethral meatus.	• Clear, amber, slightly aromatic urine with no hematuria • Pink urethral meatus with no discharge or inflammation
Nervous system	• Note level of consciousness and mental status.	• Client alert and oriented to person, place, and time • No confusion, lethargy, seizures, or motor or sensory deficits

Skills laboratory guide: Physical assessment   *continued*

BODY AREA	SPECIAL CONSIDERATIONS	NORMAL FINDINGS
Inspection, palpation, percussion, auscultation *continued*		
Musculoskeletal system	• Note bone tenderness or pain, particularly in the sternum. • Note joint range of motion (ROM), particularly in the hand, wrist, and knee joints. • Palpate joints for tenderness, pain, and swelling.	• Full active ROM in all joints bilaterally • No joint or bone pain, tenderness, or swelling
Inspection		
Lymph nodes	• Note visible lymph node enlargement and overlying skin color of head, neck, axillary, epitrochlear, inguinal, and popliteal nodes. Look for erythema or increased vascularity.	• No visible nodes; no erythema or increased vascularity
Palpation		
Lymph nodes	• Palpate lightly with pads of the index and middle fingers over skin surface of head, neck, axillary, epitrochlear, inguinal and popliteal nodes. • Palpate head, neck, axillary, and epitrochlear nodes with client seated; inguinal nodes, with client supine; popliteal nodes, with client supine or standing. • Note size, shape, surface, consistency, symmetry, mobility, color, tenderness, temperature, pulsations, and temperature of palpable nodes. In children under age 12, lymph nodes are frequently palpable; in elderly clients, nodes decrease in size and number. • Transilluminate any abnormal lump. • Auscultate for bruits in pulsating nodes.	• No palpable nodes; no tenderness or heat • Superficial nodes, if palpable, should be less than 1⅛″ (3 cm), firm, oval or round, well defined, mobile, nontender, symmetrical, nonpulsating, and should have the same temperature as surrounding tissue.
Advanced assessment skills: Percussion and palpation		
Spleen	• Percuss the lowest ICS in the left anterior axillary line during normal breathing and during a deep breath. • Percuss in several directions from areas of tympany to areas of dullness. • Press inward below the left costal margin as the client takes a deep breath.	• Dullness to pecussion in the left upper quadrant between the 6th and 10th ribs; no change with inspiration • Nonpalpable, nontender spleen

• Have the students document their findings on the Skills Laboratory Assessment Guide. Then have the paired students critique each other's assessment techniques and findings.

• Using a case study of a client with an immune or blood disorder, have the students develop a nursing care plan.

Student study questions and answers

The following questions are taken from text page 585 of Chapter 19, Immune System and Blood. Their answers are based on information in that chapter.

1. What are the organs and tissues that make up the immune system? What are their functions?

Answer

• Central lymphoid organs—the bone marrow and thymus—play an important role in developing B cells and T cells, the primary cells of the immune system.

• Lymph nodes, most abundant in the head, neck, axillae, abdomen, pelvis, and groin, help remove and destroy antigens circulating in the blood and lymph.

• The spleen, located in the left upper abdominal quadrant beneath the diaphragm, gathers and isolates worn-out erythrocytes, stores blood and platelets, and filters and removes foreign materials, old cells, and cellular debris.

• Other lymphoid tissues—the tonsils, adenoids, appendix, and Peyer's patches (intestinal lymphoid tissue)—remove foreign materials and debris in much the same way as lymph nodes.

2. The body's first line of defense against microorganisms is a series of physical, chemical, and mechanical barriers known as protective surface phenomena. How would placement of an indwelling urinary catheter compromise this defense?

Answer

The urinary tract is sterile except for the distal end of the urethra and the urethral meatus. In this area, protective surface phenomena include urine flow, low urine pH, the immunoglobulin secretory IgA, and the bactericidal effects of prostatic fluid (in men), which inhibit bacterial colonization. A series of sphincters also protects the urinary tract by impeding bacterial migration. Placement of an indwelling urinary catheter eliminates the antibacterial effect of urine, keeps the sphincters open at all times, and provides a surface along which microbes can migrate.

3. How do normal lymph node palpation findings differ for a child under age 12, an adult, and an adult age 75?

Answer

In a child under age 12, the lymph nodes commonly are palpable, particularly in the cervical and inguinal areas, and may measure 3/8″ to 1⅛″ (1 to 3 cm). Moderate numbers of cool, firm, movable, painless nodes indicate past infection.

In a healthy adult under age 75, the lymph nodes usually are not palpable, unless the client is very thin.

In an adult over age 75, lymph nodes are smaller and fewer in number. They usually are not palpable unless the client is very thin.

4. Why is an individual with decreased circulating WBCs, particularly granulocytes, unable to manifest the characteristic signs and symptoms of infection?

Answer

Granulocytes—particularly neutrophils and basophils—play a vital role in the inflammatory response, the body's first cellular defense against infectious organisms. In response to invasion of organisms, basophils secrete heparin, histamine, and kinins. These substances promote vasodilation and increased capillary permeability, leading to increased blood flow to the affected tissues. Neutrophils and other granulocytes then migrate to the invasion site and phagocytize—engulf, ingest, and digest—the organisms. These processes produce the characteristic signs and symptoms of the inflammatory response: heat, redness, swelling, and pain. An insufficient level of circulating granulocytes compromises this response and thus masks the signs and symptoms of infection.

5. Ms. Polly Wagner, age 30, comes to the clinic this morning complaining of fatigue, weakness, and intermittent epistaxis (nosebleed), which is not active at present. You take her vital signs and find that her temperature is 100.2° F (38.9° C); pulse rate is 100 beats/minute; respiratory rate is 22 breaths/minute; and blood pressure is 96/64 mm Hg. The physician orders a complete blood count, which reveals a hemoglobin of 10 g/dl, a hematocrit of 29%, and a platelet count of 25,000/mm^3. How would you report the following information related to Ms. Wagner?
• history (subjective) assessment data
• physical (objective) assessment data
• assessment techniques and any special equipment used
• two appropriate nursing diagnoses
• documentation of your findings.

Answer

History (subjective) assessment data
• Female, age 30
• Complaining of fatigue, weakness, and intermittent nosebleeds

Physical (objective) assessment data
• T 100.2° F (38.9° C), P 100, R 22, BP 96/64
• Hemoglobin 10 g/dl, hematocrit 29%, platelet count 25,000/mm^3

Assessment techniques and equipment
• Interview the client about past health history, current health history, current medications, occupational patterns, and stress and coping patterns.
• Inspect the skin and mucosa for color, presence of petechiae and purpura, and open sores or nodules.
• Palpate lymph nodes for swelling and tenderness.
• Using a stethoscope, auscultate the precordium for heart sounds, and the abdomen for bowel sounds.
• Note respiratory rate and character, and the presence of adventitious breath sounds.
• Palpate and percuss the liver and spleen for enlargement and tenderness.
• Palpate the rectal vault with a gloved and well-lubricated index finger. Note sphincter tone and local inflammation or tenderness.

Two appropriate nursing diagnoses
• Potential for injury related to bleeding
• Impaired home maintenance management related to fatigue and weakness

Documentation of findings
• S—Female, age 30, complaining of fatigue, weakness, and intermittent nosebleeds
• O—T 100.2° F, P 100, R 22, BP 96/64. Hemoglobin 10 g/dl, hematocrit 29%, platelet count 25,000/mm^3
• A—Potential for injury related to bleeding

Questions, answers, and rationales

1. Louisa Bryant, age 72, has been receiving chemotherapy with cisplatin to treat ovarian cancer. During a regular visit, she tells the nurse that she has been having frequent nosebleeds. Which cells are primarily responsible for clotting?
(a) Erythrocytes
(b) Lymphocytes
(c) Thrombocytes
(d) Granulocytes
Correct answer: (c), see text page 551. Thrombocytes (platelets) protect vascular surfaces and aggregate to promote coagulation, which stops blood loss.

2. During the health history, the nurse assesses Ms. Bryant for problems associated with excessive bleeding. Which history question would elicit symptoms of anemia?
(a) "Do you have any joint pain?"
(b) "Do you ever feel tired and weak?"
(c) "Do you have any sores that will not heal?"
(d) "Have you noticed any change in skin texture?"
Correct answer: (b), see text page 560. Exertional fatigue and weakness suggest moderate anemia; constant or extreme fatigue and weakness suggest severe anemia.

3. The nurse assesses Ms. Bryant's skin for other signs of bleeding. Petechiae are most likely to occur in which area?
(a) Face
(b) Chest
(c) Waist
(d) Back
Correct answer: (c), see text page 560. Petechiae are most likely to occur where clothing constricts circulation, such as the waist and wrists.

4. The nurse also inspects Ms. Bryant's skin for signs of anemia. This hematologic disorder may cause which color change?
(a) Erythema
(b) Plethora
(c) Vitiligo
(d) Pallor
Correct answer: (d), see text page 567. Pallor may indicate anemia or another blood disorder that disrupts oxygen delivery.

5. Because the nurse suspects that Ms. Bryant has a clotting disorder and anemia, the nurse should defer which part of the physical assessment?
(a) Rectal examination
(b) Joint assessment
(c) Ophthalmoscopy
(d) Muscle strength assessment
Correct answer: (a), see text page 569. The internal examination of the anus and rectal vault should be deferred if the nurse suspects or knows that the client has a clotting disorder with insufficient platelets ($50,000/mm^3$) or granulocytes ($1,000/mm^3$).

6. The nurse reviews Ms. Bryant's laboratory test results. Which test would confirm a clotting disorder?
(a) Bone marrow aspiration
(b) Platelet count
(c) Erythrocyte fragility
(d) Leukocyte count
Correct answer: (b), see text page 579. This test assesses the number of platelets in a blood sample and evaluates the production of platelets, which are vital to clotting.

7. Chemotherapy with cisplatin may cause which other adverse reaction?
(a) Leukopenia
(b) Polycythemia
(c) Hypergammaglobulinemia
(d) Hypoprothrombinemia
Correct answer: (a), see text page 563. Antineoplastic agents, such as cisplatin, may cause leukopenia, granulocytopenia, thrombocytopenia, and anemia.

8. Frank Stanton, age 8, is brought to the emergency department (ED) with an allergic reaction to a bee sting. Which leukocytes respond to an allergic reaction?
(a) Eosinophils
(b) Neutrophils
(c) Monocytes
(d) Lymphocytes
Correct answer: (a), see text pages 548 and 551. Eosinophils, which are a type of phagocytic granulocyte, modulate allergic responses and defend against parasites.

9. Which leukocytes respond to an allergic reaction by releasing histamine?
(a) Eosinophils
(b) Neutrophils
(c) Basophils
(d) Lymphocytes
Correct answer: (c), see text pages 548 and 551. Basophils are granulocytes that release histamine and other vasoactive amines in acute allergic reactions.

10. Stan Green, age 32, is admitted to the hospital with pneumonia secondary to acquired immunodeficiency syndrome (AIDS). When inspecting Mr. Green's oral mucosa, the nurse is likely to see which sign of AIDS?
(a) Bleeding gums
(b) Lacy white plaques
(c) Gingival recession
(d) Tonsillar hypertrophy
Correct answer: (b), see text page 568. Lacy white plaques on the buccal mucosa may be caused by hairy leukoplakia, which is associated with AIDS.

11. The nurse assesses Mr. Green's superficial lymph nodes. Which technique should the nurse use to palpate these lymph nodes?
(a) Gently palpate using the pads of the index and middle fingers.
(b) Deeply palpate using the entire hand.
(c) Deeply palpate using bimanual technique.
(d) Lightly palpate using bimanual technique.
Correct answer: (a), see text page 572. To palpate superficial lymph nodes, the nurse should use the pads of the index and middle fingers, applying gentle pressure in a rotary motion.

12. Where should the nurse palpate to assess the preauricular lymph node?
(a) In front of the ear
(b) Under the mandible
(c) Behind the neck
(d) Behind the ear
Correct answer: (a), see text page 570. The nurse should assess the preauricular node by palpating in front of the client's ear.

13. Which lymph node may be palpated under the chin?
(a) Parotid
(b) Submental
(c) Mastoid
(d) Superficial cervical
Correct answer: (b), see text page 570. The submental node may be palpated under the chin.

14. Where should the nurse palpate to assess the posterior cervical lymph nodes?
(a) Along the anterior surface of the trapezius muscle
(b) Along the anterior surface of the sternocleidomastoid muscle
(c) Along the posterior surface of the scalene muscle
(d) Along the posterior surface of the omohyoid muscle
Correct answer: (a), see text page 570. The nurse may palpate the posterior cervical nodes along the anterior surface of the trapezius muscle.

15. Lori Arden brings her daughter Patty, age 5, to the physician's office to investigate a lump on her neck. Palpation detects a superficial cervical node that is nontender and movable, and measures 2 cm. What is the most likely cause of this finding?
(a) Acute infection
(b) Metastatic disease
(c) Past infection
(d) Developmental stage
Correct answer: (d), see text page 573. In a client under age 12, lymph nodes commonly can be palpated. Normally, these nodes measure 1 to 3 cm (about an inch or less) and are nontender and movable.

16. Which physical finding is abnormal in an adult, but may be normal in a child of Patty's age?
(a) Palpable spleen tip
(b) Tender inguinal nodes
(c) Pale conjunctivae
(d) Palpable tender liver
Correct answer: (a), see text page 575. Although the spleen must be enlarged approximately three times normal size to be palpable in an adult, the tip of the spleen normally may be palpable at the left costal margin in a child.

17. Marion Clark, age 74, has metastatic breast cancer. When palpating Ms. Clark's lymph nodes in the affected area, how should the nurse expect them to feel?
(a) Tender
(b) Round
(c) Movable
(d) Hard
Correct answer: (d), see text page 573. Metastasized cancer usually affects nodes unilaterally, causing them to become discrete, nontender, firm or hard, and fixed.

18. In a healthy elderly client, the lymph nodes normally display which age-related change?
(a) Increased number and size
(b) Decreased number and size
(c) Decreased number and increased size
(d) Increased number and decreased size
Correct answer: (b), see text page 575. Normally, the number and size of lymph nodes decrease with age as lymphoid capabilities decline and fatty degeneration and fibrosis take place.

19. Tom Castleberry, age 38, is admitted to the ED after an automobile accident in which he sustained blunt trauma to the abdomen. When assessing the spleen for enlargement, the nurse should percuss in which area?
(a) Left axillary line
(b) Right upper quadrant
(c) Left lower quadrant
(d) Epigastric area
Correct answer: (a), see text page 575. The nurse should percuss the lowest intercostal space in the left axillary line.

20. Percussion over the spleen normally elicits which sound?
(a) Tympany
(b) Dullness
(c) Resonance
(d) Hyperresonance
Correct answer: (b), see text page 575. On percussion, the spleen normally produces dullness.

21. Where should the nurse attempt to palpate the spleen?
(a) In the left lower quadrant
(b) Below the left costal margin
(c) Over the costal angle
(d) At the left axillary line
Correct answer: (b), see text page 575. The nurse should palpate below the left costal margin to attempt to assess the spleen.

22. During spleen palpation, which assessment finding is normal in an adult?
(a) Palpable spleen
(b) Palpable tip of spleen
(c) Palpable spleen during inspiration
(d) Nonpalpable spleen
Correct answer: (d), see text page 575. The spleen normally is not palpable; it must be enlarged approximately three times normal size to be palpable.

Test bank for Chapter 19, Immune System and Blood

1. Louisa Bryant, age 72, has been receiving chemotherapy with cisplatin to treat ovarian cancer. During a regular visit, she tells the nurse that she has been having frequent nosebleeds. Which cells are primarily responsible for clotting?
(a) Erythrocytes
(b) Lymphocytes
(c) Thrombocytes
(d) Granulocytes

2. During the health history, the nurse assesses Ms. Bryant for problems associated with excessive bleeding. Which history question would elicit symptoms of anemia?
(a) "Do you have any joint pain?"
(b) "Do you ever feel tired and weak?"
(c) "Do you have any sores that will not heal?"
(d) "Have you noticed any change in skin texture?"

3. The nurse assesses Ms. Bryant's skin for other signs of bleeding. Petechiae are most likely to occur in which area?
(a) Face
(b) Chest
(c) Waist
(d) Back

4. The nurse also inspects Ms. Bryant's skin for signs of anemia. This hematologic disorder may cause which color change?
(a) Erythema
(b) Plethora
(c) Vitiligo
(d) Pallor

5. Because the nurse suspects that Ms. Bryant has a clotting disorder and anemia, the nurse should defer which part of the physical assessment?
(a) Rectal examination
(b) Joint assessment
(c) Ophthalmoscopy
(d) Muscle strength assessment

6. The nurse reviews Ms. Bryant's laboratory test results. Which test would confirm a clotting disorder?
(a) Bone marrow aspiration
(b) Platelet count
(c) Erythrocyte fragility
(d) Leukocyte count

7. Chemotherapy with cisplatin may cause which other adverse reaction?
(a) Leukopenia
(b) Polycythemia
(c) Hypergammaglobulinemia
(d) Hypoprothrombinemia

8. Frank Stanton, age 8, is brought to the emergency department (ED) with an allergic reaction to a bee sting. Which leukocytes respond to an allergic reaction?
(a) Eosinophils
(b) Neutrophils
(c) Monocytes
(d) Lymphocytes

9. Which leukocytes respond to an allergic reaction by releasing histamine?
(a) Eosinophils
(b) Neutrophils
(c) Basophils
(d) Lymphocytes

10. Stan Green, age 32, is admitted to the hospital with pneumonia secondary to acquired immunodeficiency syndrome (AIDS). When inspecting Mr. Green's oral mucosa, the nurse is likely to see which sign of AIDS?
(a) Bleeding gums
(b) Lacy white plaques
(c) Gingival recession
(d) Tonsillar hypertrophy

11. The nurse assesses Mr. Green's superficial lymph nodes. Which technique should the nurse use to palpate these lymph nodes?
(a) Gently palpate using the pads of the index and middle fingers.
(b) Deeply palpate using the entire hand.
(c) Deeply palpate using bimanual technique.
(d) Lightly palpate using bimanual technique.

12. Where should the nurse palpate to assess the pre-auricular lymph node?
(a) In front of the ear
(b) Under the mandible
(c) Behind the neck
(d) Behind the ear

13. Which lymph node may be palpated under the chin?
(a) Parotid
(b) Submental
(c) Mastoid
(d) Superficial cervical

14. Where should the nurse palpate to assess the posterior cervical lymph nodes?
(a) Along the anterior surface of the trapezius muscle
(b) Along the anterior surface of the sternocleidomastoid muscle
(c) Along the posterior surface of the scalene muscle
(d) Along the posterior surface of the omohyoid muscle

15. Lori Arden brings her daughter Patty, age 5, to the physician's office to investigate a lump on her neck. Palpation detects a superficial cervical node that is nontender and movable, and measures 2 cm. What is the most likely cause of this finding?
(a) Acute infection
(b) Metastatic disease
(c) Past infection
(d) Developmental stage

16. Which physical finding is abnormal in an adult, but may be normal in a child of Patty's age?
(a) Palpable spleen tip
(b) Tender inguinal nodes
(c) Pale conjunctivae
(d) Palpable tender liver

17. Marion Clark, age 74, has metastatic breast cancer. When palpating Ms. Clark's lymph nodes in the affected area, how should the nurse expect them to feel?
(a) Tender
(b) Round
(c) Movable
(d) Hard

18. In a healthy elderly client, the lymph nodes normally display which age-related change?
(a) Increased number and size
(b) Decreased number and size
(c) Decreased number and increased size
(d) Increased number and decreased size

19. Tom Castleberry, age 38, is admitted to the ED after an automobile accident in which he sustained blunt trauma to the abdomen. When assessing the spleen for enlargement, the nurse should percuss in which area?
(a) Left axillary line
(b) Right upper quadrant
(c) Left lower quadrant
(d) Epigastric area

20. Percussion over the spleen normally elicits which sound?
(a) Tympany
(b) Dullness
(c) Resonance
(d) Hyperresonance

21. Where should the nurse attempt to palpate the spleen?
(a) In the left lower quadrant
(b) Below the left costal margin
(c) Over the costal angle
(d) At the left axillary line

22. During spleen palpation, which assessment finding is normal in an adult?
(a) Palpable spleen
(b) Palpable tip of spleen
(c) Palpable spleen during inspiration
(d) Nonpalpable spleen

20

Endocrine System

Overview

Because the endocrine system helps regulate important body functions, including tissue growth and development, reproduction, energy production, metabolism, and the ability to adapt to stress, endocrine dysfunction can produce a wide range of systemic signs and symptoms. To prepare the nurse to assess this complex body system, Chapter 20 describes endocrine anatomy and physiology, pertinent health history questions, appropriate physical assessment techniques, and relevant laboratory tests. Here are the chapter highlights:

- The endocrine system includes the pituitary gland, thyroid gland, parathyroid glands, adrenal glands, islets of Langerhans in the pancreas, gonads (ovaries and testes), thymus, and pineal gland.
- Hormones, the functional units of the endocrine system, regulate most major body functions and maintain homeostasis with nervous system actions mainly through the hypothalamus.
- Because endocrine system problems may affect any body system, the nurse should use a holistic approach when obtaining a health history.
- During the health history, the nurse should ask about medication use, which may indicate that the client is being treated for an endocrine disorder or that the client is using drugs that may affect hormone levels and cause endocrine dysfunction.
- Physical assessment of the endocrine system involves measuring the client's height, weight, and vital signs and using inspection, palpation, and auscultation.

- When inspecting a client with an endocrine problem, the nurse should focus on the client's general appearance, speech, and body development; skin, hair, and nails; head and neck; chest; genitalia; and extremities.
- If a thyroid disorder is suspected, the nurse should palpate and auscultate the thyroid gland.
- Laboratory studies used to assess endocrine function include electrolytes, blood chemistries, hematology and urine tests, and measurements of individual hormones.
- The nurse should use health history, physical assessment, and laboratory study data to develop a nursing care plan.
- For more information about endocrine system assessment, see pages 101PG through 104PG of the Photo Gallery in the text.

Suggested lecture topics

- Review endocrine system anatomy and physiology, including developmental variations. (For visual aids, see the transparency master *Structures of the endocrine system* and pages 101PG through 102PG in the text.)
- Discuss health history questions important to endocrine system assessment, explaining their rationales.
- Using a student, demonstrate thyroid palpation. (For visual aids, see page 103PG in the text.)
- Discuss normal assessment findings for an adult client and variations in pediatric, pregnant, and elderly clients.
- Discuss common abnormal findings for an endocrine system assessment. (For visual aids, see page 104PG in the text.)

Suggested critical thinking activities

- Pair the students and have them perform an endocrine assessment, including history and physical assessment, on each other.
- Have the students document their findings on the Skills Laboratory Assessment Guide. Then have them critique each other's assessment techniques and documentation.
- Using a case study of a client with an endocrine disorder, have the students develop a nursing care plan.

Student study questions and answers

The following study questions are taken from text page 608 of Chapter 20, Endocrine System. Their answers are based on information in that chapter.

1. Which glands make up the endocrine system? What are the major functions of each gland?

Answer

Endocrine system glands include the pituitary gland, thyroid gland, parathyroid glands, adrenal glands, pancreas, gonads (testes in males and ovaries in females), thymus, and pineal gland.

The anterior lobe of the pituitary gland produces six hormones: somatropin, thyroid stimulating hormone, adrenocorticotropic hormone, follicle-stimulating hormone, luteinizing hormone, and prolactin. The posterior pituitary stores and releases oxytocin and vasopressin. The thyroid gland produces the hormones thyroxine, triiodothyronine, and thyrocalcitonin. The parathyroids produce parathyroid hormone. The adrenal glands produce the catecholamines epinephrine and norepinephrine, the glucocorticoids cortisol, cortisone, and corticosterone as well as aldosterone, androgen, and estrogen. The pancreas produces insulin, glucagon, and somatostatin. The gonads produce testosterone in the male and the estrogens estrone and estradiol as well as progesterone in the female. The thymus produces thymosin and thymopoietin. The pineal gland produces melatonin.

2. What are five skin abnormalities that should alert you to possible endocrine disorders, and what specific endocrine disorders are usually associated with each abnormality?

Answer

Hyperpigmentation of joints, genitalia, buccal mucosa, palmar creases, recent scars, and sun-exposed body areas occurs with Addison's disease. Gray-brown pigmentation of the neck and axillae (acanthosis nigricans) may be associated with polycystic ovaries, growth hormone excess, or Cushing's syndrome. Dry, coarse, rough, and scaly skin can indicate hypothyroidism or hypoparathyroidism. Coarse,

---

Skills laboratory guide: Health history

To collect information about the client's endocrine system, ask questions about health and illness patterns, health promotion and protection patterns, and role and relationship patterns. Sample questions from each category are listed below.

HEALTH AND ILLNESS PATTERNS

- Do you feel tired, lethargic, or weak?
- Have you noticed any muscle twitching?
- Do you feel any numbness or tingling in your arms or legs?
- What was your growth pattern?
- Does anyone in your family have diabetes mellitus, thyroid disease, hypertension (high blood pressure), or elevated blood fats?
- Have you noticed any changes in your skin, such as acne, increased or decreased oiliness or dryness, or change in color?
- Have you ever had seizures?

HEALTH PROMOTION AND PROTECTION PATTERNS

- Have you been sleeping more or less than usual?
- What type of exercise do you engage in? How regularly do you exercise? Have you had any difficulty exercising lately?
- Have you been feeling under more stress lately? Can you talk about what may be causing this stress? Does your current problem seem to be related to this stress?
- What is your approximate yearly or monthly household income? Do you have health insurance?
- What type of work do you do? What are your normal work or school hours? Do you have enough time for breaks and meals?

ROLE AND RELATIONSHIP PATTERNS

- What is your image of yourself? Do you think that the problem you are experiencing will get better or worse? What bothers you most about your problem?
- Do you have family members or close friends that you can ask for help when you need it?

---

leathery, moist skin and enlarged sweat glands usually occur in acromegaly. Yellowish nodules on extensor surfaces of the elbows and knees and on the buttocks typically occur in severe hypertriglyceridemia.

3. What are the essential steps in palpating the thyroid gland? What palpation findings should you expect in a normal thyroid? What findings would be considered abnormal?

Answer

To palpate the thyroid gland using the anterior approach, the nurse faces the client and locates the cricoid cartilage with the pads of the index and middle fingers, then palpates the thyroid isthmus just below the cricoid cartilage while the client swallows. To palpate the anterior of the right lobe, the nurse uses the right hand to displace the trachea to the right. To palpate the posterior of the right lobe, the nurse grasps

Skills laboratory guide: Physical assessment

This chart guides the student during assessment by identifying body areas, special considerations and techniques to be used, and normal findings.

BODY AREA	SPECIAL CONSIDERATIONS	NORMAL FINDINGS
Inspection		
Vital signs, height, and weight	• Compare findings with the client's baseline measurements. The normal growth rate averages 3″ (7.6 cm) per year between ages 1 and 7, and 2″ (5 cm) per year between ages 8 and 15. • Compare the client's anthropomorphic measurements to a standard height-weight chart.	• Appropriate vital signs, height, and weight for client's age and sex
General appearance	• Note general appearance and mental and emotional status. Note affect, speech, level of consciousness (LOC), orientation, appropriateness and neatness of dress and grooming, and activity level. • Evaluate general body development, including posture, body build, body proportions, and body fat distribution. In an infant, the distance from the top of the head to the pubis is normally 70% of overall height; at age 2, 60%; at age 10, 52%. An elderly client normally loses about 3″ in height by age 70.	• Appropriate appearance, alert, and cooperative • Appropriate affect; clear speech; oriented to person, place, and time; well-groomed and well-dressed; appropriate activity level • Erect posture; appropriate body build; proportional body parts; normal body fat distribution for sex • No moon facies, buffalo hump, or kyphosis
Skin, hair, and nails	• Note skin color, lesions, areas of increased or decreased pigmentation, texture, temperature, and hydration. An elderly client normally has dry, thin skin and decreased temperature. • Note hair amount, distribution, condition, and texture. A pregnant client may have increased pigmentation—for example, linea negra, mask of pregnancy, or darker areolae—and altered hair growth and texture. • Assess nails for cracking, peeling, separation from nail bed, clubbing, infection, discoloration, length, and thickness.	• Uniform skin color; no hyperpigmentation, hypopigmentation, or discoloration • Warm, dry skin • No skin coarseness; scales; thinness; excessive moisture, warmth, or dryness; purplish striae; edema; or bruises • Medium-textured, evenly distributed hair • No hair coarseness, dryness, brittleness, thinness, silkiness, alopecia, or hirsutism • Firm nails that adhere well to nail beds • No nail thickness, thinness, brittleness, or increased pigmentation
Head and neck	• Assess eye shape and symmetry, noting periorbital edema, eyelid tremors or incomplete closure, and exophthalmos. • Note tongue size, lesions, position, and unusual movements. • Examine neck first with it held straight, then slightly extended, and finally while the client swallows water. Check neck symmetry, contour, and position, and tracheal position.	• Symmetrical, clear, bright eyes with no periorbital edema, eyelid tremors or incomplete closure, or exophthalmos • Midline, appropriately-sized tongue with no lesions, tremors, or fasciculations • Symmetrical neck and trachea with no masses
Chest	• Note size, shape, symmetry, and any deformities. In females, note breast size, shape, pigmentation, and symmetry, and nipple discharge. In males, note gynecomastia and nipple discharge. A pregnant client will have increased breast size and may have nipple discharge.	• Symmetrical chest with no deformities • In females, symmetrical breast size and shape with no hyperpigmentation or nipple discharge • In males, no gynecomastia or nipple discharge
Genitalia	• Note development of external genitalia, particularly the clitoris (in females) and testes (in males).	• No clitoral enlargement • No abnormally small testes
Extremities	• Check for tremors by having client stretch both arms out in front with palms down and fingers separated. Then place a sheet of paper on the outstretched fingers and watch for trembling. • Check leg muscle strength by having client sit on the edge of the examination table and extend the legs horizontally. • Note hand-grasp strength, muscle strength, and symmetry. Note leg muscle development, symmetry, color, and hair distribution. • Examine feet for size; note any lesions, corns, or calluses.	• Symmetrical extremities • Strong hand grasp bilaterally with no tremors or atrophy • Strong legs bilaterally with no discoloration or abnormal hair distribution • Foot size in proportion to body; no lesions, corns, or calluses

Skills laboratory guide: Physical assessment *continued*

BODY AREA	SPECIAL CONSIDERATIONS	NORMAL FINDINGS
Palpation		
Thyroid	• Palpate the thyroid using the anterior or posterior approach. With either approach, have the client swallow as you palpate the thyroid isthmus just below the cricoid cartilage. • Have the client tilt the head to the side you are assessing, when using the posterior approach. • Note thyroid size, shape, symmetry of lobes, consistency, nodules, and mobility if gland is palpable.	• Nonpalpable, nontender thyroid gland
Face	• Elicit Chvostek's sign by tapping the facial nerve; note facial muscle contraction toward the ear.	• No facial muscle contraction
Arm	• Elicit Trousseau's sign by placing a blood pressure cuff on the client's arm and inflating it above the client's systolic pressure; note carpal spasms.	• No carpal spasms
Auscultation		
Thyroid	• Auscultate the thyroid if it is enlarged. • Detect systolic bruits by having the client hold his or her breath as you listen over the thyroid with the stethoscope bell.	• No bruits

the sternocleidomastoid muscle with the left hand and palpates the lobe between the fingers. To palpate the left lobe, the nurse uses the left hand to move the thyroid cartilage and the right hand to palpate.

To palpate the thyroid gland using the posterior approach, the nurse uses the same technique as the anterior approach, except that the client must tilt the head slightly to the side being assessed and the nurse must use the opposite hand for palpation.

Although the isthmus may be palpable, the thyroid gland normally is not palpable, except in a client with an extremely thin neck. The normal thyroid gland is butterfly-shaped with symmetrical lobes and feels smooth, firm, well defined, and nontender. As the client swallows, it should rise above the cartilage.

Abnormal findings include a palpable thyroid that is enlarged, asymmetrical, irregularly shaped, tender, or nodular, or has bruits.

4. When assessing a client for a potential endocrine problem, why should you assess body systems, such as the nervous and reproductive systems?

Answer
When assessing the endocrine system, the nurse also should assess the nervous and reproductive systems because disorders in these body systems may affect the endocrine system and because endocrine disorders may affect these systems.

The nervous system plays a major role in hormone regulation, directly controlling production of antidiuretic hormone (ADH) and oxytocin through the hypothalamus in the brain. The hypothalamus also has a role in control of pituitary hormones and production of the catecholamines epinephrine and norepinephrine. Because the hypothalamus controls the autonomic nervous system, it regulates the hormones epinephrine and norepinephrine. Nervous system manifestations of endocrine disorders may include changes in mental and emotional status, speech, level of consciousness, orientation, or behavior; the presence of tremors; muscle weakness or wasting; numbness; or tingling.

The reproductive system depends on the endocrine system to function smoothly. The gonads (testes in males and ovaries in females) are endocrine glands that are part of the reproductive system. The endocrine system produces the gonadal hormones (testosterone in males and estrogen in females) that are responsible for secondary sex characteristic development and for reproduction. Reproductive system manifestations of endocrine disorders may include an enlarged clitoris in females and small testes and infertility in males.

5. Mrs. Maria DelaCruz, age 74, was admitted with complaints of polyuria, polydipsia, and polyphagia. Her skin turgor is poor as evidenced by tenting, she is obese, and she states that her mother has diabetes. On admission, her blood glucose level measured 436 mg/dl. After receiving insulin to lower her blood glucose level, she was started on low-dose oral hypoglycemic therapy. How should you document the following information related to a nursing assessment of Mrs. DelaCruz?
- history (subjective) assessment data
- physical (objective) assessment data
- assessment techniques and equipment used
- two appropriate nursing diagnoses
- documentation of your findings.

Answer

History (subjective) assessment data
- Complains of polyuria, polydipsia, and polyphagia
- States mother has diabetes

Physical (objective) assessment data
- Female, age 74, obese
- Poor skin turgor as evidenced by tenting
- Blood glucose level 436 mg/dl on admission

Assessment techniques and equipment used
- Interview the client about current health status, past health status, family health status, exercise and activity, nutrition, and social support patterns.
- Measure the client's vital signs, height, and weight.
- Inspect the client's general appearance and all body structures and systems.
- Palpate the thyroid.
- Equipment should include a tape measure, scale with height-measuring device, stethoscope, watch with second hand, and blood pressure cuff.

Two appropriate nursing diagnoses
- Knowledge deficit related to oral hypoglycemic therapy
- Altered nutrition: more than body requirements, related to obesity

Documentation of findings
- S—Client complains of polyuria, polydipsia, and polyphagia. States her mother has diabetes.
- O—Obese female appears stated age of 74. Poor skin turgor. Blood glucose level 436 mg/dl.
- A—Knowledge deficit related to oral hypoglycemic therapy

Questions, answers, and rationales

1. Barbara Schultz, age 62, seeks care for unintentional weight gain and weakness—possible signs and symptoms of hypothyroidism. To assess for additional symptoms of hypothyroidism, the nurse could ask which health history question?
(a) "Have you noticed an increase in the amount of urine you pass?"
(b) "Have any noticed any muscle twitching?"
(c) "Do you feel any numbness or tingling in your arms or legs?"
(d) "Do you usually feel cold when other people in the same room are comfortable?"
Correct answer: (d), see text page 593. Heat intolerance commonly is associated with hyperthyroidism; cold intolerance, with hypothyroidism.

2. If Ms. Schultz has hypothyroidism, the nurse is likely to notice which change in her voice?
(a) Hoarse voice
(b) High-pitched voice
(c) Soft voice
(d) Deep voice
Correct answer: (a), see text pages 599 and 602. Signs and symptoms of hypothyroidism include sparse, brittle, coarse hair; muscle stiffness; diminished hearing; constipation; hoarseness, and slowed cognitive activities.

3. During the physical assessment, the nurse inspects Ms. Schultz's hair. Which assessment finding suggests hypothyroidism?
(a) Coarse, brittle hair
(b) Thick, oily hair
(c) Thick, dry hair
(d) Thin, fine, oily hair
Correct answer: (a), see text pages 599 and 602. Hypothyroidism may cause hair to become sparse (especially at the eyebrows), coarse, dry, and brittle.

4. The nurse prepares to palpate Ms. Schultz's thyroid gland. To palpate the client's thyroid isthmus, where should the nurse position the fingers?
(a) Below the hyoid bone
(b) Above the thyroid cartilage
(c) Below the cricoid cartilage
(d) Next to the tracheal rings
Correct answer: (c), see text page 600. The nurse assesses the thyroid isthmus by palpating just below the cricoid cartilage, using the pads of the index and middle fingers.

5. When attempting to palpate the thyroid gland, the nurse should give Ms. Schultz which instruction?
(a) Hyperextend the neck.
(b) Hold the breath.
(c) Relax the neck.
(d) Swallow.
Correct answer: (d), see text page 600. The client should swallow during thyroid palpation. Swallowing raises the larynx, trachea, and thyroid gland, but not the nodes or other structures.

6. Ms. Schultz is scheduled for laboratory tests to assess her thyroid hormone levels. Based on their structure, thyroid hormones fall into which classification?
(a) Polypeptides
(b) Steroids
(c) Tropins
(d) Amines
Correct answer: (d), see text page 590. Thyroid hormones are classified as amines, which are derived from tyrosine (an essential amino acid found in most proteins).

7. Joan Martin, age 37, seeks care for unintentional weight loss and menstrual irregularities—possible signs of hyperthyroidism. During the assessment, the nurse remains alert for related signs or symptoms. Which health history finding suggests hyperthyroidism?
(a) Nervousness
(b) Constipation
(c) Cold intolerance
(d) Decreased appetite
Correct answer: (a), see text page 603. Hyperthyroidism also may cause fatigue, nervousness, heat intolerance, and increased appetite.

8. If Ms. Martin has hyperthyroidism, the nurse is likely to detect which finding when assessing her eyes?
(a) Diplopia
(b) Papilledema
(c) Exophthalmos
(d) Unequal pupils
Correct answer: (c), see text pages 599 and 603. Exophthalmos (eyeball protrusion) and incomplete eyelid closure, usually bilateral, are associated with severe hyperthyroidism.

9. Palpation reveals an enlarged thyroid gland. Because this gland is enlarged, the nurse should use which technique to assess it further?
(a) Percussion
(b) Auscultation
(c) Ballottement
(d) Deep palpation
Correct answer: (b), see text page 601. The nurse should auscultate an enlarged thyroid gland to detect systolic bruits, which may indicate hyperthroidism.

10. Lou Brock, age 77, comes to the clinic for a regular check-up. He has had diabetes mellitus for more than 20 years. Which sign or symptom commonly is associated with diabetes mellitus?
(a) Polyuria
(b) Hirsutism
(c) Diaphoresis
(d) Nervousness
Correct answer: (a), see text page 602. Classic signs and symptoms of diabetes mellitus include fatigue, loss of strength, weight loss, bloating, fullness, impotence, polyuria, and polydypsia.

11. Which drug could cause severe adverse reactions in a diabetic client such as Mr. Brock?
(a) Bumetanide
(b) Furosemide
(c) Propranolol
(d) Clonidine
Correct answer: (c), see text page 594. Propranolol and other beta blockers may cause severe adverse reactions for a diabetic client by masking signs and symptoms of hypoglycemia, impairing glucose tolerance, inhibiting insulin release, and causing hyperglycemic reactions.

12. When assessing Mr. Brock, the nurse should consider which finding a normal result of aging?
(a) 3″ loss in chest circumference
(b) 3″ loss in body height
(c) 3″ loss in arm length
(d) 3″ loss in leg length
Correct answer: (b), see text page 603. With age, a person normally loses about 3″ in height by age 70.

13. Mary Stewart, age 54, seeks care for rib fractures. Her medical history reveals osteoporosis and hypertension. The nurse obtains a complete drug history on admission. Which drug can cause cushingoid signs and symptoms?
(a) Ketoconazole
(b) Furosemide
(c) Prednisone
(d) Phenytoin
Correct answer: (c), see text page 594. Corticosteroids, such as prednisone and methylprednisolone, may cause cushingoid fat distribution.

14. When performing a physical assessment of Ms. Stewart, the nurse inspects her skin. Which skin change would suggest Cushing's syndrome?
(a) Thinning
(b) Purple striae
(c) Coarse, dry skin
(d) Bronze skin coloration
Correct answer: (b), see text page 603. Cushing's syndrome may cause purple striae on the arms, breasts, abdomen, and thighs.

15. Glen Brown, age 58, is admitted to the critical care unit for testing of suspected pheochromocytoma. Pheochromocytoma produces an excess of which hormones?
(a) Steroids
(b) Estrogens
(c) Catecholamines
(d) Glucocorticoids
Correct answer: (c), see text page 587. A pheochromocytoma is a tumor of the adrenal medulla that secretes excessive catecholamines at inappropriate times.

16. The nurse performs a complete physical assessment before Mr. Brown undergoes testing. Which assessment finding commonly is associated with pheochromocytoma?
(a) Hypertension
(b) Hypoglycemia
(c) Bradycardia
(d) Electrolyte imbalance
Correct answer: (a), see text page 598. Hypertension develops in many endocrine disorders, particularly pheochromocytoma.

17. While Kate Smithers, age 51, is recovering from a thyroidectomy, the nurse periodically assesses for signs and symptoms of hypoparathyroidism, which may result from injury to the parathyroid gland during thyroid surgery. Which assessment finding suggests this endocrine disorder?
(a) Cold insensitivity
(b) Confusion
(c) Polydipsia
(d) Polyuria
Correct answer: (b), see text page 602. Hypoparathyroidism may produce lethargy, irritability, emotional lability, impaired memory, and confusion.

18. The nurse also evaluates Ms. Smithers's electrolyte levels regularly. Hypoparathyroidism is likely to affect which electrolyte?
(a) Sodium
(b) Calcium
(c) Chloride
(d) Potassium
Correct answer: (b), see text page 600. Hypocalcemia may result from deficient or insufficient parathormone secretion from hypoparathyroidism or surgical removal of the parathyroid glands.

19. When the nurse applies a blood pressure cuff and inflates it above Ms. Smithers's systolic pressure, the client displays carpal spasm. What is this finding called?
(a) Romberg sign
(b) Ortolani's sign
(c) Trousseau's sign
(d) Trendelenberg's sign
Correct answer: (c), see text page 601. The nurse elicits Trousseau's sign by placing a blood pressure cuff on the client's arm and inflating it above the client's systolic pressure. In a positive test, the client exhibits carpal spasm in 3 minutes.

20. The nurse attempts to elicit Chvostek's sign in Ms. Smithers. To do this, the nurse should tap over which nerve?
(a) Facial
(b) Abducen
(c) Trigeminal
(d) Spinoaccessory
Correct answer: (a), see text page 601. To elicit Chvostek's sign, the nurse taps the facial nerve in front of the ear. If the facial muscles contract toward the ear, the test is positive for hypocalcemia.

Test bank for Chapter 20, Endocrine System

1. Barbara Schultz, age 62, seeks care for unintentional weight gain and weakness—possible signs and symptoms of hypothyroidism. To assess for additional symptoms of hypothyroidism, the nurse could ask which health history question?
(a) "Have you noticed an increase in the amount of urine you pass?"
(b) "Have any noticed any muscle twitching?"
(c) "Do you feel any numbness or tingling in your arms or legs?"
(d) "Do you usually feel cold when other people in the same room are comfortable?"

2. If Ms. Schultz has hypothyroidism, the nurse is likely to notice which change in her voice?
(a) Hoarse voice
(b) High-pitched voice
(c) Soft voice
(d) Deep voice

3. During the physical assessment, the nurse inspects Ms. Schultz's hair. Which assessment finding suggests hypothyroidism?
(a) Coarse, brittle hair
(b) Thick, oily hair
(c) Thick, dry hair
(d) Thin, fine, oily hair

4. The nurse prepares to palpate Ms. Schultz's thyroid gland. To palpate the client's thyroid isthmus, where should the nurse position the fingers?
(a) Below the hyoid bone
(b) Above the thyroid cartilage
(c) Below the cricoid cartilage
(d) Next to the tracheal rings

5. When attempting to palpate the thyroid gland, the nurse should give Ms. Schultz which instruction?
(a) Hyperextend the neck.
(b) Hold the breath.
(c) Relax the neck.
(d) Swallow.

6. Ms. Schultz is scheduled for laboratory tests to assess her thyroid hormone levels. Based on their structure, thyroid hormones fall into which classification?
(a) Polypeptides
(b) Steroids
(c) Tropins
(d) Amines

7. Joan Martin, age 37, seeks care for unintentional weight loss and menstrual irregularities—possible signs of hyperthyroidism. During the assessment, the nurse remains alert for related signs or symptoms. Which health history finding suggests hyperthyroidism?
(a) Nervousness
(b) Constipation
(c) Cold intolerance
(d) Decreased appetite

8. If Ms. Martin has hyperthyroidism, the nurse is likely to detect which finding when assessing her eyes?
(a) Diplopia
(b) Papilledema
(c) Exophthalmos
(d) Unequal pupils

9. Palpation reveals an enlarged thyroid gland. Because this gland is enlarged, the nurse should use which technique to assess it further?
(a) Percussion
(b) Auscultation
(c) Ballottement
(d) Deep palpation

10. Lou Brock, age 77, comes to the clinic for a regular check-up. He has had diabetes mellitus for more than 20 years. Which sign or symptom commonly is associated with diabetes mellitus?
(a) Polyuria
(b) Hirsutism
(c) Diaphoresis
(d) Nervousness

11. Which drug could cause severe adverse reactions in a diabetic client such as Mr. Brock?
(a) Bumetanide
(b) Furosemide
(c) Propranolol
(d) Clonidine

12. When assessing Mr. Brock, the nurse should consider which finding a normal result of aging?
(a) 3″ loss in chest circumference
(b) 3″ loss in body height
(c) 3″ loss in arm length
(d) 3″ loss in leg length

13. Mary Stewart, age 54, seeks care for rib fractures. Her medical history reveals osteoporosis and hypertension. The nurse obtains a complete drug history on admission. Which drug can cause cushingoid signs and symptoms?
(a) Ketoconazole
(b) Furosemide
(c) Prednisone
(d) Phenytoin

14. When performing a physical assessment of Ms. Stewart, the nurse inspects her skin. Which skin change would suggest Cushing's syndrome?
(a) Thinning
(b) Purple striae
(c) Coarse, dry skin
(d) Bronze skin coloration

15. Glen Brown, age 58, is admitted to the critical care unit for testing of suspected pheochromocytoma. Pheochromocytoma produces an excess of which hormones?
(a) Steroids
(b) Estrogens
(c) Catecholamines
(d) Glucocorticoids

16. The nurse performs a complete physical assessment before Mr. Brown undergoes testing. Which assessment finding commonly is associated with pheochromocytoma?
(a) Hypertension
(b) Hypoglycemia
(c) Bradycardia
(d) Electrolyte imbalance

17. While Kate Smithers, age 51, is recovering from a thyroidectomy, the nurse periodically assesses for signs and symptoms of hypoparathyroidism, which may result from injury to the parathyroid gland during thyroid surgery. Which assessment finding suggests this endocrine disorder?
(a) Cold insensitivity
(b) Confusion
(c) Polydipsia
(d) Polyuria

18. The nurse also evaluates Ms. Smithers's electrolyte levels regularly. Hypoparathyroidism is likely to affect which electrolyte?
(a) Sodium
(b) Calcium
(c) Chloride
(d) Potassium

19. When the nurse applies a blood pressure cuff and inflates it above Ms. Smithers's systolic pressure, the client displays carpal spasm. What is this finding called?
(a) Romberg sign
(b) Ortolani's sign
(c) Trousseau's sign
(d) Trendelenberg's sign

20. The nurse attempts to elicit Chvostek's sign in Ms. Smithers. To do this, the nurse should tap over which nerve?
(a) Facial
(b) Abducen
(c) Trigeminal
(d) Spinoaccessory

21

Complete and Partial Assessments

Overview

Chapter 21 describes how to perform a complete assessment by integrating health history, physical assessment, and laboratory study review in a format of brevity, accuracy, and consistency. The chapter also explains how and when to perform a properly focused partial assessment. Here are the chapter highlights:

• The most important part of the nursing assessment, the health history provides information about the client and helps guide physical assessment.

• The complete health history includes biographic data, health and illness patterns, health promotion and protection patterns, role and relationship patterns, and a summary of health history data.

• The nurse may perform a complete physical assessment during a client's first visit to an outpatient setting or as a periodic checkup after the first visit.

• After conducting a general survey and measuring the client's height, weight, and vital signs, the nurse can begin the "hands on" part of the complete physical assessment. This involves assessing each body structure and system in an integrated fashion, using a body region approach rather than a body system approach.

• During a complete physical assessment, a systematic head-to-toe approach helps the nurse ensure consistency of assessments and aids documentation. It also minimizes the number of changes in nurse-client positioning, avoids tiring the client, allows the nurse to work more efficiently, and ensures that no assessment area is overlooked.

• The partial assessment focuses on a specific client concern or problem. It may be performed in many different health care settings.

• A partial health history is appropriate for an outpatient, an inpatient (as in an emergency department), or a client in distress. It requires complete biographical data and detailed information on the client's reason for seeking health care, and allows for additional health history topics.

• Usually, the nurse performs a partial physical assessment to evaluate specific symptoms reported in the health history. Such an assessment would include a general survey, vital sign measurements, and assessment of specific body structures and systems. This type of assessment is particularly useful when tracking the progress of a client with a particular problem.

• Proper documentation is essential for organizing complete or partial assessment data. To document the physical assessment, the nurse should organize and record findings by body system.

Suggested lecture topics

• Discuss the components of a complete health history, providing sample questions for each component.

Skills laboratory guide: Complete physical assessment

Use this laboratory guide with the *Performing physical assessments* chart on pages 614 to 631 of the text. Like the text chart, this assessment guide is organized by body region from head to toe. Refer to the text chart for specific assessment steps, normal findings, and special considerations. Use this guide when conducting your own assessments, filling in the blanks with appropriate data. Before beginning the detailed physical assessment, however, remember to record your general survey data and the client's height, weight, and vital signs.

BODY AREA	DOCUMENTATION
Head and neck	
Eyes and ears	
Posterior thorax	
Anterior thorax	
Abdomen	
Upper extremities	
Lower extremities	
Nervous system	
Reproductive system	

- Review the basic approach to complete physical assessment, including preparation; the general survey; measurement of height, weight, and vital signs; and a detailed assessment of each body region.
- Discuss how to document a complete physical assessment.
- Using case studies of clients with different chief complaints, explain the best approach to partial assessment of each client.

Suggested critical thinking activities

- Pair the students by sex and have them perform a complete assessment on each other, including a health history and physical assessment.
- Have the students document their findings on the *Skills Laboratory Guide: Complete physical assessment.*
- Have the class critique each student's documentation for completeness and clarity.
- Using case studies of clients with different complaints, have the students describe the partial assessment components for each client.

Student study questions and answers

The following questions are taken from text pages 634 and 635 of Chapter 21, Complete and Partial Assessments. Their answers are based on information in that chapter.

1. When should you perform a complete and a partial health history? What information should you obtain during each type of history?

Answer
The nurse should obtain a complete health history when time and the client's condition allow, such as on an initial visit to an outpatient facility. The complete health history consists of five basic components: biographic data, health and illness patterns, health promotion and protection patterns, role and relationship patterns, and a summary of health history data.

The nurse should perform a partial health history when the client is in distress or otherwise unable to withstand an extended interview, when time is limited, or when the assessment is a follow-up to a complete assessment. This type of history focuses on the client's biographic data and reason for seeking health care. Other health history components, such as past health status and family health status, are combined as needed.

2. What body systems and structures should you evaluate when performing a complete physical assessment of the anterior thorax, posterior thorax, and abdomen?

Answer
Assessment of the anterior thorax evaluates the skin, respiratory system, cardiovascular system, musculoskeletal system, breasts, nipples, and axillae. Posterior thorax assessment evaluates the skin, respiratory system, musculoskeletal system, and urinary system. Abdominal assessment evaluates the skin, gastrointestinal system, immune system, blood, urinary system, and cardiovascular system.

3. What organizational approach would you take to a complete physical assessment? How does this compare with the organizational approach you would use to document physical assessment findings?

Answer
After gathering the appropriate equipment and preparing the examination room, the nurse should begin the complete physical assessment with a general survey that gathers basic information about the client's overall health and mental status. Next, the nurse should measure and record the client's height, weight, and vital signs. Then, the nurse should assess each body structure and system, moving from head to toe and using the body region approach, rather than the body system approach that is used to document assessment findings.

4. During the complete physical assessment, which physical assessment techniques are used on which parts of the body?

Answer
- Inspection. The nurse uses this technique for all body structures and systems. Although internal organs cannot be seen, the nurse inspects appropriate external areas (such as symmetry of chest expansion and accessory muscle use for the respiratory system) to help assess organ or system function.
- Palpation. The nurse uses this technique for the head and face, neck, ears, anterior and posterior thorax, breasts, axillae, abdomen, reproductive system, rectum, and extremities. As needed, the nurse uses light, deep, or rebound palpation, as well as simply touching areas of concern, such as a joint or a skin lesion.
- Percussion. The nurse uses this technique to assess the sinuses, lungs, abdomen, costovertebral angle, and deep tendon reflexes. Depending on the location, the nurse percusses with the fingers, fist, or a rubber hammer.
- Auscultation. The nurse uses a stethoscope to auscultate the cardiovascular and respiratory systems and the abdomen.

5. Assessment of pediatric and elderly clients requires certain modifications from the usual adult assessment. For instance, one area involving major differences is the eyes. What are the important special considerations to keep in mind when performing an eye assessment in pediatric and elderly clients?

Answer
For a pediatric client, the nurse should remember the following special considerations:
• In an infant, visual acuity assessment is not possible. Instead, the blink reflex is assessed. For a child age 30 to 42 months, the nurse should assess visual acuity with a Denver Eye Screening Exam (DESE); for a child age 7 and under, with the Snellen E chart or the DESE.
• Visual acuity varies with age; for example, 20/30 is normal for a toddler.
• Early detection of color blindness is especially important for a pediatric client. It allows the child to learn to compensate for the problem and alerts teachers to the child's needs.
• A pediatric client who fails the six cardinal positions of gaze test, the cover-uncover test, or the corneal light reflex test requires immediate referral to an ophthalmologist for evaluation and possible correction of strabismus (crossed eyes).

For an elderly client, the nurse should remember the following special considerations:
• Lens elasticity decreases with age, commonly causing presbyopia, which reduces near vision.
• Peripheral vision also normally decreases with age.
• With age, the eyelashes thin, and the eyes may appear lackluster.
• An elderly client may have a thickened bulbar conjunctiva on the nasal side (pinguecula) or a thin, grayish ring around the cornea (arcus senilus).
• A client over age 85 may show almost no pupil reaction to accommodation.

Questions, answers, and rationales

1. Janet Graves, age 32, is scheduled for a complete annual assessment. What is the most important part of the complete assessment?
(a) Health history
(b) General survey
(c) Vital sign measurements
(d) Height and weight measurements
Correct answer: (a), see text page 611. The most important part of the complete assessment, the health history provides the nurse with a focus for the assessment.

2. How much time should the nurse allow to obtain a complete history from Ms. Graves?
(a) 10 to 15 minutes
(b) 15 to 30 minutes
(c) 30 to 60 minutes
(d) 60 to 90 minutes
Correct answer: (c), see text page 612. A complete health history should take about ½ hour to 1 hour to obtain.

3. Whether performing a complete or a partial assessment, the nurse always should include which component of the health history?
(a) Role and relationship patterns
(b) Summary of health history data
(c) Health promotion and protection patterns
(d) Reason for seeking health care
Correct answer: (d), see text page 633. For a complete assessment, the nurse includes all five components of the health history; for a partial assessment, just biographic data and the reason for seeking health care.

4. To prepare for the complete physical assessment, the nurse gathers all appropriate supplies and equipment. Which item is not needed to assess the typical adult?
(a) Goniometer
(b) Paper clip
(c) Reflex hammer
(d) Denver Eye Screening Examination
Correct answer: (d), see text pages 612 and 617. Complete physical assessment of an adult normally requires a standard Snellen eye chart; of a child age 7 or under, a Snellen E chart.

5. Before the physical assessment, what should the nurse tell Ms. Graves to do?
(a) "Assume whatever position makes you most comfortable."
(b) "Remain dressed, and we'll uncover each area as it is assessed."
(c) "Empty your bladder and provide a urine specimen."
(d) "Drink a glass of water so we can obtain a urine specimen after the examination."
Correct answer: (c), see text page 612. After gathering the necessary equipment, the nurse should instruct the client to empty the bladder (and provide a urine specimen, if needed), remove all clothing, and put on a gown.

6. During the complete physical assessment, what should the nurse do to prevent contamination of the client or another client?
(a) Wear gloves.
(b) Obtain specimens.
(c) Wear a gown and mask.
(d) Wash hands frequently.
Correct answer: (a), see text page 612. To prevent contamination of the client, other clients, or the nurse, gloves should be worn when examining the mucous membranes, genitals, rectum, or any areas with lesions or signs of infection or infestation.

7. The nurse begins the complete physical assessment with a general survey. Which of the following areas is not part of the general survey?
(a) Facial expression, contour, and symmetry
(b) Tone, clarity, and strength of speech
(c) Dress, grooming, and personal hygiene
(d) Height, weight, and vital signs
Correct answer: (d), see text page 613. Height, weight, and vital signs are considered separate from the general survey.

8. To minimize position changes and perform the physical assessment efficiently, how should the nurse proceed?
(a) By body system
(b) By body structure
(c) By body region
(d) According to the client's preference
Correct answer: (c), see text page 613. To minimize changes in nurse-client positioning and to allow efficient performance of the physical assessment, the nurse should work from head to toe by body region.

9. How should the nurse document physical assessment findings for Ms. Graves?
(a) By structure
(b) By function
(c) By region
(d) By system
Correct answer: (d), see text page 613. To allow easier access to more concise assessment data for the health care team, the nurse should organize and record assessment findings by body system.

10. When documenting complete assessment findings, the nurse should include which data?
(a) All data (normal and abnormal findings)
(b) Positive findings only
(c) Negative findings only
(d) General findings only
Correct answer: (a), see text page 613. The nurse should document all data specifically and completely, including normal and abnormal findings.

11. Which documentation statement suggests an abnormal finding for Ms. Graves?
(a) Tympanic membranes shiny and pink
(b) Anteroposterior diameter 1:2
(c) Right breast slightly larger than left
(d) Bowel sounds auscultated in all four quadrants
Correct answer: (a), see text page 632. On otoscopic assessment, the tympanic membranes normally appear pearly gray.

12. Donna Barenborn, age 27, and her family have just moved into the area. She brings her son Joshua, age 3 months, to the pediatrician for his initial visit. The nurse performs a complete assessment, beginning with the head and neck. Which finding is considered abnormal for a child of this age?
(a) Fine, thin hair
(b) Soft, yet firm, fontanels
(c) Smooth, well-separated sutures
(d) Palpable lymph nodes ⅛″ across
Correct answer: (c), see text page 614. In an infant, the sutures should be smooth and not override one another or feel separated.

13. To inspect Joshua's nostrils, how should the nurse proceed?
(a) Use an ophthalmoscope handle with a nasal attachment.
(b) Transilluminate the nostrils.
(c) Use a nasal speculum.
(d) Use only a flashlight.
Correct answer: (d), see text page 615. The nurse should use only a flashlight to inspect an infant's or toddler's nostrils; a nasal speculum is too sharp.

14. As part of Joshua's assessment, the nurse measures the anteroposterior and lateral diameters of his thorax. What is the normal ratio of anteroposterior-to-lateral diameter in an infant?
(a) 1:1
(b) 1:3
(c) 2:1
(d) 3:1
Correct answer: (a), see text pages 619 and 620. An infant's anteroposterior diameter may equal or exceed the lateral diameter; a toddler's should be smaller than the lateral diameter.

15. Seven months pregnant, Peggy Darnell, age 21, comes to the clinic for her first prenatal visit. The nurse practitioner performs a complete physical assessment. Which assessment finding is abnormal in a pregnant client?
(a) Darkened nipples
(b) Enlarged breasts
(c) Nipple retraction
(d) Purplish streaks
Correct answer: (c), see text pages 622. Nipple retraction, dimpling, and flattening are abnormalities in any client.

16. Leonard Cuthbert, age 44, undergoes a complete physical assessment as a prerequisite for a new job. Because Mr. Cuthbert is Black, the nurse can expect to see which normal variation when inspecting his eyes?
(a) Hyperemic blood vessels
(b) Small, dark spots on the sclera
(c) Thin, grayish ring in the cornea
(d) Thickened bulbar conjunctiva on the nasal side
Correct answer: (b), see text pages 618. A Black client may have small, dark spots on the sclera and a gray-blue cornea.

17. On admission to a life-care community, Edgar Minton, age 85, has a complete assessment in the health care department. When the nurse touches Mr. Minton in different areas with a cotton swab and a sharp object to assess his nervous system function, which finding is considered normal and age-related?
(a) Correct identification of sensation, but not location
(b) Correct identification of location, but not sensation
(c) Correct, but slowed, identification of location and sensation
(d) Inability to perceive sensation in a particular area
Correct answer: (b), see text pages 627. This nervous system test may take more time for an elderly client.

18. John Winthrop, age 36, is admitted to the emergency department (ED) with a fractured tibia caused by a fall. The nurse performs a partial assessment. What is the focus of the partial assessment?
(a) Reason for seeking health care
(b) Client's overall health status
(c) Results of diagnostic studies
(d) Client's past medical history
Correct answer: (a), see text page 633. The partial assessment focuses on a specific client concern or problem.

19. What are the components of the partial physical assessment?
(a) General survey, vital sign measurements, and assessment of specific body structures and systems
(b) Vital sign measurements, height and weight measurements, and assessment of specific body structures and systems
(c) General survey, vital sign measurements, and a review of all body systems
(d) Height and weight measurements and vital sign measurements
Correct answer: (a), see text page 633. No matter what the client's condition, a partial assessment should include a general survey, vital sign measurements, and evaluation of certain body structures and systems.

20. When performing any partial physical assessment, the nurse may use a checklist. Which assessment is not commonly included to evaluate basic structures and systems?
(a) Assess level of consciousness.
(b) Palpate for pretibial edema.
(c) Auscultate the abdomen.
(d) Percuss the costovertebral angles.
Correct answer: (d), see text page 633. Unless the client's reason for seeking care suggests a urinary disorder, the nurse does not usually assess the kidneys by percussing the costovertebral angles.

Test bank for Chapter 21, Complete and Partial Assessments

1. Janet Graves, age 32, is scheduled for a complete annual assessment. What is the most important part of the complete assessment?
(a) Health history
(b) General survey
(c) Vital sign measurements
(d) Height and weight measurements

2. How much time should the nurse allow to obtain a complete history from Ms. Graves?
(a) 10 to 15 minutes
(b) 15 to 30 minutes
(c) 30 to 60 minutes
(d) 60 to 90 minutes

3. Whether performing a complete or a partial assessment, the nurse always should include which component of the health history?
(a) Role and relationship patterns
(b) Summary of health history data
(c) Health promotion and protection patterns
(d) Reason for seeking health care

4. To prepare for the complete physical assessment, the nurse gathers all appropriate supplies and equipment. Which item is not needed to assess the typical adult?
(a) Goniometer
(b) Paper clip
(c) Reflex hammer
(d) Denver Eye Screening Examination

5. Before the physical assessment, what should the nurse tell Ms. Graves to do?
(a) "Assume whatever position makes you most comfortable."
(b) "Remain dressed, and we'll uncover each area as it is assessed."
(c) "Empty your bladder and provide a urine specimen."
(d) "Drink a glass of water so we can obtain a urine specimen after the examination."

6. During the complete physical assessment, what should the nurse do to prevent contamination of the client or another client?
(a) Wear gloves.
(b) Obtain specimens.
(c) Wear a gown and mask.
(d) Wash hands frequently.

7. The nurse begins the complete physical assessment with a general survey. Which of the following areas is not part of the general survey?
(a) Facial expression, contour, and symmetry
(b) Tone, clarity, and strength of speech
(c) Dress, grooming, and personal hygiene
(d) Height, weight, and vital signs

8. To minimize position changes and perform the physical assessment efficiently, how should the nurse proceed?
(a) By body system
(b) By body structure
(c) By body region
(d) According to the client's preference

9. How should the nurse document physical assessment findings for Ms. Graves?
(a) By structure
(b) By function
(c) By region
(d) By system

10. When documenting complete assessment findings, the nurse should include which data?
(a) All data (normal and abnormal findings)
(b) Positive findings only
(c) Negative findings only
(d) General findings only

11. Which documentation statement suggests an abnormal finding for Ms. Graves?
(a) Tympanic membranes shiny and pink
(b) Anteroposterior diameter 1:2
(c) Right breast slightly larger than left
(d) Bowel sounds auscultated in all four quadrants

12. Donna Barenborn, age 27, and her family have just moved into the area. She brings her son Joshua, age 3 months, to the pediatrician for his initial visit. The nurse performs a complete assessment, beginning with the head and neck. Which finding is considered abnormal for a child of this age?
(a) Fine, thin hair
(b) Soft, yet firm, fontanels
(c) Smooth, well-separated sutures
(d) Palpable lymph nodes ⅛″ across

13. To inspect Joshua's nostrils, how should the nurse proceed?
(a) Use an ophthalmoscope handle with a nasal attachment.
(b) Transilluminate the nostrils.
(c) Use a nasal speculum.
(d) Use only a flashlight.

14. As part of Joshua's assessment, the nurse measures the anteroposterior and lateral diameters of his thorax. What is the normal ratio of anteroposterior-to-lateral diameter in an infant?
(a) 1:1
(b) 1:3
(c) 2:1
(d) 3:1

15. Seven months pregnant, Peggy Darnell, age 21, comes to the clinic for her first prenatal visit. The nurse practitioner performs a complete physical assessment. Which assessment finding is abnormal in a pregnant client?
(a) Darkened nipples
(b) Enlarged breasts
(c) Nipple retraction
(d) Purplish streaks

16. Leonard Cuthbert, age 44, undergoes a complete physical assessment as a prerequisite for a new job. Because Mr. Cuthbert is black, the nurse can expect to see which normal variation when inspecting his eyes?
(a) Hyperemic blood vessels
(b) Small, dark spots on the sclera
(c) Thin, grayish ring in the cornea
(d) Thickened bulbar conjunctiva on the nasal side

17. On admission to a life-care community, Edgar Minton, age 85, has a complete assessment in the health care department. When the nurse touches Mr. Minton in different areas with a cotton swab and a sharp object to assess his nervous system function, which finding is considered normal and age-related?
(a) Correct identification of sensation, but not location
(b) Correct identification of location, but not sensation
(c) Correct, but slowed, identification of location and sensation
(d) Inability to perceive sensation in a particular area

18. John Winthrop, age 36, is admitted to the emergency department (ED) with a fractured tibia caused by a fall. The nurse performs a partial assessment. What is the focus of the partial assessment?
(a) Reason for seeking health care
(b) Client's overall health status
(c) Results of diagnostic studies
(d) Client's past medical history

19. What are the components of the partial physical assessment?
(a) General survey, vital sign measurements, and assessment of specific body structures and systems
(b) Vital sign measurements, height and weight measurements, and assessment of specific body structures and systems
(c) General survey, vital sign measurements, and a review of all body systems
(d) Height and weight measurements and vital sign measurements

20. When performing any partial physical assessment, the nurse may use a checklist. Which assessment is not commonly included to evaluate basic structures and systems?
(a) Assess level of consciousness.
(b) Palpate for pretibial edema.
(c) Auscultate the abdomen.
(d) Percuss the costovertebral angles.

22

Perinatal and Neonatal Assessment

Overview

Complete and accurate assessment forms the basis for nursing care for a client during pregnancy and after delivery, and for her neonate. To prepare the nurse to perform these assessments competently, Chapter 22 discusses the essentials of prenatal, postpartum, and neonatal assessments, including health history questions, physical assessment steps, and documentation of findings. Here are the chapter highlights:

• Prenatal assessment begins when the client first suspects she may be pregnant and continues through labor and delivery. The nurse's assessment includes a thorough health history, focusing on questions related to the pregnancy and the client's overall health status, and physical assessment, covering all maternal body systems as well as an evaluation of fetal growth and well-being.

• Postpartum assessment involves the physiologic and psychological changes as the client's body returns to its pre-pregnant state as well as the mother's and family's adjustments to these changes.

• Neonatal assessment begins immediately after delivery and continues throughout the infant's time in the nursery. A complete assessment includes a perinatal history, determination of gestational age, physical assessment—including evaluation of neonatal reflexes—and behavioral assessment.

• For more information about perinatal and neonatal assessments, see pages 105PG through 112PG of the Photo Gallery in the text.

Suggested lecture topics

• Discuss health history questions important to prenatal, postpartum, and neonatal assessments, explaining the rationales for asking them.

• Using audiovisual aids, describe normal findings in prenatal, postpartum, and neonatal assessments. (For visual aids, see the transparency master *Assessing the fundus* on page 248 and pages 105PG through 112PG in the text.)

• Using simulators, demonstrate physical assessment of prenatal, postpartum, and neonatal clients.

• Discuss abnormal assessment findings in prenatal, postpartum, and neonatal clients.

Suggested critical thinking activities

• Pair the students and have them obtain and document a simulated prenatal and postpartum history from each other. Then have them critique each other's assessment techniques and documentation.

• Using case studies of prenatal, postpartum, and neonatal clients, have the students develop a nursing care plan for each.

• Have the students document their case study findings on the Skills Laboratory Assessment Guide.

Skills laboratory guide: Health history

To collect information about the client's pregnancy or delivery, ask questions about health and illness patterns, health promotion and protection patterns, and role and relationship patterns. Sample questions from each category are listed below.

PRENATAL HEALTH HISTORY	POSTPARTUM HEALTH HISTORY
Health and illness patterns	**Health and illness patterns**
• When was the first day of your last menstrual period? Was this period like the previous ones? • Have you had uterine or pelvic surgery or injury? • Have you had a sexually transmitted disease? • Have you been pregnant before? If so, how would you describe the pregnancy and its outcome? • Is your blood Rh-negative? • Has anyone in your family experienced any complications during pregnancy, labor, or delivery? • Has anyone in your family had hypertension, diabetes mellitus, gestational diabetes, obesity, or heart disease?	• How do you feel? Are you experiencing any specific problems you would like to discuss? • How is your energy level? • Do you have any pain or discomfort in your abdominal or genital areas? • Do you have any discomfort in your breasts or nipples? • Do you have difficulty urinating? • Have you had a bowel movement yet? • Do you have any weakness or decreased sensations in your legs and feet?
Health promotion and protection patterns	**Health promotion and protection patterns**
• Are you currently taking any prescription or over-the-counter medications? • Are you currently using any street drugs or alcohol? • Did you use a contraceptive before this pregnancy? If so, which type? When did you stop using it? • Do you smoke cigarettes? • How would you describe your stress level? • What type of work do you do? What sort of environment do you work in? • Have you thought about what type of delivery you would like? Have you attended any prenatal classes?	• How much sleep are you getting? • Have you been walking? • Do you feel that the baby is increasing your stress? • Do you know the signs and symptoms of postpartum problems that require immediate medical attention? • Have you scheduled a follow-up examination? • Do you have a car seat to take the baby home from the hospital?
Role and relationship patterns	**Role and relationship patterns**
• How do you feel about being pregnant? • Do you feel that you are receiving sufficient support from your family and friends during your pregnancy?	• How do you feel about the new baby and your role as mother? • How is your relationship with your partner? • Do you feel that you are receiving enough help and support from family and friends?

Student study questions and answers

The following study questions are taken from text page 647 of Chapter 22, Perinatal and Neonatal Assessment. Their answers are based on information in that chapter.

1. Mrs. Graves, age 28, is 7 months pregnant. She expresses distress about the stretch marks on her abdomen. What information should you give her?

Answer
The nurse should explain that the stretch marks, or striae gravidarum, appear as the abdominal skin stretches to accommodate the growing fetus. The nurse also should reassure the client that stretch marks usually fade gradually after delivery.

2. Which prenatal health history questions help assess both maternal and fetal health?

Answer
• Have you had uterine or pelvic surgery or injury?
• Have you ever had a sexually transmitted disease? If so, which one and when? What treatment did you receive?
• Have you been pregnant before? If so, how would you describe the pregnancy and its outcome? How long did the pregnancy and labor last? What type of delivery was it? Did you suffer any complications during pregnancy, labor, or delivery or have any problems after delivery? What was the infant's birth weight and overall health?
• Have you ever had an abortion?
• Is your blood Rh negative?
• Has anyone in your family ever experienced any complications during pregnancy, labor, or delivery?

Skills laboratory guide: Physical assessment

This chart guides the student during assessment by identifying body areas, special considerations and techniques to be used, and normal findings.

BODY AREA	SPECIAL CONSIDERATIONS	NORMAL FINDINGS
Prenatal physical assessment		
Inspection		
Skin	• Note hyperpigmentation on face (chloasma), abdomen (linea nigra), areolae, nipples, and vulva.	• Presence or absence of chloasma and linea nigra, and darkening of areolae, nipples, and vulva
Respiratory	• Note breathing pattern, respiratory rate, and dyspnea on exertion.	• Increased respiratory rate • Use of thoracic muscles for breathing • Slight dyspnea on exertion
Breasts	• Note breast size, shape, symmetry, venous pattern, and striae. Note nipple size, shape, and discharge.	• Enlarged, symmetrical breasts with increased venous pattern and possible striae • Enlarged, erect nipples with colostrum discharge
Abdomen	• Note size, shape, and presence of striae gravidarum.	• Round, symmetrical abdomen with striae
Musculoskeletal	• Note posture and gait.	• Erect posture; coordinated gait • Slight lordosis late in pregnancy
Arms and legs	• Note varicosities and peripheral edema.	• Venous varicosities possible in the legs • Hand, finger, and leg edema possible
Palpation		
Thyroid	• Attempt to palpate thyroid gland.	• Thyroid may be palpable
Abdomen	• Estimate uterine size after 12th week. Palpate from above the uterus where the abdomen is soft down to firm uterine edge; measure to notch at inferior edge of symphysis pubis.	• Approprate uterine size for week of gestation (12 to 13 weeks, above symphysis pubis; 16 weeks, between symphysis pubis and umbilicus; 20 weeks, at umbilicus)
Auscultation		
Cardiovascular	• Note accentuated heart sounds, systolic murmur, displaced point of maximum intensity (PMI).	• Accentuated heart sounds, possibly with systolic murmur • Laterally displaced PMI from 5th intercostal space at midclavicular line
Abdomen	• Note bowel sounds. • Note fetal heart sounds with Doppler above symphysis pubis at midline (early in pregnancy) or through fetal back (late in pregnancy).	• Decreased bowel sounds • Normal fetal heart rate of 120 to 160 beats/minute, varying with age of fetus
Postpartum physical assessment		
Inspection		
Breasts	• Note signs of infection, bleeding, crusting, engorgement, increased vascularity, and redness.	• Increased vascularity; no signs of infection, bleeding, crusting, or engorgement
Perineum and rectum	• Examine perineum and episiotomy site for erythema, edema, ecchymoses, or hematoma. • Note character and amount of vaginal drainage. • Note hemorrhoids.	• No erythema, edema, ecchymoses, or hematoma • Lochia rubra, 1 to 3 days postpartum; lochia serosa, 4 to 10 days postpartum; lochia alba, after 10 days postpartum • No hemorrhoids
Legs	• Note peripheral edema, varicosities, and signs of thrombophlebitis, such as Homan's sign.	• No edema, varicosities, or signs of thrombophlebitis • No Homan's sign
Palpation		
Breasts	• Note warm areas, tenderness, enlargement, or firmness.	• Soft, nontender breasts with no enlargement or warm areas

continued

Skills laboratory guide: Physical assessment *continued*

BODY AREA	SPECIAL CONSIDERATIONS	NORMAL FINDINGS
Postpartum physical assessment *continued*		
Palpation *continued*		
Abdomen	• Assess muscle tone and fundal height.	• Soft abdomen with decreased muscle tone • Firm fundus below umbilicus, immediately postpartum; above symphysis pubis, up to 10 days postpartum; non-palpable fundus, 10 to 14 days postpartum
Arms and legs	• Check peripheral pulses and temperature.	• Palpable pedal pulses; normal temperature
Neonatal physical assessment		
Inspection		
Respirations	• Note respiratory rate and rhythm. Brief (15-second) apnea is common.	• Irregular, shallow respirations, ranging from 30 to 60 breaths/minute
General appearance	• Note overall skin color. • Assess level of consciousness and muscle tone. • Measure weight and height. Most neonates lose 10% of birth weight in the first 3 to 4 days after birth.	• No jaundice, pallor, cyanosis, or ruddy discoloration • Alertness and symmetrical extremity movement • Average weight between 5 lb, 8 oz and 8 lb, 13 oz (2500 to 4000 g) • Average height between 18" and 22" (45 to 55 cm)
Skin and hair	• Note skin color and condition. Vernix caseosa normally is present immediately after birth and diminishes after several days. Acrocyanosis or mottling are common in the first 24 hours after birth; milia often occur across the nose, cheeks, and chin for the first several weeks after birth. • Note hair and lanugo distribution.	• Appropriate skin color for neonate's race, ranging from pink in Caucasian neonates to creamy tan in darker-skinned, Black, Hispanic, or Asian neonates • Some head hair; lanugo on face, shoulders, and back
Head	• Measure head circumference. • Inspect and measure fontanels. • Check overall facial appearance and symmetry. • Note size and shape of eyes and ear position. Nystagmus and strabismus are common in the first 2 to 3 months. Because of immature lacrimal glands, tears or discharge may appear. • Note nose shape and position, nasal patency, and drainage. Because neonates are obligatory nose-breathers, check nostril patency by occluding one nostril at a time and noting signs of respiratory distress, such as sternal retraction.	• Head circumference 12 ¾" to 14½" (32 to 36 cm) • Diamond-shaped anterior fontanel, 1⅛" to 1⅝" (3 to 4 cm) long by ¾" to 1⅛" (2 to 3 cm) wide • Closed posterior fontanel possible at birth • Appropriately placed, proportionate, symmetrical facial features • Symmetrical eyes framed by eyebrows and eyelashes; round, firm eyeballs • Symmetrical ear pinnas aligned with outer canthus of eyes • Midline, flat, broad nose; patent nostrils with no drainage
Chest	• Measure chest circumference at nipple line. • Note symmetry of nipples and chest movement. Breast engorgement may occur in either sex related to maternal estrogen in utero.	• Chest circumference 12" to 13" (30 to 33 cm) or ¾" to 1½" less than head circumference • Rounded chest with symmetrical movements and nipples
Abdomen	• Note size and shape of abdomen. • Note location and condition of umbilical cord stump. • Note passage of meconium.	• Round, dome-shaped abdomen • Soft, moist, white umbilical stump midline at lower abdomen with no bleeding or signs of infection • Meconium stool within 24 hours of birth
Back	• Note spinal position and alignment of shoulders, scapulae, and iliac crests.	• Straight spine; shoulders, scapulae, and iliac crests in planar alignment
Extremities	• Note arm and leg position and movements. • Perform Ortolani's maneuver to test hip joint stability.	• Full range of motion with all four extremities moving spontaneously and equally • No Ortolani's sign
Anus and genitalia	• Note anal patency and ability to urinate. • In males, check for undescended testicles, foreskin patency, and location of urinary meatus. In females, note discharge. Pseudomenstruation (blood-tinged discharge) may be present.	• Patent anus • Urination within 24 hours of birth • In males: descended testicles, difficult-to-retract foreskin covering glans penis, urinary meatus at tip of penis. In females: slightly edematous genitalia, presence of smegma

Skills laboratory guide: Physical assessment *continued*

BODY AREA	SPECIAL CONSIDERATIONS	NORMAL FINDINGS
Neonatal physical assessment *continued*		
Palpation		
Head	• Palpate anterior and posterior fontanels.	• Open anterior fontanel for 18 months after birth • Closed posterior fontanel at birth, or flat and open for up to 3 months after birth
Chest	• Palpate for signs of fracture, such as crepitus.	• Rounded chest with no signs of fracture
Abdomen	• Palpate the abdomen.	• Soft abdomen with no masses
Back	• Palpate spine of prone neonate.	• Intact spine with no indentations or dimpling
Auscultation		
Cardiovascular	• Assess pulse rate and heart sounds. • Auscultate apical pulse with a stethoscope for 1 minute.	• Pulse rate 120 to 160 beats/minute at rest; 180 beats/minute during crying and motor activity; 100 beats/minute during deep sleep • Higher-pitched, shorter, and louder heart sounds than in adult
Abdomen	• Auscultate for bowel sounds.	• Bowel sounds present 1 to 2 hours after birth
Reflex assessment		
Sucking, or rooting, reflex	• Touch the neonate's lip, cheek, or corner of mouth.	• Head turning toward stimulus and opening of mouth with sucking activity
Extrusion reflex	• Touch or depress the neonate's tongue.	• Tongue forced outward
Tonic neck, or "fencing," reflex	• With neonate in supine position, turn the head from midline to one side.	• Extremity extension on side toward which neonate is turned; reflex of opposite extremities
Palmar grasp reflex	• Apply pressure to the neonate's palm.	• Fingers curling around your finger
Plantar grasp reflex	• Apply pressure to base of the neonate's toes.	• Toes curling downward
Moro, or "startle," reflex	• Apply a sudden stimulus, such as a hand clap, when the neonate is lying quietly.	• Symmetrical, embracing motion
Stepping, or "walking," reflex	• Hold the neonate vertically and allow the soles of the feet to touch a table surface.	• Stepping that simulates walking

• Has anyone in your family had hypertension, diabetes mellitus, gestational diabetes, obesity, or heart disease?
• Are you currently taking any prescription or over-the-counter medications?
• Are you currently using any street drugs or alcohol?
• Do you smoke cigarettes?
• What is your typical daily diet?
• What type of work do you do?

3. How would you compare normal prenatal changes in the abdomen and breasts with postpartum changes?

Answer
As pregnancy progresses, striae gravidarum typically appear on the abdomen as the abdominal skin stretches to accommodate the growing fetus. The umbilicus may flatten or protrude. The uterus displaces the colon laterally upward and posteriorly, thereby repositioning the appendix. Peristalsis slows during pregnancy, so bowel sounds may decrease. In about the 8th week of pregnancy, the breasts begin to enlarge. The nipples become larger and more erect, and Montgomery's tubercles become more prominent. Colostrum, the precursor of milk, may be expressed as early as the 24th week of pregnancy. Striae on the breasts may become more visible as vascularity and venous engorgement increase.

After delivery, the abdomen is soft, lacking appreciable muscle tone. Muscle tone usually returns to the prepregnant level by 6 weeks postpartum. Immediately after delivery, the fundus should be firm and positioned at the umbilicus. As normal involution progresses, the fundus moves from the umbilicus to just above the symphysis pubis. Throughout the postpartum period, the uterus should remain rounded and firm. After delivery, the breasts should be soft and nontender. However, many women experience engorgement caused by the increased vascularity that prepares for lactation. Engorged breasts become enlarged, firm, and usually tender.

4. Which aspects of general appearance are vital to the neonatal physical assessment?

Answer
Important aspects of the neonate's general appearance include overall skin color, muscle tone, level of consciousness, weight, and height.

5. Which reflexes help assess the neonate's neuromuscular system and how are they elicited?

Answer
The sucking or rooting reflex is elicited by touching the neonate's lip, cheek, or corner of the mouth; the extrusion reflex, by touching or depressing the neonate's tongue; the tonic neck reflex, by turning the supine neonate's head from midline to one side; the palmar grasp reflex, by applying pressure to the neonate's palm; the plantar grasp reflex, by applying pressure to the base of the neonate's toes; the Moro reflex, by applying a sudden stimulus, such as a hand clap, when the neonate is lying quietly; the stepping reflex, by holding the neonate vertically and allowing the soles of the feet to touch a table surface.

Questions, answers, and rationales

1. Megan Stewart, age 23, has missed two menstrual periods and has had a positive home pregnancy test. After laboratory tests confirm her pregnancy, she schedules a complete prenatal examination. When assessing Ms. Stewart's head and neck, the nurse should consider which finding normal?
(a) Displaced trachea
(b) Distended neck veins
(c) Palpable thyroid gland
(d) Bounding carotid pulsations
Correct answer: (c), see text page 639. In about 50% of all pregnant women, the thyroid gland enlarges because of increased vascularity and hyperplasia of this glandular tissue.

2. As the pregnancy progresses, the nurse can expect to see which change in Ms. Stewart's respiratory system?
(a) Abdominal breathing
(b) Accessory muscle use
(c) Increased respiratory rate
(d) Decreased respiratory rate
Correct answer: (c), see text page 639. The growing fetus elevates the diaphragm, causing an increased maternal respiratory rate.

3. The nurse auscultates Ms. Stewart's heart. During pregnancy, which heart sound normally is heard?
(a) S_3
(b) S_4
(c) Systolic murmur
(d) Diastolic murmur
Correct answer: (c), see text page 639. During pregnancy, blood volume normally increases by 30% to 50%, causing a systolic murmur in about 90% of all pregnant women.

4. The nurse also inspects and palpates Ms. Stewart's breasts. Which breast change is considered normal during pregnancy?
(a) Venous engorgement
(b) Orange peel skin
(c) Retraction
(d) Dimpling
Correct answer: (a), see text page 639. During pregnancy, the breasts display increased vascularity and venous engorgement.

5. During the assessment, the nurse auscultates the abdomen. By which week of gestation should fetal heart sounds normally be audible with a Doppler system?
(a) Second
(b) Fourth
(c) Eighth
(d) Tenth
Correct answer: (d), see text page 639. Fetal heart sounds cay be heard with a Doppler system as early as the tenth gestational week.

6. For a client in early pregnancy, where is the best place to listen for fetal heart sounds?
(a) Above the symphysis pubis
(b) Below the symphysis pubis
(c) Above the umbilicus
(d) At the umbilicus
Correct answer: (a), see text page 639. In early pregnancy, the fetal heart beat is loudest in the area of maximum intensity, just above the mother's symphysis pubis at midline.

7. The nurse assesses Ms. Stewart's musculoskeletal system to obtain baseline data. Later in pregnancy, the client is likely to display which change?
(a) Kyphosis
(b) Lordosis
(c) Scoliosis
(d) Kyphoscoliosis
Correct answer: (b), see text page 639. To compensate for changes in the center of gravity caused by the gravid uterus, the client may throw her shoulders backward and hyperextend her vertebral column, producing lordosis.

8. Three days ago, Jane Shaw, age 28, delivered a healthy, 8-pound baby boy. Now the nurse is performing a postpartum assessment. Which finding suggests breast engorgement?
(a) Firm, tender breasts
(b) Soft, nodular breasts
(c) Soft, warm breasts
(d) Red, warm breasts
Correct answer: (a), see text page 642. Engorged breasts become enlarged, firm, and usually tender.

9. Before palpating Ms. Shaw's fundus, what should the nurse tell her to do?
(a) Empty her bladder.
(b) Try to have a bowel movement.
(c) Assume a sitting position.
(d) Change her perineal pad.
Correct answer: (a), see text page 642. Because urine in the bladder causes the fundus to rise or be displaced from midline, the nurse should instruct the client to urinate before fundal assessment.

10. Where should the nurse expect to palpate Ms. Shaw's fundus?
(a) Above the umbilicus
(b) At the umbilicus
(c) Below the umbilicus
(d) Nowhere (It should be nonpalpable.)
Correct answer: (c), see text page 642. Upon delivery, the fundus can be palpated at the umbilicus. For 10 to 14 days later, it can be palpated below the umbilicus.

11. Palpation reveals a boggy fundus. What should the nurse do?
(a) Recheck the fundus in one hour.
(b) Call the physician immediately.
(c) Document this finding, which is normal.
(d) Massage the fundus and watch for drainage.
Correct answer: (d), see text page 642. The nurse should massage a boggy fundus gently and observe for lochia drainage. Massage helps the uterus return to its normal size and helps remove any clots and other matter that remain.

12. The nurse also assesses Ms. Shaw's perineum. At 3 days postpartum, the client should display which type of lochia?
(a) Lochia rubra
(b) Lochia serosa
(c) Lochia alba
(d) Lochia negra
Correct answer: (a), see text page 642. Lochia rubra (dark-red vaginal drainage) occurs during the first 3 days after delivery.

13. During Ms. Shaw's assessment, the nurse performs a vascular check. Which test helps detect thrombophlebitis?
(a) Test for Homan's sign
(b) Capillary refill test
(c) Retrograde filling test
(d) Straight leg raising test
Correct answer: (a), see text page 642. Pain in the calf during dorsiflexion of the foot is a positive Homan's sign and indicates thrombophlebitis.

14. The nurse also performs a complete assessment of Ms. Shaw's neonate, Bobby. When assessing Bobby's respirations, which finding is considered normal?
(a) Irregular, shallow, respirations at a rate of 30 to 60 breaths/minute
(b) Regular, deep, respirations at a rate of 30 to 60 breaths/minute
(c) Regular, shallow, respirations at a rate of 12 to 20 breaths/minute
(d) Irregular, deep, respirations at a rate of 12 to 20 breaths/minute
Correct answer: (a), see text page 644. A neonate's respirations normally are irregular and shallow and occur at a rate of 30 to 60 breaths/minute, sometimes with brief apnea.

15. When auscultating Bobby's breath sounds, the nurse should consider which ones normal?
(a) Vesicular
(b) Bronchovesicular
(c) Brochial
(d) Tracheal
Correct answer: (c), see text page 644. Auscultated breath sounds normally are bronchial and loud in a neonate.

16. When auscultating Bobby's heart sounds, the nurse should report which rate to the physician?
(a) 160 to 180 beats/minute
(b) 120 to 160 beats/minute
(c) 100 to 120 beats/minute
(d) Less than 100 beats/minute
Correct answer: (d), see text page 644. The normal heart rate is 120 to 160 beats/minute. It increases to 180 beats/minute during crying and motor activity and decreases to 100 beats/minute during deep sleep.

17. Upon weighing Bobby, the nurse finds that he has lost ½ lb. since his birth 3 days ago. At this age, what is the maximum weight loss that is considered normal?
(a) 10%
(b) 15%
(c) 20%
(d) 25%
Correct answer: (a), see text page 644. A neonate may lose up to 10% of birth weight within the first 3 or 4 days of life.

18. The nurse assesses Bobby's anterior and posterior fontanels. How soon after birth does the posterior fontanel normally close?
(a) 3 months
(b) 6 months
(c) 12 months
(d) 18 months
Correct answer: (a), see text page 644. The triangle-shaped posterior fontanel may be closed at birth (from molding) but can remain palpable for about 3 months.

19. During the assessment, Ms. Shaw asks the nurse, "When will Bobby's umbilical stump fall off?" How should the nurse respond?
(a) "In about 3 days"
(b) "In about 1 week"
(c) "In about 2 weeks"
(d) "In about 4 weeks"
Correct answer: (c), see text page 645. The umbilical stump progressively shrinks, turns black, and detaches in approximately 2 weeks.

20. Which technique can the nurse use to assess Bobby's hip joint stability?
(a) Ortolani's maneuver
(b) Apley's maneuver
(c) Test for McMurray's sign
(d) Walking reflex test
Correct answer: (a), see text page 645. Clicking or popping during Ortolani's maneuver may indicate an unstable hip joint.

21. Bobby voids immediately after the assessment. After the first few days after birth, how frequently does a neonate normally void?
(a) 2 to 6 times daily
(b) 5 to 10 times daily
(c) 15 to 20 times daily
(d) 20 to 30 times daily
Correct answer: (c), see text page 645. Urine voided in the first few days may be scant and infrequent (2 to 6 times daily); however, as dietary intake increases, the frequency of daily voiding also increases (15 to 20 times daily).

Test bank for Chapter 22, Perinatal and Neonatal Assessment

1. Megan Stewart, age 23, has missed two menstrual periods and has had a positive home pregnancy test. After laboratory tests confirm her pregnancy, she schedules a complete prenatal examination. When assessing Ms. Stewart's head and neck, the nurse should consider which finding normal?
(a) Displaced trachea
(b) Distended neck veins
(c) Palpable thyroid gland
(d) Bounding carotid pulsations

2. As the pregnancy progresses, the nurse can expect to see which change in Ms. Stewart's respiratory system?
(a) Abdominal breathing
(b) Accessory muscle use
(c) Increased respiratory rate
(d) Decreased respiratory rate

3. The nurse auscultates Ms. Stewart's heart. During pregnancy, which heart sound normally is heard?
(a) S_3
(b) S_4
(c) Systolic murmur
(d) Diastolic murmur

4. The nurse also inspects and palpates Ms. Stewart's breasts. Which breast change is considered normal during pregnancy?
(a) Venous engorgement
(b) Orange peel skin
(c) Retraction
(d) Dimpling

5. During the assessment, the nurse auscultates the abdomen. By which week of gestation should fetal heart sounds normally be audible with a Doppler system?
(a) Second
(b) Fourth
(c) Eighth
(d) Tenth

6. For a client in early pregnancy, where is the best place to listen for fetal heart sounds?
(a) Above the symphysis pubis
(b) Below the symphysis pubis
(c) Above the umbilicus
(d) At the umbilicus

7. The nurse assesses Ms. Stewart's musculoskeletal system to obtain baseline data. Later in pregnancy, the client is likely to display which change?
(a) Kyphosis
(b) Lordosis
(c) Scoliosis
(d) Kyphoscoliosis

8. Three days ago, Jane Shaw, age 28, delivered a healthy, 8-pound baby boy. Now the nurse is performing a postpartum assessment. Which finding suggests breast engorgement?
(a) Firm, tender breasts
(b) Soft, nodular breasts
(c) Soft, warm breasts
(d) Red, warm breasts

9. Before palpating Ms. Shaw's fundus, what should the nurse tell her to do?
(a) Empty her bladder.
(b) Try to have a bowel movement.
(c) Assume a sitting position.
(d) Change her perineal pad.

10. Where should the nurse expect to palpate Ms. Shaw's fundus?
(a) Above the umbilicus
(b) At the umbilicus
(c) Below the umbilicus
(d) Nowhere (It should be nonpalpable.)

11. Palpation reveals a boggy fundus. What should the nurse do?
(a) Recheck the fundus in one hour.
(b) Call the physician immediately.
(c) Document this finding, which is normal.
(d) Massage the fundus and watch for drainage.

12. The nurse also assesses Ms. Shaw's perineum. At 3 days postpartum, the client should display which type of lochia?
(a) Lochia rubra
(b) Lochia serosa
(c) Lochia alba
(d) Lochia negra

13. During Ms. Shaw's assessment, the nurse performs a vascular check. Which test helps detect thrombophlebitis?
(a) Test for Homan's sign
(b) Capillary refill test
(c) Retrograde filling test
(d) Straight leg raising test

14. The nurse also performs a complete assessment of Ms. Shaw's neonate, Bobby. When assessing Bobby's respirations, which finding is considered normal?
(a) Irregular, shallow, respirations at a rate of 30 to 60 breaths/minute
(b) Regular, deep, respirations at a rate of 30 to 60 breaths/minutes
(c) Regular, shallow, respirations at a rate of 12 to 20 breaths/minute
(d) Irregular, deep, respirations at a rate of 12 to 20 breaths/minute

15. When auscultating Bobby's breath sounds, the nurse should consider which ones normal?
(a) Vesicular
(b) Bronchovesicular
(c) Brochial
(d) Tracheal

16. When auscultating Bobby's heart sounds, the nurse should report which rate to the physician?
(a) 160 to 180 beats/minute
(b) 120 to 160 beats/minute
(c) 100 to 120 beats/minute
(d) Less than 100 beats/minute

17. Upon weighing Bobby, the nurse finds that he has lost ½ lb. since his birth 3 days ago. At this age, what is the maximum weight loss that is considered normal?
(a) 10%
(b) 15%
(c) 20%
(d) 25%

18. The nurse assesses Bobby's anterior and posterior fontanels. How soon after birth does the posterior fontanel normally close?
(a) 3 months
(b) 6 months
(c) 12 months
(d) 18 months

19. During the assessment, Ms. Shaw asks the nurse, "When will Bobby's umbilical stump fall off?" How should the nurse respond?
(a) "In about 3 days"
(b) "In about 1 week"
(c) "In about 2 weeks"
(d) "In about 4 weeks"

20. Which technique can the nurse use to assess Bobby's hip joint stability?
(a) Ortolani's maneuver
(b) Apley's maneuver
(c) Test for McMurray's sign
(d) Walking reflex test

21. Bobby voids immediately after the assessment. After the first few days after birth, how frequently does a neonate normally void?
(a) 2 to 6 times daily
(b) 5 to 10 times daily
(c) 15 to 20 times daily
(d) 20 to 30 times daily

Quiz Bank

Quiz bank for Chapter 1, Assessment and the Nursing Process

Matching related elements

Match the steps of the nursing process in the left column with the corresponding definition in the right column.

1. Assessment
2. Nursing diagnosis
3. Planning
4. Implementation
5. Evaluation

(a) Identification of an actual or potential client health problem
(b) Collection and organization of data
(c) Determination of a client's status in relation to set goals
(d) Development of goals
(e) Performance of interventions

True or false

1. A sign is an indication of disease perceived subjectively by the client.
   ☐ True   ☐ False
2. Nursing interventions are actions used to implement the care plan.
   ☐ True   ☐ False
3. Physical assessment findings provide subjective data.
   ☐ True   ☐ False
4. A nursing diagnosis identifies the client's actual or potential medical problem.
   ☐ True   ☐ False

Quiz bank for Chapter 2, Nursing and Medicine: A Collaborative Approach

Matching related elements

Match the term in the left column with the corresponding definition in the right column.

1. Health
2. Health problem
3. Health promotion
4. Holism
5. Illness

(a) Actions taken to develop resources or maintain well-being
(b) Optimal physical, social, and emotional functioning
(c) Anything that impairs an individual's physical, social, or emotional functioning
(d) Impairment of an individual's ability to adapt to environmental stressors
(e) View of health that encompasses man, environment, family, and community

True or false

1. Collaboration involves joint communication and decision-making between nurses and physicians.
   ☐ True   ☐ False
2. A model is a body of knowledge that can be applied to a professional practice.
   ☐ True   ☐ False
3. A theory is the framework used to describe a profession.
   ☐ True   ☐ False
4. Phenomena are individual or group responses to actual or potential health problems.
   ☐ True   ☐ False

Quiz bank for Chapter 3, The Health History

Matching related elements

Match the interviewing technique in the left column with the corresponding definition in the right column.

1. Closed-ended question
2. Open-ended question
3. Reflection
4. Restating
5. Validation
6. Clarification

(a) Technique of returning a verbal message using the same words in which it was sent
(b) Confirmation of information to ensure the questioner's understanding
(c) Paraphrasing or rewording another's idea
(d) Question that elicits facts with a one- or two-word response
(e) Technique that elicits additional information to make something clear or understandable
(f) Question that elicits perceptions and feelings

True or false

1. Acquired roles are functions or behavior patterns determined by biological or societal expectations.
   ☐ True ☐ False
2. Assimilation is the loss of cultural identity when an individual becomes part of a different, dominant culture.
   ☐ True ☐ False
3. Ethnicity is an affiliation with a group of people classified according to common racial, national, religious, linguistic, or cultural background.
   ☐ True ☐ False
4. Culture is an integrated system of learned behavior that is biologically inherited.
   ☐ True ☐ False

Quiz bank for Chapter 4, Physical Assessment Skills

Matching related elements

Match the assessment technique in the left column with the corresponding definition in the right column.

1. Auscultation
2. Palpation
3. Inspection
4. Percussion
5. Ballottement

(a) Assessing a floating structure by bouncing it and feeling it rebound
(b) Listening for sounds produced by various body structures
(c) Using the sense of touch to feel pulsations and vibrations and assess body structures
(d) Using sight, hearing, and smell to make observations
(e) Tapping on the skin surface to assess organs and fluid accumulation

True or false

1. Immediate percussion is performed by striking the fingers directly on the body surface.
   ☐ True ☐ False
2. Mediate percussion is performed by striking a finger of one hand against a finger of the other.
   ☐ True ☐ False
3. A pleximeter may be used for direct percussion.
   ☐ True ☐ False
4. A plexor is a mediating device used to perform indirect percussion.
   ☐ True ☐ False

Quiz bank for Chapter 5, Activities of Daily Living and Sleep Patterns

Matching related elements

Match the sleep problem in the left column with the corresponding definition in the right column.

1. Insomnia
2. Narcolepsy
3. Parasomnia
4. Enuresis
5. Somnambulism
6. Bruxism

(a) Sleepwalking
(b) Abnormal sleep tendencies and pathological manifestations of REM sleep
(c) Involuntary urination during sleep
(d) Dysfunction of sleep, sleep stages, or partial arousals
(e) Teeth grinding during sleep
(f) Disorder of initiating and maintaining sleep

True or false

1. Night terrors are bad dreams that do not cause arousal.
   ☐ True   ☐ False
2. Rapid eye movement (REM) sleep is characterized by dreaming.
   ☐ True   ☐ False
3. Sleep apnea is transient failure to breathe during sleep.
   ☐ True   ☐ False
4. Biological rhythms are intrinsic clocks that adjust to the environment to maintain a person's internal balance.
   ☐ True   ☐ False

Quiz bank for Chapter 6, Nutritional Status

Matching related elements

Match the nutrition-related disorder in the left column with the corresponding definition in the right column.

1. Anorexia nervosa
2. Bulimia
3. Kwashiorkor
4. Marasmus
5. Pica

(a) Disorder involving severe self-limitation of food intake
(b) Disorder marked by periods of starvation and excessive food intake
(c) Semistarvation caused by inadequate caloric intake
(d) Disease related to protein deficiency
(e) Craving for substances not normally considered food

True or false

1. Anabolism is the phase of cell metabolism in which complex substances are broken down into simpler ones.
   ☐ True   ☐ False
2. Glycogenesis is the process by which glycogen is reconverted to glucose.
   ☐ True   ☐ False
3. Lipogenesis is the transformation of excess hormones into fatty acids.
   ☐ True   ☐ False
4. Nitrogen balance is the state of equilibrium in which nitrogen intake equals nitrogen excretion.
   ☐ True   ☐ False

Quiz bank for Chapter 7, Skin, Hair, and Nails

Matching related elements

Match the sign or symptom in the left column with the corresponding definition in the right column.

1. Alopecia
2. Anhidrosis
3. Ecchymosis
4. Hirsutism
5. Intertrigo
6. Pruritus

(a) Itching that usually leads to scratching
(b) Masculine distribution of body hair in a woman
(c) Abnormally decreased perspiration
(d) Erythematous irritation involving skin folds
(e) Partial or complete hair loss
(f) Irregularly shaped hemorrhagic area; bruise

True or false

1. An annular lesion occurs along the course of a cutaneous nerve.
   ☐ True   ☐ False
2. A pedunculated lesion has a stalk or stem.
   ☐ True   ☐ False
3. Morphology refers to the clinical description of a lesion.
   ☐ True   ☐ False

Quiz bank for Chapter 8, Head and Neck

Matching related elements

Match the anatomical structure in the left column with the corresponding definition in the right column.

1. Choanae
2. Frenulum
3. Papillae
4. Suture
5. Turbinates
6. Uvula

(a) Immovable joint between the cranial bones
(b) Funnel-shaped openings between the nasopharynx and nasal cavity
(c) Bony internal nasal wall
(d) Small, nipple-shaped projections on the tongue
(e) Band of tissue that attaches the posterior tongue to the floor of mouth
(f) Small, cone-shaped mass that hangs from the soft palate

True or false

1. The nasolabial folds are the creases that extend from the angle of the nose to the corner of the mouth.
   ☐ True   ☐ False
2. Frontal sinus palpation normally elicits tenderness.
   ☐ True   ☐ False
3. The normal color of healthy oral mucosa is red.
   ☐ True   ☐ False
4. The parotid glands drain through Stensen's ducts.
   ☐ True   ☐ False

Quiz bank for Chapter 9, Eyes and Ears

Matching related elements

Match the eye or ear disorder in the left column with the corresponding definition in the right column.

1. Strabismus
2. Cataract
3. Diplopia
4. Hordeolum
5. Vertigo
6. Tinnitus

(a) Sensation of movement of self or surroundings
(b) Infection of the meibomian glands of the eyelid
(c) Ringing sound in one or both ears
(d) Double vision
(e) Progressive loss of lens transparency in the eye
(f) Crossed eyes

True or false

1. A conductive hearing loss commonly results from damage to inner ear structures.
   ☐ True   ☐ False
2. Myopia is a refractive error resulting from eyeball elongation.
   ☐ True   ☐ False
3. In miosis, the sphinctor muscle of the iris contracts, causing the pupils to constrict.
   ☐ True   ☐ False
4. In the accommodation reflex, the eyes adjust for near vision by pupillary dilation and eye convergence.
   ☐ True   ☐ False

Quiz bank for Chapter 10, Respiratory System

Matching related elements

Match the auscultatory findings in the left column with the corresponding description in the right column.

1. Bronchophony
2. Egophony
3. Rhonchi
4. Wheezes
5. Crackles

(a) Increased referred voice sounds in which "e" sounds like "a"
(b) Increased referred voice sounds in which the word "ninety-nine" reverberates clearly over consolidation areas and sounds muffled over others
(c) Relatively low-pitched musical sounds produced by air passing through narrowed airways
(d) Short, moist, explosive sounds produced by air passing through liquid in the airways
(e) Bubbling sounds produced by air passing through fluid-filled airways

True or false

1. Respiratory acidosis results from increased excretion of carbon dioxide by the lungs.
   ☐ True   ☐ False
2. Metabolic alkalosis may result from excess retention of bicarbonate.
   ☐ True   ☐ False
3. External respiration occurs via hypoventilation, perfusion, and infusion.
   ☐ True   ☐ False
4. Internal respiration refers to gas exchange between red blood cells and tissue cells.
   ☐ True   ☐ False

Quiz bank for Chapter 11, Cardiovascular System

Matching related elements

Match the heart sound in the left column with the corresponding definition in the right column.

1. S_1
2. S_2
3. S_3
4. S_4
5. Pericardial friction rub
6. Snap
7. Ejection click

(a) Early diastolic sound associated with myocardial infarction

(b) High-pitched abnormal sound auscultated medial to the apex just after S_2

(c) Late diastolic sound associated with hypertension

(d) High-pitched systolic and diastolic sound heard best at the left sternal border

(e) Normal diastolic sound caused by closure of the aortic and pulmonic valves

(f) High-pitched abnormal sound auscultated at the apex during mid- to late systole

(g) Normal systolic heart sound caused by closure of the mitral and tricuspid valves

True or false

1. Afterload is the volume of blood in the ventricles after diastole.
   ☐ True   ☐ False
2. Diastole is the ventricular filling phase of the cardiac cycle.
   ☐ True   ☐ False
3. Pulse pressure is the difference between the apical pulse rate and radial pulse rate.
   ☐ True   ☐ False
4. Stroke volume is the heart rate multiplied by the amount of blood ejected with each contraction.
   ☐ True   ☐ False

Quiz bank for Chapter 12, Female and Male Breasts

Matching related elements

Match the anatomical structures in the left column with the corresponding definition in the right column.

1. Areola
2. Acini cells
3. Tail of Spence
4. Montgomery's tubercles
5. Cooper's ligaments

(a) Milk-producing breast structures

(b) Pigmented circular area surrounding the nipple

(c) Fibrous tissue bands that support each breast

(d) Breast tissue extension from upper outer quadrant toward the axilla

(e) Elevated, small, round papules on the areolar surface

True or false

1. During a lumpectomy, the surgeon removes diseased breast tissue and surrounding lymph nodes.
   ☐ True   ☐ False
2. Colostrum is thin, yellowish, serous fluid that contains immunologically active substances, white blood cells, water, protein, fat, and carbohydrates.
   ☐ True   ☐ False
3. Enlargement of one or both male breasts is called gynecomastia.
   ☐ True   ☐ False
4. Breast cancer usually produces a tender breast mass.
   ☐ True   ☐ False

Quiz bank for Chapter 13, Gastrointestinal System

Matching related elements

Match the gastrointestinal (GI) sign or symptom in the left column with the corresponding definition in the right column.

1. Ascites
2. Dyspepsia
3. Dysphagia
4. Encopresis
5. Hematemesis
6. Melena

(a) Bloody vomitus
(b) Black, tarry, stool
(c) Collection of fluid in the abdominal cavity
(d) Indigestion
(e) Fecal incontinence
(f) Difficulty swallowing

True or false

1. The nurse should palpate the abdomen before auscultating for bowel sounds.
   ☐ True   ☐ False
2. Borborygmi is an abdominal sound caused by hyperperistalsis.
   ☐ True   ☐ False
3. The gallbladder lies in the left upper quadrant.
   ☐ True   ☐ False
4. Abdominal percussion normally produces resonance.
   ☐ True   ☐ False

Quiz bank for Chapter 14, Urinary System

Matching related elements

Match the urinary disorder in the left column with the corresponding definition in the right column.

1. Calculus
2. Enuresis
3. Oliguria
4. Polyuria
5. Pyuria

(a) Pus in the urine
(b) Pathologic stone formed of mineral salts
(c) Involuntary urination during sleep
(d) Reduced ability to form and eliminate urine
(e) Excretion of an abnormally large urine volume

True or false

1. Through diffusion, molecules move from an area of greater concentration to one of lesser concentration.
   ☐ True   ☐ False
2. Hydrogen ion concentration is measured by pH, which reflects a solution's acidity or alkalinity.
   ☐ True   ☐ False
3. Insensible fluid loss is water lost through evaporation.
   ☐ True   ☐ False

Quiz bank for Chapter 15, Female Reproductive System

Matching related elements

Match the reproductive system disorder in the left column with the corresponding definition in the right column.

1. Anovulation
2. Cervical ectropion
3. Systocele
4. Dysmenorrhea
5. Dyspareunia
6. Rectocele
7. Vaginitis

(a) Rectal herniation through the posterior vaginal wall
(b) Menstrual discomfort
(c) Painful or difficult sexual intercourse
(d) Inflammation of the vaginal mucosa
(e) Lack of ovulation
(f) Eversion of the epithelium onto the cervix
(g) Bladder herniation through the anterior vaginal wall

True or false

1. Parity reflects the number of pregnancies.
   ☐ True   ☐ False
2 The climacteric is the last menstrual period.
   ☐ True   ☐ False
3. Menarche is the onset of menstrual periods.
   ☐ True   ☐ False
4. Osteoporosis (loss of bone density) occurs most frequently in menopausal women.
   ☐ True   ☐ False

Quiz bank for Chapter 16, Male Reproductive System

Matching related elements

Match the reproductive system disorder in the left column with the corresponding definition in the right column.

1. Cryptorchidism
2. Epispadias
3. Hydrocele
4. Hypospadias
5. Phimosis
6. Paraphimosis

(a) Opening on the urethral meatus on the dorsal surface of the penis
(b) Spermatic fluid collection in the tunica vaginalis of the scrotum
(c) Inability of the retracted prepuce to move back over the glans penis
(d) Failure of testes to descend into the scrotum
(e) Urethral meatus opening on the ventral surface of the penis
(f) Abnormal tightness of the prepuce, preventing its retraction from the glans penis

True or false

1. Circumcision requires surgical removal of the prepuce of the penis.
   ☐ True   ☐ False
2. Testosterone is produced in the prostate gland.
   ☐ True   ☐ False
3. The life span of sperm is less than 24 hours at body temperature.
   ☐ True   ☐ False
4. Penile erection is controlled by the sympathetic nervous system.
   ☐ True   ☐ False

Quiz bank for Chapter 17, Nervous System

Matching related elements

Match the neurologic signs and symptoms in the left column with the corresponding definition in the right column.

1. Anosmia   (a) Loss of ability to move

2. Aphasia   (b) Weakness

3. Ataxia   (c) Inabilty to understand or use language

4. Dysesthesia   (d) Disturbance of sensation characterized by tingling, prickling, or numbness

5. Paresis   (e) Loss of sense of smell

6. Paralysis   (f) Unsteady gait

7. Paresthesia   (g) Unpleasant abnormal sensation or pain

True or false

1. Vestibular function reflects the sense of equilibrium, which originates in the middle ear.
   ☐ True   ☐ False
2. Decerebrate positioning is characterized by flexion and adduction of the arms and extension of the legs.
   ☐ True   ☐ False
3. Proprioception is the ability to know the position of a body part without having to look at it.
   ☐ True   ☐ False
4. A client with paraplegia displays paralysis on one side of the body.
   ☐ True   ☐ False

Quiz bank for Chapter 18, Musculoskeletal System

Matching related elements

Match the body movement in the left column with the corresponding definition in the right column.

1. Circumduction   (a) Moving in a circular fashion

2. Abduction   (b) Moving toward midline

3. Extension   (c) Moving away from midline

4. Pronation   (d) Increasing the joint angle

5. Supination   (e) Turning upward

6. Adduction   (f) Turning downward

7. Flexion   (g) Decreasing the joint angle

True or false

1. The nurse uses a goniometer to measure muscle strength.
   ☐ True   ☐ False
2. Crepitus occurs when irregular bone edges rub together.
   ☐ True   ☐ False
3. Lordosis is an exaggerated convexity of the lumbar spine.
   ☐ True   ☐ False
4. In a client with varus, part of a limb is turned inward toward midline.
   ☐ True   ☐ False

Quiz bank for Chapter 19, Immune System and Blood

Matching related elements

Match the following term in the left column with the corresponding definition in the right column.

1. Antibody
2. Antigen
3. Eosinophil
4. Basophil
5. Reticulocyte
6. Thrombocyte

(a) Granulocyte that contains serotonin and histamine
(b) Foreign substance that elicits an immune response
(c) Immature red blood cell with a meshlike network
(d) Granulocyte that responds to allergens and parasites
(e) Immunoglobulin synthesized in response to an antigen
(f) Disk-shaped cell essential for coagulation

True or false

1. Autoimmunity refers to the body's natural response to foreign antigens.
   ☐ True   ☐ False
2. Immunosuppression may result from radiation or drugs.
   ☐ True   ☐ False
3. Phagocytosis is the process by which a cell engulfs and destroys foreign material.
   ☐ True   ☐ False
4. Hemostasis refers to maintenance of equilibrium within the body.
   ☐ True   ☐ False

Quiz bank for Chapter 20, Endocrine System

Matching related elements

Match the endocrine disorder in the left column with the corresponding cause in the right column.

1. Acromegaly
2. Addison's disease
3. Cretinism
4. Cushing's syndrome
5. Pheochromocytoma

(a) Deficient thyroid hormone secretion in children
(b) Excess corticosteroid production
(c) Decreased cortisol and aldosterone secretion
(d) Tumor of the adrenal medulla that secretes excess catecholamines
(e) Excess growth hormone production in adults

True or false

1. The catecholamines epinephrine and norepinephrine are the functioning units of the autonomic nervous system.
   ☐ True   ☐ False
2. A steroid is a type of hormone formed as a protein derived from cholesterol.
   ☐ True   ☐ False
3. Glands synthesize and release chemical substances that regulate body processes.
   ☐ True   ☐ False
4. Hormones are produced by endocrine glands to regulate the functions of organs.
   ☐ True   ☐ False

Quiz bank for Chapter 21, Complete and Partial Assessments

Matching related elements

Match the test or assessment technique in the left column with the corresponding body structure or system it assesses in the right column.

1. Cover-uncover test
2. Romberg test
3. Weber's test
4. Palpation for tactile fremitus
5. Palpation for capillary refill
6. Palpation from the forehead to the posterior triangle of the neck

(a) Respiratory system
(b) Ears
(c) Immune system
(d) Eyes
(e) Nervous system
(f) Cardiovascular system

True or false

1. Complete assessments are performed more commonly than partial assessments because they provide more data.
   ☐ True   ☐ False
2. A partial assessment usually is used to monitor a client with a particular problem.
   ☐ True   ☐ False
3. The nurse should perform a complete physical assessment by body system.
   ☐ True   ☐ False
4. The nurse should document physical assessment findings by body system.
   ☐ True   ☐ False

Quiz bank for Chapter 22, Perinatal and Neonatal Assessment

Matching related elements

Match the perinatal or neonatal skin change in the left column with the corresponding definition in the right column.

1. Chloasma
2. Linea nigra
3. Milia
4. Striae gravidarum
5. Vernix caseosa

(a) Tiny, white papules on the nose, cheeks, and chin
(b) White, cheeselike sebaceous deposit over the skin
(c) Brownish pigmentation of the face
(d) Pinkish white or red lines on the breasts, abdomen, thighs, and buttocks
(e) Black line on the abdomen from the umbilicus to the pubis

True or false

1. The nurse can elicit the extrusion reflex by touching the neonate's lip, cheek, or corner of the mouth.
   ☐ True   ☐ False
2. The nurse can elicit the Moro reflex by turning the supine neonate's head from midline to one side.
   ☐ True   ☐ False
3. The nurse can elicit the "fencing" reflex by clapping the hands suddenly when the neonate is lying quietly.
   ☐ True   ☐ False
4. The nurse can elicit the stepping reflex by applying pressure to the base of the neonate's toes.
   ☐ True   ☐ False

Answers to quiz bank for Chapter 1, Assessment and the Nursing Process

Matching related elements
1. (b); 2. (a); 3. (d); 4. (e); 5. (c) (page 3)
True or false
1. False; 2. True; 3. False; 4. False (page 3)

Answers to quiz bank for Chapter 2, Nursing and Medicine: A Collaborative Approach

Matching related elements
1. (b); 2. (c); 3. (a); 4. (e); 5. (d) (page 21)
True or False
1. True; 2. False; 3. False; 4. True (page 21)

Answers to quiz bank for Chapter 3, The Health History

Matching related elements
1. (d); 2. (f); 3. (a); 4. (c); 5. (b); 6. (e) (page 35)
True or false
1. False; 2. True; 3. True; 4. False (page 35)

Answers to quiz bank for Chapter 4, Physical Assessment Skills

Matching related elements
1. (b); 2. (c); 3. (d); 4. (e); 5. (a) (page 72)
True or false
1. True; 2. True; 3. False; 4. False (page 72)

Answers to quiz bank for Chapter 5, Activities of Daily Living and Sleep Patterns

Matching related elements
1. (f); 2. (b); 3. (d); 4. (c); 5. (a); 6. (e) (page 105)
True or false
1. False (page 105); 2. True (page 105); 3. True (page 115); 4. True (page 105)

Answers to quiz bank for Chapter 6, Nutritional Status

Matching related elements
1. (a); 2. (b); 3. (d); 4. (c); 5. (e) (page 124)
True or false
1. False; 2. False; 3. False; 4. True (page 124)

Answers to quiz bank for Chapter 7, Skin, Hair, and Nails

Matching related elements
1. (e); 2. (c); 3. (f); 4. (b); 5. (d); 6. (a) (page 154)
True or false
1. False (page 154); 2. True (page 154); 3. True (page 167)

Answers to quiz bank for Chapter 8, Head and Neck

Matching related elements
1. (b); 2. (e); 3. (d); 4. (a); 5. (c); 6. (f) (page 183)
True or false
1. True (page 183); 2. False (page 193); 3. False (page 195); 4. True (page 185)

Answers to quiz bank for Chapter 9, Eyes and Ears

Matching related elements
1. (f) (page 217); 2. (e) (page 207); 3. (d) (page 207); 4. (b) (page 207); 5. (a) (page 207); 6. (c) (page 207)
True or false
1. False; 2. True; 3. True; 4. False (page 207)

Answers to quiz bank for Chapter 10, Respiratory System

Matching related elements
1. (b) (page 244); 2. (a) (page 244); 3. (e) (page 245); 4. (c) (page 245); 5. (d) (page 244)
True or false
1. False; 2. True; 3. False; 4. True (page 244)

Answers to quiz bank for Chapter 11, Cardiovascular System

Matching related elements
1. (g); 2. (e); 3. (a); 4. (c); 5. (d); 6. (b); 7. (f) (page 283)
True or false
1. False (page 283); 2. True (page 283); 3. False (page 283); 4. False (page 284)

Answers to quiz bank for Chapter 12, Female and Male Breasts

Matching related elements
1. (b) (page 335); 2. (a) (page 336); 3. (d) (page 335); 4. (e) (page 336); 5. (c) (page 336)
True or false
1. False (page 335); 2. True (page 335); 3. True (page 335); 4. False (page 349)

Answers to quiz bank for Chapter 13, Gastrointestinal System

Matching related elements
1. (c); 2. (d); 3. (f); 4. (e); 5. (a); 6. (b) (page 355)
True or false
1. False (page 365); 2. True (pages 355 and 368); 3. False (page 366); 4. False (page 368)

Answers to quiz bank for Chapter 14, Urinary System

Matching related elements
1. (b); 2. (c); 3. (d); 4. (e); 5. (a) (page 386)
True or false
1. True; 2. True; 3. True (page 386)

Answers to quiz bank for Chapter 15, Female Reproductive System

Matching related elements
1. (e); 2. (f); 3. (g); 4. (b); 5. (c); 6. (a); 7. (d) (page 414)
True or false
1. False; 2. False; 3. True; 4. True (page 414)

Answers to quiz bank for Chapter 16, Male Reproductive System

Matching related elements
1. (d); 2. (a); 3. (b); 4. (e); 5. (f); 6. (c) (page 443)
True or false
1. True (page 443); 2. False (page 445); 3. False (page 445); 4. False (page 443)

Answers to quiz bank for Chapter 17, Nervous System

Matching related elements
1. (e); 2. (c); 3. (f); 4. (g); 5. (b); 6. (a); 7. (d) (page 463)
True or false
1. False; 2. False; 3. True; 4. False (page 463)

Answers to quiz bank for Chapter 18, Musculoskeletal System

Matching related elements
1. (a); 2. (c); 3. (d); 4. (f); 5. (e); 6. (b); 7. (g) (page 516)
True or false
1. False; 2. True; 3. False; 4. True (page 511)

Answers to quiz bank for Chapter 19, Immune System and Blood

Matching related elements
1. (e) (page 548); 2. (b) (page 548); 3. (d) (page 548); 4. (a) (page 548); 5. (c) (page 549); 6. (f) (page 549)
True or false
1. False (page 548); 2. True (page 548); 3. True (page 549); 4. False (page 548)

Answers to quiz bank for Chapter 20, Endocrine System

Matching related elements
1. (e); 2. (c); 3. (a); 4. (b); 5. (d) (page 587)
True or false
1. True; 2. True; 3. True; 4. True (page 587)

Answers to quiz bank for Chapter 21, Complete and Partial Assessments

Matching related elements
1. (d) (page 617); 2. (e) (page 629); 3. (b) (page 619); 4. (a) (page 620); 5. (f) (page 626); 6. (c) (page 614)
True or false
1. False (page 633); 2. True (page 633); 3. False (page 613); 4. True (page 613)

Answers to quiz bank for Chapter 22, Perinatal and Neonatal Assessment

Matching related elements
1. (c); 2. (e); 3. (a); 4. (d); 5. (b) (page 637)
True or false
1. False; 2. False; 3. False; 4. False (page 646)

Skills laboratory assessment guide

Use this form to document health history and physical assessment findings in conjunction with the *Skills laboratory guide: Health history* and *Skills laboratory guide: Physical assessment* in the clinical laboratory. Modify the headings as needed to reflect unusual assessments. For example, substitute neurologic functions for inspection, palpation, percussion, and auscultation during nervous system assessment.

HEALTH HISTORY FINDINGS

Health and illness patterns

Health promotion and protection patterns

Role and relationship patterns

continued

Skills laboratory assessment guide *continued*

PHYSICAL ASSESSMENT FINDINGS

Inspection

Palpation

Percussion

Auscultation

The nursing process and scientific method

The nursing process incorporates elements of the scientific method, as shown below.

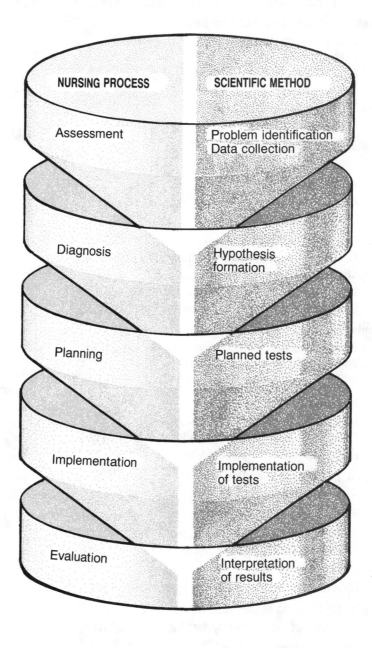

NURSING PROCESS	SCIENTIFIC METHOD
Assessment	Problem identification Data collection
Diagnosis	Hypothesis formation
Planning	Planned tests
Implementation	Implementation of tests
Evaluation	Interpretation of results

Light palpation

To perform light palpation, press gently on the skin, indenting it ½″ to ¾″ (1 to 2 cm). Use the lightest touch possible; too much pressure blunts your sensitivity. You may close your eyes to concentrate on what your fingers are feeling.

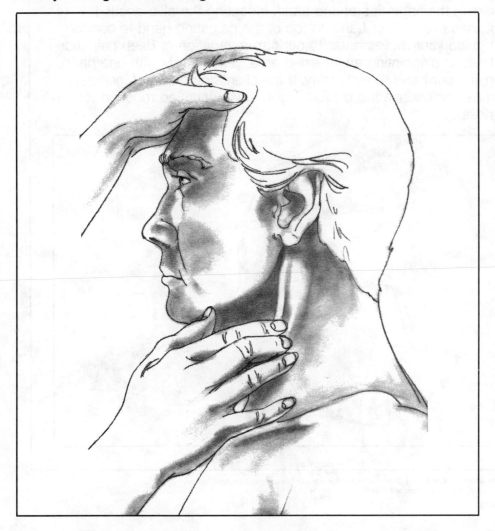

Morton: *Health Assessment in Nursing* (2nd ed.). ©1993, Springhouse Corporation. All rights reserved.
For use with Chapter 4, Physical Assessment Skills.

Deep palpation

To perform deep palpation (bimanual palpation), apply heavy pressure with the fingertips of one hand, indenting the skin about 1½″ (4 cm). Place your other hand on top of the palpating hand to control and guide your movements. To perform a variation of deep palpation that allows pinpointing an inflamed area, press firmly with one hand, then lift your hand away quickly. If the client complains of increased pain as you release the pressure, you have identified rebound tenderness.

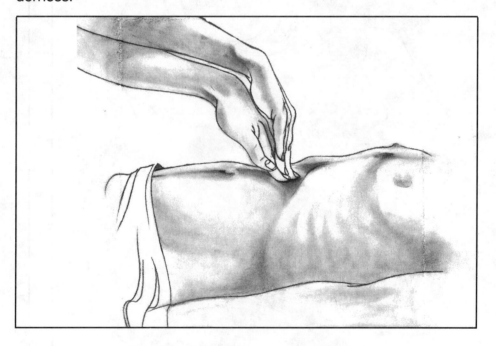

Morton: *Health Assessment in Nursing* (2nd ed.). ©1993, Springhouse Corporation. All rights reserved.
For use with Chapter 4, Physical Assessment Skills.

Light and deep ballottement

To perform light ballottement, apply light, rapid pressure from quadrant to quadrant of the client's abdomen. Keep your hand on the skin surface to detect any tissue rebound.

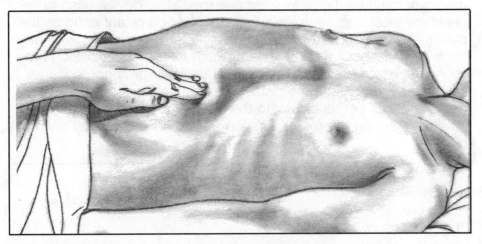

To perform deep ballottement, apply abrupt, deep pressure; then release the pressure, but maintain fingertip contact with the skin.

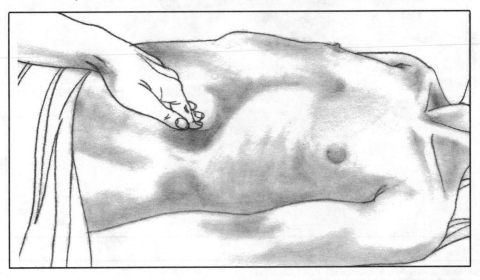

Indirect percussion

To perform indirect percussion, use the middle finger of your non-dominant hand as the pleximeter (the mediating device used to receive the taps) and the middle finger of your dominant hand as the plexor (the device used to tap the pleximeter). Place the pleximeter finger firmly against a body surface, such as the upper back. With your wrist flexed loosely, use the tip of your plexor finger to deliver a crisp blow just beneath the distal joint of the pleximeter. Be sure to hold the plexor perpendicular to the pleximeter. Tap lightly and quickly, removing the plexor as soon as you have delivered each blow.

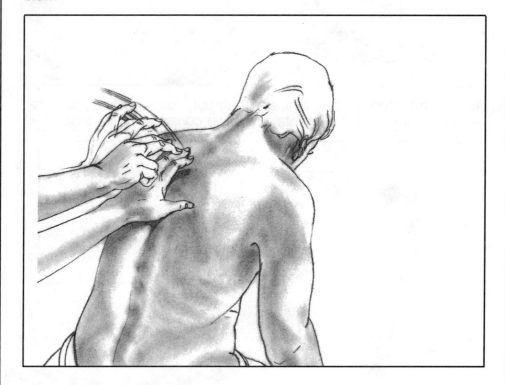

Morton: *Health Assessment in Nursing* (2nd ed.). ©1993, Springhouse Corporation. All rights reserved.
For use with Chapter 4, Physical Assessment Skills.

Direct percussion

To perform direct percussion, tap your hand or fingertip directly against the body surface. This method helps assess an adult's sinuses for tenderness or elicit sounds in a child's thorax.

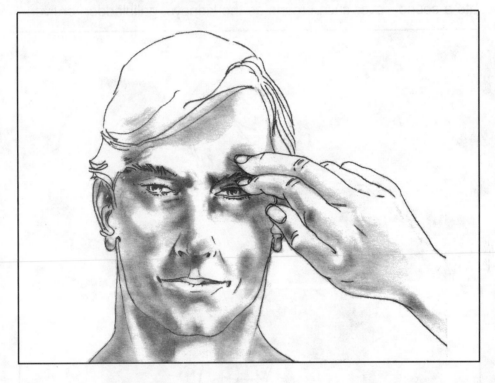

Blunt percussion

To perform blunt percussion, strike the ulnar surface of your fist against the body surface. Alternatively, you may use both hands by placing the palm of one hand over the area to be percussed, then making a fist with the other hand and using it to strike the back of the first hand. Both techniques aim to elicit tenderness — *not* to create a sound — over such organs as the kidneys, gallbladder, or liver.

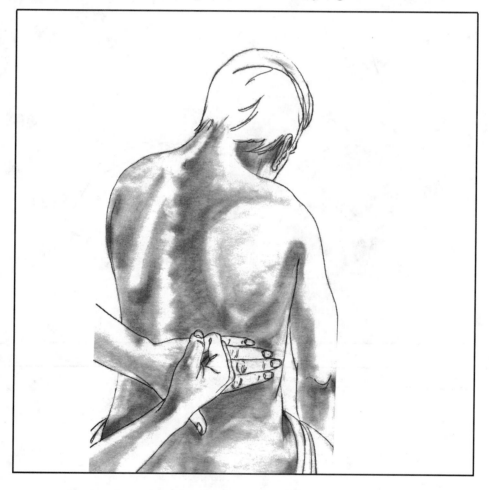

Anatomy of the skin

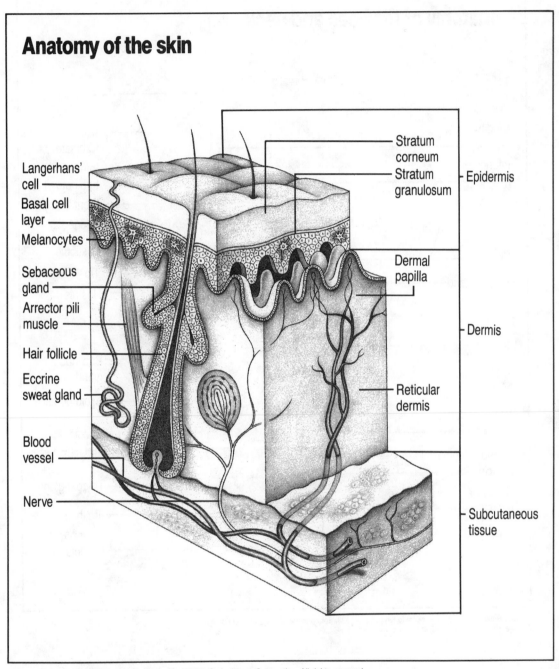

Langerhans'
cell

Basal cell
layer

Melanocytes

Sebaceous
gland

Arrector pili
muscle

Hair follicle

Eccrine
sweat gland

Blood
vessel

Nerve

Stratum
corneum

Stratum
granulosum

Dermal
papilla

Reticular
dermis

Epidermis

Dermis

Subcutaneous
tissue

Morton: *Health Assessment in Nursing* (2nd ed.). ©1993, Springhouse Corporation. All rights reserved.
For use with Chapter 7, Skin, Hair, and Nails.

Anatomy of the head and neck

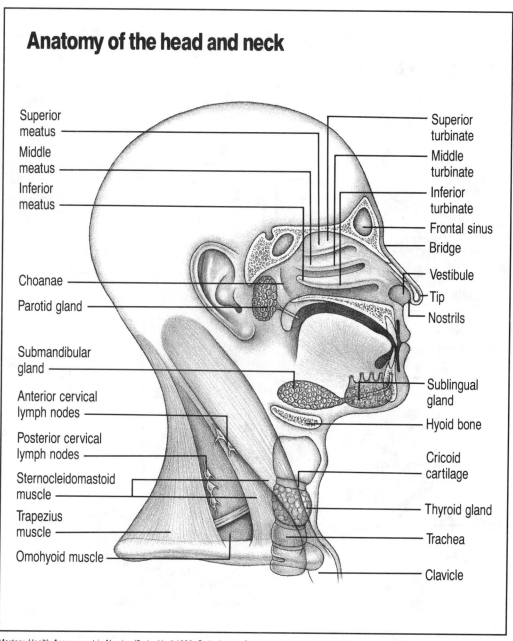

Superior meatus

Middle meatus

Inferior meatus

Choanae

Parotid gland

Submandibular gland

Anterior cervical lymph nodes

Posterior cervical lymph nodes

Sternocleidomastoid muscle

Trapezius muscle

Omohyoid muscle

Superior turbinate

Middle turbinate

Inferior turbinate

Frontal sinus

Bridge

Vestibule

Tip

Nostrils

Sublingual gland

Hyoid bone

Cricoid cartilage

Thyroid gland

Trachea

Clavicle

Morton: *Health Assessment in Nursing* (2nd ed.). ©1993, Springhouse Corporation. All rights reserved.
For use with Chapter 8, Head and Neck.

Structures of the mouth

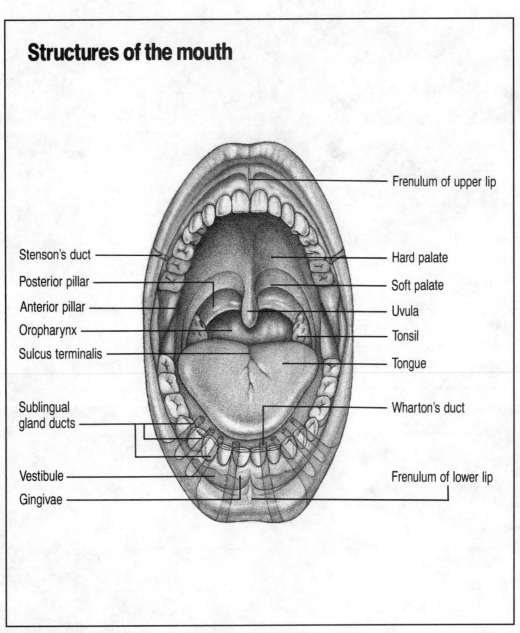

Stenson's duct

Posterior pillar

Anterior pillar

Oropharynx

Sulcus terminalis

Sublingual gland ducts

Vestibule

Gingivae

Frenulum of upper lip

Hard palate

Soft palate

Uvula

Tonsil

Tongue

Wharton's duct

Frenulum of lower lip

Extraocular and intraocular structures

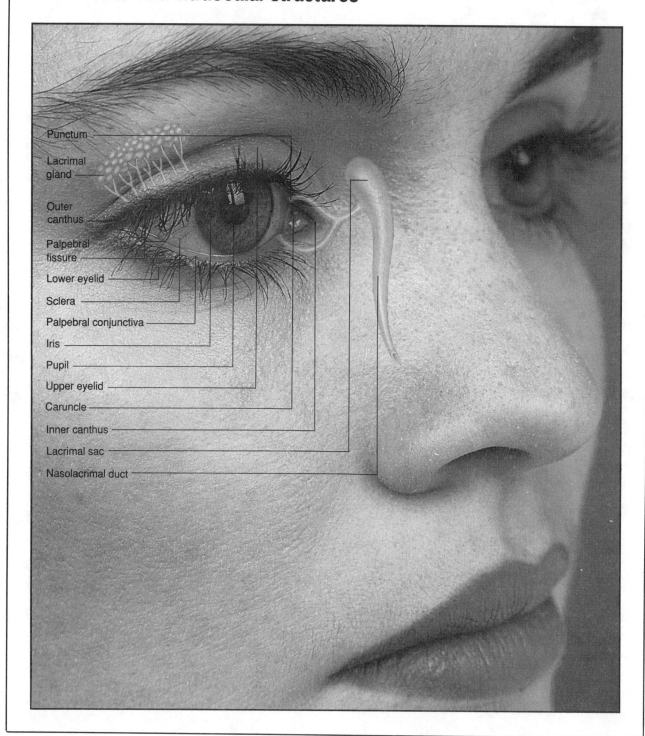

Punctum

Lacrimal gland

Outer canthus

Palpebral fissure

Lower eyelid

Sclera

Palpebral conjunctiva

Iris

Pupil

Upper eyelid

Caruncle

Inner canthus

Lacrimal sac

Nasolacrimal duct

Inspecting the conjunctivae

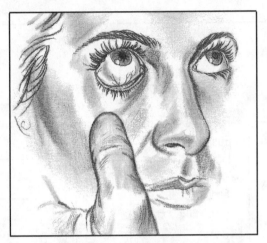

Bulbar conjunctiva

To inspect the bulbar conjunctiva, gently separate the eyelids with your thumb or index finger. Ask the client to look up, down, left, and right as you examine the eye.

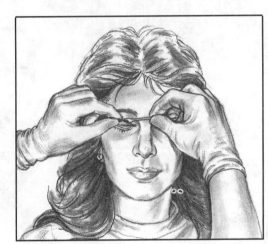

Palpebral conjunctiva

To examine the upper conjunctiva, hold the upper eyelashes and press on the tarsal border with a cotton-tipped applicator to evert the eyelid. Ask the client to look down. Hold the lashes to the brow and examine the conjunctiva, which should be pink and free from swelling.

To return the eyelid to its normal position, release the eyelashes and ask the client to look upward. If this does not invert the eyelid, grasp the eyelashes and gently pull them forward.

Morton: *Health Assessment in Nursing* (2nd ed.). ©1993, Springhouse Corporation. All rights reserved.
For use with Chapter 9, Eyes and Ears.

Structures of the ear

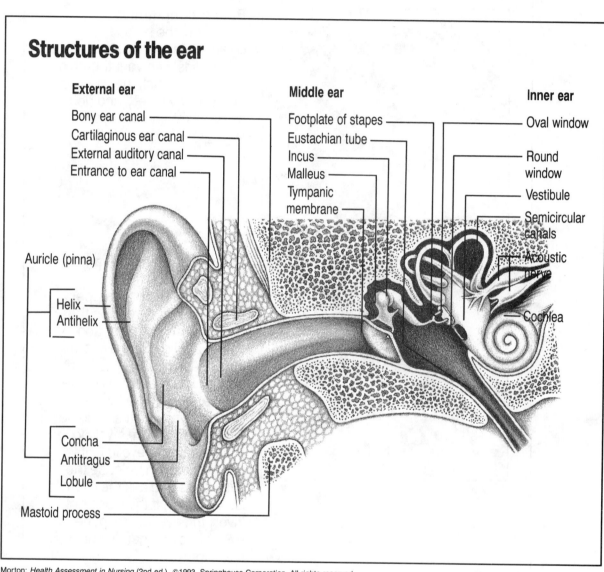

External ear

Bony ear canal
Cartilaginous ear canal
External auditory canal
Entrance to ear canal

Auricle (pinna)

Helix
Antihelix

Concha
Antitragus
Lobule

Mastoid process

Middle ear

Footplate of stapes
Eustachian tube
Incus
Malleus
Tympanic membrane

Inner ear

Oval window
Round window
Vestibule
Semicircular canals
Acoustic nerve
Cochlea

Otoscopic view of the tympanic membrane

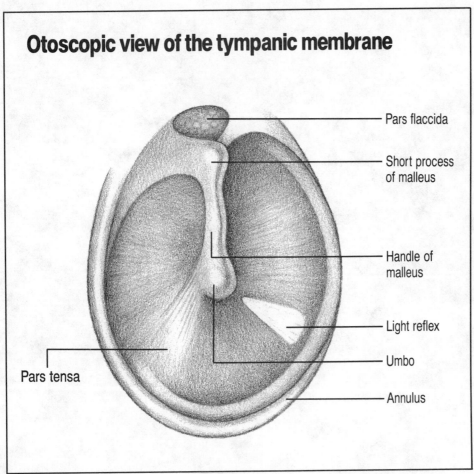

Pars flaccida

Short process
of malleus

Handle of
malleus

Light reflex

Umbo

Annulus

Pars tensa

Structures of the respiratory system

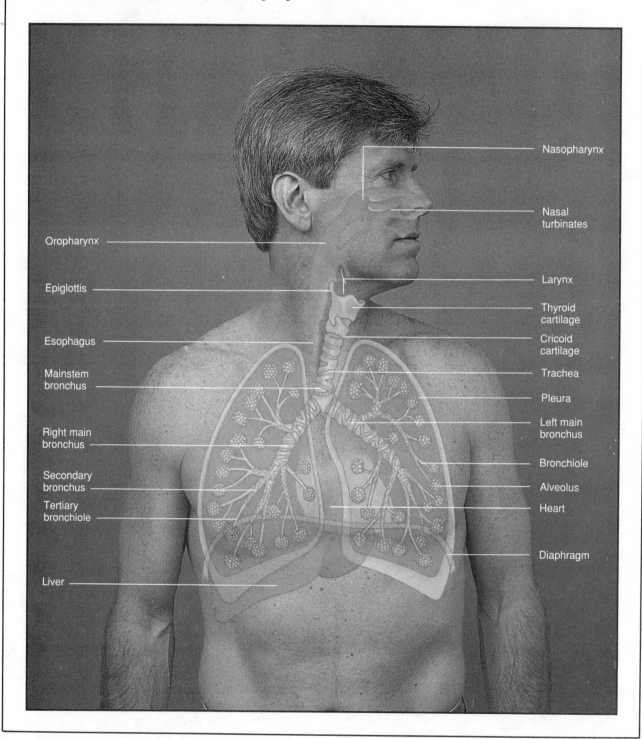

Nasopharynx

Nasal turbinates

Oropharynx

Larynx

Epiglottis

Thyroid cartilage

Esophagus

Cricoid cartilage

Mainstem bronchus

Trachea

Pleura

Right main bronchus

Left main bronchus

Bronchiole

Secondary bronchus

Alveolus

Tertiary bronchiole

Heart

Diaphragm

Liver

Thorax palpation

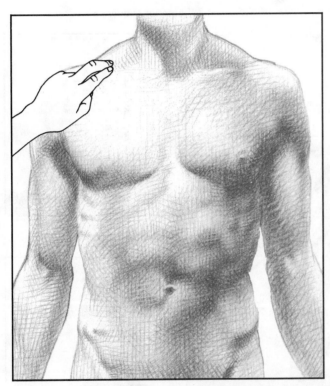

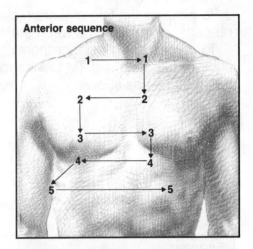

Anterior sequence

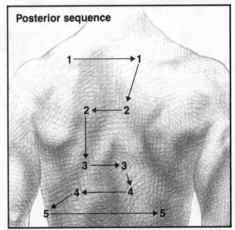

Posterior sequence

Using the fingertips and palmar surfaces of one or both hands, the nurse should palpate the thorax systematically and in a circular motion, alternating palpation from one side of the thorax to the other. To palpate the anterior thorax, begin in the supraclavicular area, as shown. Then follow the sequence, as illustrated, progressing to the infraclavicular, sternal, xiphoid, rib, and axillary areas. Begin posterior palpation in the supraclavicular area, move to the area between the scapulae (interscapular), then below the scapulae (infrascapular), and down to the lateral walls of the thorax.

Morton: *Health Assessment in Nursing* (2nd ed.). ©1993, Springhouse Corporation. All rights reserved.
For use with Chapter 10, Respiratory System.

Thorax percussion

When percussing a client's thorax, the nurse should always use mediate percussion and follow the same sequence, comparing sound variations from one side to the other.

To percuss the anterior thorax, place your hands over the lung apices in the supraclavicular area. Then proceed downward, moving from side to side at 1½" to 2" (3- to 5-cm) intervals.

To percuss the lateral thorax, start at the axilla and move down the side of the rib cage, percussing between the ribs as shown.

To percuss the posterior thorax, progress in a zigzag fashion from the suprascapular to the interscapular to infrascapular areas, avoiding the vertebral column and the scapulae as shown.

Anterior sequence

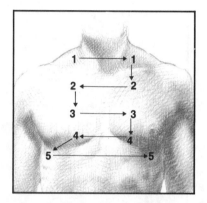

Left lateral sequence

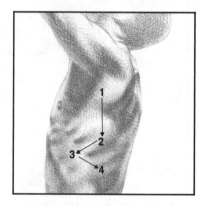

Posterior sequence

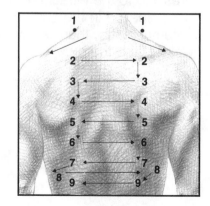

Percussion

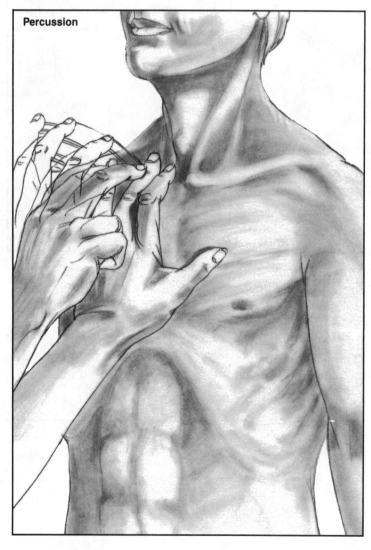

Cardiovascular structures

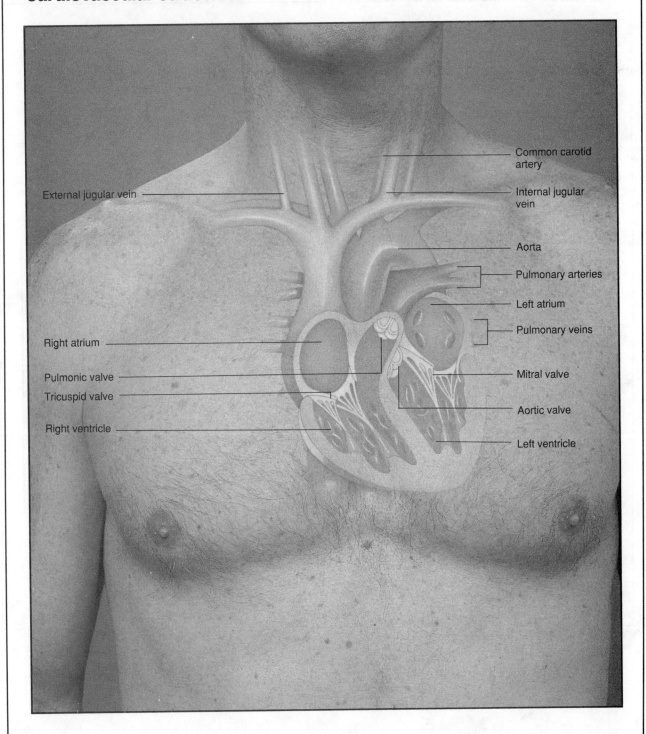

Common carotid artery

Internal jugular vein

External jugular vein

Aorta

Pulmonary arteries

Left atrium

Pulmonary veins

Right atrium

Pulmonic valve

Tricuspid valve

Mitral valve

Aortic valve

Right ventricle

Left ventricle

Precordium inspection and palpation

To detect normal and abnormal pulsations over the precordium, the nurse should inspect and palpate six different areas according to the following guidelines.

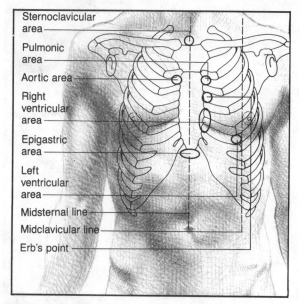

Locate the six precordial areas by using the anatomic landmarks named for the underlying structures.

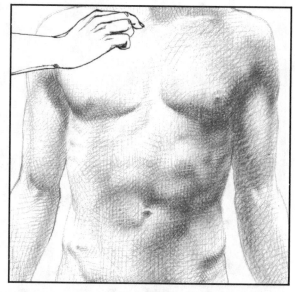

Then palpate (or inspect) the precordium in the following sequence: the sternoclavicular area, aortic area, pulmonic area, right ventricular area, left ventricular area, and epigastric area.

Cardiac auscultation

Auscultation is the most important technique used to assess the cardiovascular system. To perform cardiac ausculation, follow these guidelines.

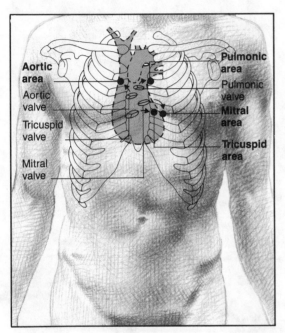

1. Locate the four different auscultation sites, as illustrated. The shaded areas indicate the auscultation sites; the arrows show the direction of the blood flow from the valve creating the sound.

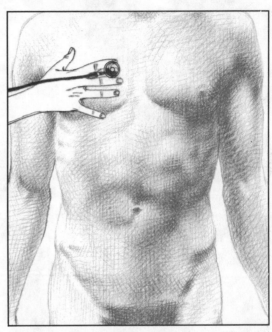

2. Then auscultate in the following sequence: the aortic area, pulmonic area, tricuspid area, and mitral area.

Quadrants of the breast and associated lymph nodes

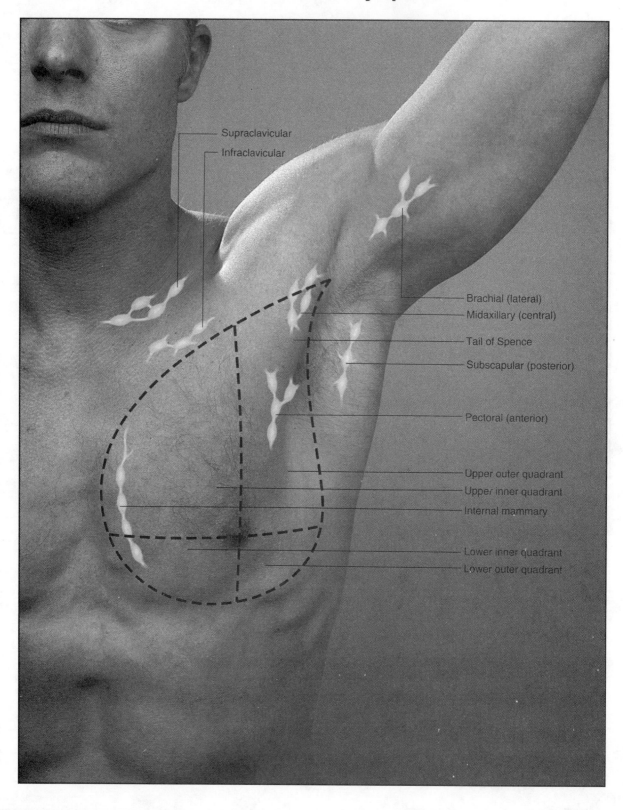

Supraclavicular

Infraclavicular

Brachial (lateral)

Midaxillary (central)

Tail of Spence

Subscapular (posterior)

Pectoral (anterior)

Upper outer quadrant

Upper inner quadrant

Internal mammary

Lower inner quadrant

Lower outer quadrant

Structures of the gastrointestinal system

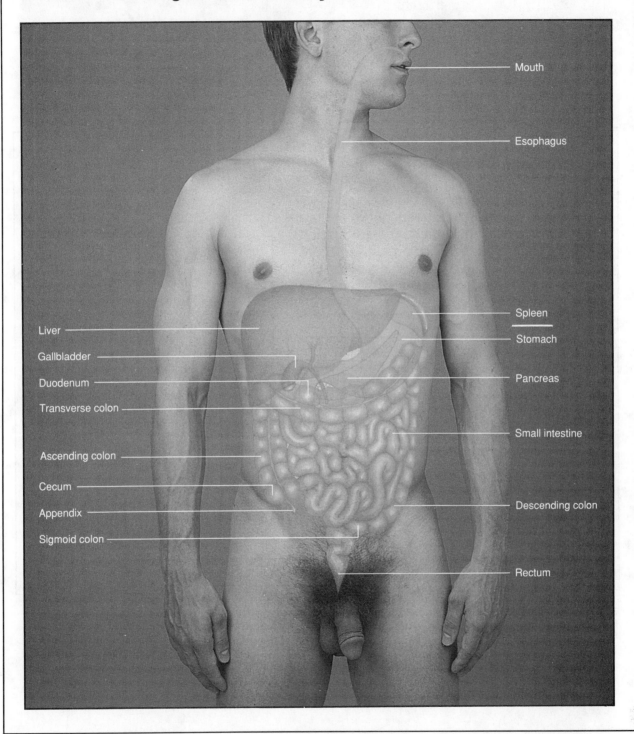

Mouth

Esophagus

Liver

Gallbladder

Duodenum

Transverse colon

Ascending colon

Cecum

Appendix

Sigmoid colon

Spleen

Stomach

Pancreas

Small intestine

Descending colon

Rectum

Morton: *Health Assessment in Nursing* (2nd ed.). ©1993, Springhouse Corporation. All rights reserved.
For use with Chapter 13, Gastrointestinal System.

Percussing the abdomen

The nurse should percuss the abdomen systematically, starting with the right upper quadrant and moving clockwise to the percussion sites in each quadrant. However, if the client complains of pain in a particular quadrant, adjust the percussion sequence to percuss that quadrant last.

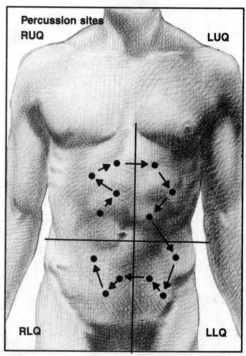

Percussion sites
RUQ | LUQ
RLQ | LLQ

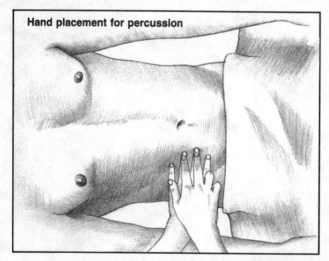

Hand placement for percussion

Structures of the central nervous system

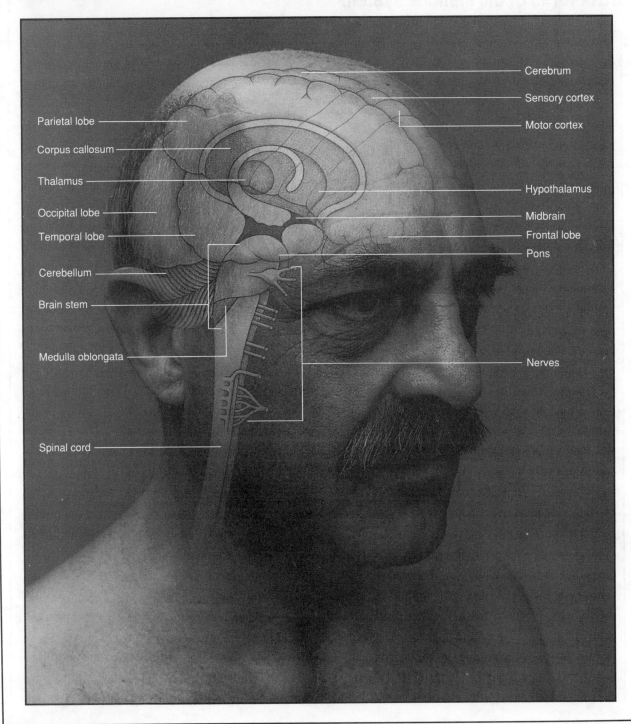

Cerebrum

Sensory cortex

Motor cortex

Parietal lobe

Corpus callosum

Thalamus

Hypothalamus

Occipital lobe

Midbrain

Temporal lobe

Frontal lobe

Pons

Cerebellum

Brain stem

Medulla oblongata

Nerves

Spinal cord

Structures of the immune system

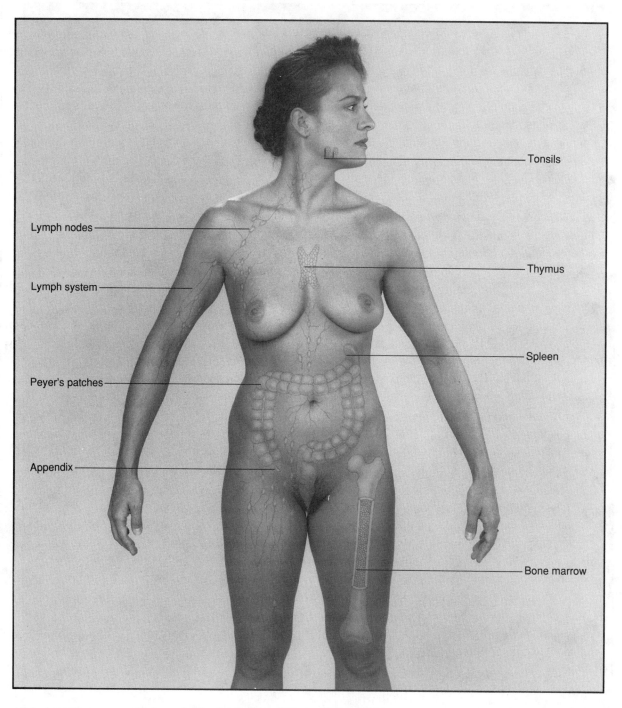

Tonsils

Lymph nodes

Lymph system

Peyer's patches

Appendix

Thymus

Spleen

Bone marrow

Structures of the endocrine system

Pineal gland

Pituitary gland

Thyroid gland

Parathyroid glands

Thymus

Adrenal gland

Pancreas

Testes

Assessing the fundus

To estimate the size of the uterus—and fetal growth—palpate and measure the fundus. Before the 12th gestational week, when the gravid uterus moves into the abdominal cavity, estimate uterine size by bimanual assessment. After the 12th week, use fundal palpation to determine fundal height.

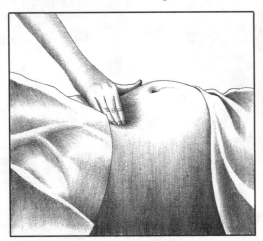

Palpating fundal height
Stand at the supine client's right side and place the palm of your left hand about 1⅛" to 1⅝" (3 to 4 cm) above where the fundus should be. Palpating toward the symphysis pubis, find the point where the soft abdomen ends and the firm, round fundal edge begins.

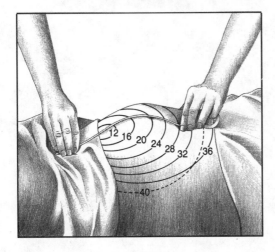

Measuring fundal height
Next, using a measuring tape, determine the distance along the anterior abdominal wall from the top of the fundus to the notch at the inferior edge of the symphysis pubis. At 12 to 13 weeks, the fundus can be felt just above the symphysis pubis; at 16 weeks, the fundus is about midway between the symphysis pubis and the umbilicus; at 20 weeks, it can be felt at the umbilical level.

Morton *Health Assessment in Nursing* (2nd ed.). ©1993, Springhouse Corporation. All rights reserved.
For use with Chapter 22, Perinatal and Neonatal Assessment.